"The compelling life and near-death story of Sean Strub, of thousands lost to HIV-AIDS, and thousands more living with it whom his activism helped save. Wow."

—Andrew Tobias, author of *The Best Little Boy in the World*

"By taking us with him on his journey from a conservative family in Iowa to the heart of a global movement for human rights, Sean Strub gives us ideas, strength, and heart in our own journey."

—Gloria Steinem

"Absorbing . . . Strub is a dispassionate, reliable guide whose directness and honesty create considerable impact. Anyone would profit from reading this book."

—Martin Duberman, author of *Stonewall* and Professor of History Emeritus at the Graduate School of the City University of New York

"This take-no-prisoners memoir has the quality of a suspenseful page-turner, and will keep you reading until the final sentence."

—John D'Emilio, author of *Intimate Matters: A History of Sexuality in America*

"From early struggles against AIDS to later collective acting up, Sean Strub's lively, gossipy memoir is also deeply moving history."

—Jonathan Ned Katz, author of *Gay American History*

"*Body Counts* is a powerful account of the epidemic's early years and the subsequent three decades. . . . A page-turner with moving insight and fresh analysis told in a compelling and highly personal style."

—Lily Tomlin

"Strub paints a striking picture. . . . A valuable document."

—*Kirkus Reviews*

"Elegantly written, moving, and powerful . . . eye-opening."

—Mary Frances Berry, Geraldine R. Segal Professor of American Social Thought, University of Pennsylvania, and Past Chair of the U.S. Commission on Civil Rights

"Direct and honest prose relates a familiar story of growing self-aware-ness, coming of age, and coming out in a fresh and compelling manner. The big surprise comes when one recognizes how dramatic the machi-nations of drug trials, power politics, and the building of a grass roots movement can be."

—Bill T. Jones

"A gripping story of a movement that changed the soul of our world."

—Kathy Boudin, Assistant Professor,
Columbia University School of Social Work

"Strub's memoir, like Strub himself, is an inspiration."

—Richard McCann, author of *Mother of Sorrows*

"A compelling page-turner . . . To understand today's HIV epidemic, read *Body Counts*."

—Rory Kennedy, filmmaker

"A wonderful storyteller, Strub does such a great job of showing how life also went on amidst so much death. I very much admire his writing—how clean and powerful it is."

—Will Schwalbe, author of *The End of Your Life Book Club*

"A critical historical voice . . . Absorbing."

—*The Cleveland Plain Dealer*

"A well-written and welcome addition to the histories of the queer and AIDS movements."

—*Gay City News*

"An eyewitness account from the inside of the epidemic."

—*Next Magazine*

"[*Body Counts*] depicts incredible acts of courage by Strub and his con-stellation of collaborators. Against thick walls of institutional homopho-bia and shrieking AIDS hysteria, they forged battles that shaped seminal moments in AIDS history. . . . Gripping."

—*Windy City Times*

BODY COUNTS

A Memoir of Activism, Sex, and Survival

Sean Strub

SEAN STRUB

SCRIBNER
New York London Toronto Sydney New Delhi

Scribner
A Division of Simon & Schuster, Inc.
1230 Avenue of the Americas
New York, NY 10020

First Scribner trade paperback edition September 2014

SCRIBNER and design are registered trademarks of The Gale Group, Inc., used under license by Simon & Schuster, Inc., the publisher of this work.

For information about special discounts for bulk purchases, please contact Simon & Schuster Special Sales at 1-866-506-1949 or business@simonandschuster.com.

The Simon & Schuster Speakers Bureau can bring authors to your live event. For more information or to book an event, contact the Simon & Schuster Speakers Bureau at 1-866-248-3049 or visit our website at www.simonspeakers.com.

Interior design by Jill Putorti
Cover design by Christopher Lin
Cover photograph by Iowa City Press-Citizen

Manufactured in the United States of America

10 9 8 7 6 5 4 3 2 1

Library of Congress Cataloging-in-Publication Data is available.

ISBN 978-1-4516-6195-8
ISBN 978-1-4516-6196-5 (pbk)
ISBN 978-1-4516-6197-2 (ebook)

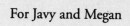

For Javy and Megan

CONTENTS

December 1989, New York City   *1*

Chapter 1: Out of Iowa   5

Chapter 2: The Way Out   23

Chapter 3: Tennessee and Me   45

Chapter 4: Sphere of Influence   49

Chapter 5: Making Movement   65

Chapter 6: Virus and Violence   83

Chapter 7: Kentucky Fried Closet   97

Chapter 8: The End of a Day Like This   109

Chapter 9: Of Mousetraps and Men   121

Chapter 10: Stigma and Solidarity   141

Chapter 11: Testing and Telling   155

Chapter 12: The Living Room   169

Chapter 13: Rolo-dead File   183

Chapter 14: Silence=Death   195

Chapter 15: Unexpected Expire   207

Chapter 16: Keith and Swen   219

Chapter 17: Cardinal Sin   227

Chapter 18: Hope Is Hope   235

Chapter 19: Running Man   239

Chapter 20: Taking the Helms   251

Chapter 21: Today Is a Good Day   259

Chapter 22: *The Night Larry Kramer Kissed Me*   265

Chapter 23: Ask and Tell   275

Chapter 24: Launch   283

Chapter 25: Firsts   289

Chapter 26: Pharma Watching   305

Chapter 27: Creating Communities   309

Chapter 28: Dark Mark   315

Chapter 29: Feeling Our Pain   325

Chapter 30: Barebacking   335

Chapter 31: Eugene and Angel   341

Chapter 32: Memento Mori   347

Chapter 33: Recall   355

Chapter 34: Lazarus   361

Chapter 35: Stephen   371

Chapter 36: Postpartum   379

Chapter 37: Naked to the World   383

Chapter 38: HIV Is Not a Crime   391

Acknowledgments   401

Index   405

An Interview with Sean Strub   421

BODY
COUNTS

DECEMBER 1989
NEW YORK CITY

I am nervously sitting in a pew near the front of St. Patrick's Cathedral in New York where John Cardinal O'Connor is about to celebrate Mass. It has been years since I attended a Catholic Mass and even longer since I took communion, the holiest of sacraments, but that is why I am here. Looking up at the cathedral's soaring nave, I remember the awe I felt as an altar boy at St. Mary's in Iowa City and, later, the anger when the Church betrayed me.

It is bitterly cold, a near record low. Many parishioners wear heavy coats as they hold hymnals in gloved hands. Slush-covered boots have left a wet trail down the long center aisle. There's a puddle under my pew. The mood in the church is tense—nothing like the droning boredom of the Masses of my youth. As the minutes pass, I think of the Jesuits who taught me as a child that a good Catholic acts upon the church's social teachings, even if that means confronting the church. My hands are trembling with the cold, my apprehension and other feelings too deep to name.

Outside St. Patrick's, forty-five hundred angry men and women have assembled, packing Fifth Avenue and chanting and waving placards that read "Curb your Dogma," "Papal Bull," and "Condoms Not

Coffins." Fists pump the air, bullhorns blare. ACT UP, the AIDS Coalition to Unleash Power, is protesting O'Connor's assault on safe sex and reproductive rights. There is an almost carnival-like spirit to the demonstration with ACT UP affinity groups, such as Church Ladies for Choice, the Hail Marys, and Speaking in Tongues, performing their protests. In ACT UP, high camp and high seriousness are uniquely compatible. An artist named Ray Navarro is dressed as Jesus Christ, swathed in a white shroud, carrying a large wooden cross over his near-skeletal shoulder. His bearded face is gaunt, and he wears a crown of thorns over his long, thinning hair. Despite the cold, Ray looks beatific. He will be dead in less than a year. Keith Haring is there, too, in a knitted cap with a long, hand-knitted scarf wrapped around his slender neck. He has two months left.

Inside the cathedral, O'Connor's Mass is interrupted again and again by ACT UP protesters. Surreptitiously spread throughout the church, they stand up and yell out their statements. My friend Michael Petrelis climbs on a pew and shouts, "O'Connor, you're killing us!" Another friend, Jamie Leo, dressed as a priest near the front of the church, offers up a prayer in protest. Two boyfriends in black leather motorcycle jackets handcuff themselves to one pew. Right after O'Connor begins his homily, thirty protesters stage a die-in, blowing whistles, throwing hundreds of condoms in the air, and going limp in the center aisle. The cops, two long lines of blue on either side of the cathedral, have their moment, binding wrists with plastic handcuffs and carrying the protesters away on stretchers, as if they were taking them to a hospital rather than to paddy wagons.

With his homily in tatters, O'Connor retreats from the altar to his thronelike chair. He sits with his head in his hands, melodramatically trying to convey spiritual pain. Photographs of the media-savvy cardinal looking tragically besieged will elicit overwhelming sympathy when they appear on the front page of Monday's newspapers.

Communion begins amid the general confusion. ACT UP protesters line up, interspersed among the regular parishioners, but when it is their turn, they make loud political pronouncements: "Safe sex is moral sex!" "I support a woman's right to choose!" "Condoms save lives!" Soon it is my turn to receive the body and blood of Christ. A small, dark-skinned priest is serving my queue; his white, green, and gold vestments are oversized and bright. He hesitates briefly, his eyes fixed on the pink triangle and Silence=Death logo visible on the T-shirt underneath my coat. Then he holds the host in the air and intones, with a strong Spanish accent, "the body of Christ."

This is the moment—my moment to confront the Church—when instead of repeating "the body of Christ" as expected, I am to make my political statement. But I have not prepared one. When I rehearsed this moment in my mind, I imagined I might break into tears or erupt in rage because no slogan—in fact, no words at all—seemed adequate.

"May the Lord bless the man I love, who died a year ago this week," I hear myself say. My voice begins as a tremble but finishes strong. Police standing a few feet away are ready to intervene, watching to see how the priest reacts. His hand jerks slightly, but he looks me in the eye and gives me the wafer.

With my heart pounding, I walk back to my pew. My mind is fixed on bodies, but not the body of Christ. I think of Michael's body and the agonizing brain infection that turned his last days into a kind of crucifixion. I think of the bodies of the protesters carried out on stretchers and those chanting outside, many struggling to survive. I think of my own body, wondering how much longer it will last.

Parishioners are staring at me, their faces disgusted or sympathetic or just plain stunned. Some have their heads bowed, hands pressed tightly in prayer like the devout at St. Mary's, their faith unshakable and unwilling to brook any criticism of the Church. They might be praying for us.

After Mass, I pass through the cathedral's heavy doors into the bright sunlight and, it seems to me, into the arms of my true community. I am exultant, in a state that feels like grace, certain that if I am to die of AIDS, I will die as a fighter, not a victim.

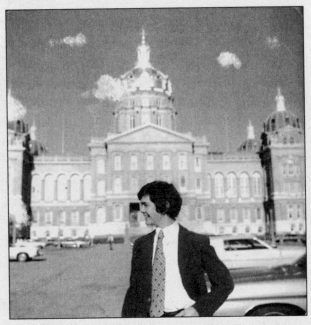

In front of the Iowa State Capitol, wearing the red jacket required
of all State Senate pages, May 1975.

CHAPTER 1

Out of Iowa

Elevator number one was "Senators Only," and my job was to move senators up to the Senate floor in the U.S. Capitol and back to their offices as quickly as possible. From 1976 to 1978, for twenty hours a week, I manually opened and closed a shiny brass accordion-style gate at each floor, always with a friendly greeting. Whenever the gate squeaked or scraped, I would squirt a little oil on its metal joints. The interior of the antique elevator cab was polished walnut and rosewood, with a hand-operated cast-iron gearshift worn smooth by many decades of constant movement forward ("Going up!") and back ("Going down!"). A small wooden folding seat was hinged against the wall, but I never used it. I preferred to stand and greet passengers eye to eye.

I had arrived in Washington from Iowa in March 1976, with a copy of Michael Harrington's *The Other America* in my suitcase, as a seventeen-year-old idealist determined to make my mark in the world. I wasn't sure what that might be, but I harbored political ambition and secretly thought I might go very far. My parents believed I went to Washington to attend Georgetown University that fall. "A fine Jesuit school," my dad called it. But for me, the main attraction was the job ferrying members of the U.S. Senate up and down. It was a plum post for an eager young politico, and the pay was good. I also liked that my elevator was on the Senate side of the Capitol, the so-called "upper chamber" of Congress.

I was on a political fast track. When I had hit adolescence, and the attention of my male peers turned to girls, mine turned to politics. That's how I lucked in to the elevator operator post. As a page in the Iowa State Senate in 1975, I often got rides from the capital in Des Moines to my parents' house in Iowa City from a journalist, Frank Nye, who lived nearby in Cedar Rapids. Shortly before Christmas in 1975, he and his wife invited me to a dinner party at their house, where I met Iowa's senator Dick Clark, one of the U.S. Senate's most liberal members. I didn't realize Clark was an elected official until the dinner conversation turned to national politics. He seemed particularly well informed, so I asked him, "Do you work in Washington?," prompting a humiliating burst of laughter from others at the table.

Despite my faux pas, Clark thought I showed promise and handed me his card with his executive assistant's name scrawled on the back. "Tell Bob I told you to call and see if we might be able to get you an appointment as a page, and maybe you could help out a bit in my office as an intern," he said. I left Clark's aide a message the next morning, saying I had already served as a page in the State Senate in Des Moines and was excited about the chance to work in Washington. When he called back, he said I was too old to be a page—the cutoff was sixteen—but he would look into another patronage position for me, which turned out to be the elevator post.

I should already have been in college at the time, but I had taken a gap year to work on the Democratic presidential campaigns leading up to the January 1976 Iowa precinct caucuses. Even though I wasn't old enough to vote, I was elected as a delegate to the state convention for U.S. Representative Morris Udall. When his campaign fizzled (he commented at the time, "the people have spoken—the bastards!"), I switched my allegiance to California's governor, Jerry Brown, a former

Jesuit seminarian who was a late entry into the race. A few weeks after my move to Washington, I took a day off from the elevator job to join Brown's campaign entourage in Maryland on May 16, 1976—my eighteenth birthday—just two days before that state's primary.

The Capitol Hill complex—which then included three House and two Senate office buildings, as well as the Capitol—had fifty-eight elevators. Most still required manual operation, which was supplied by politically well-connected teenagers. Members of Congress and staff treated us like mascots, though we were hardly pampered. If the Senate worked late into the night, we did as well. One perk was that we could wander through parts of the Capitol that the public never sees. Another elevator operator, Jay, and I made good use of his knowledge of the meandering labyrinth of passageways, tunnels, and hidden staircases and his cache of master keys. Once, we climbed the steep steps to the dome and smoked a quick joint while enjoying a spectacular 360-degree view of the city. During the day, we slipped past velvet-roped brass stanchions forbidding public passage as though we owned the place, and at night, we wandered through the several levels of underground tunnels, noiseless except for the sounds of our footsteps echoing off overhanging steam pipes. One night when the Senate was working very late, we sneaked into the engineer's office and cranked up the heat in the Senate chamber until the senators were so miserable that they adjourned, releasing us from our posts.

I couldn't imagine anything more exciting for an ambitious political junkie than employment literally a few steps away from the Senate chamber. I got a daily contact high as I angled to meet as many powerful political figures as I possibly could, and I let myself imagine that I was nearly as much a part of the political process as they were. I knew several members of Congress had served as pages, worked in the mailroom, or run an elevator in the Capitol when they were young. If being in the right place at the right time mattered, I would make sure I was in the right places at *all* the right times.

Washington was definitely that place in the spring of 1976, full of promise and drama for a teenager with a political consciousness shaped by Watergate, the Vietnam War, feminism, and social-justice movements. The voting age had dropped from twenty-one to eighteen, the Equal Rights Amendment had passed Congress, and the 1973 *Roe* v. *Wade* Supreme Court decision had energized the women's rights movement. It had been only two years since Gerald Ford had assumed the presidency in the wake of Richard Nixon's resignation, declaring, "Our long national nightmare is over." Jimmy Carter, the little-known former Georgia governor, campaigned for the Democratic presidential nomination in 1976 with a promise—"I will never lie to you"—that was emblematic of a hopeful new era.

When I saw the White House, the Washington Monument, and the Capitol building for the first time, I felt as if I had reached the center of the universe. The red, white, and blue logos for the upcoming bicentennial celebration were plastered all over town. The freshman class in Congress at the time was full of young reform-minded liberals known as the "Watergate babies," elected in the Democratic landslide of 1974 and driving a progressive national agenda. Across the country, Americans felt corruption skulking out the window and a fresh breeze of clean politics coming through the door.

My interest in politics was partly a geographic coincidence. In 1967, when I was nine, my family moved from an isolated rural area north of Iowa City, where we kept horses and sheep, to an affluent neighborhood in Iowa City adjacent to the sprawling University of Iowa campus and its huge medical center. The parents of most of the kids in the neighborhood were college professors or doctors at the UI hospital. While my fourth-grade classmates at Lincoln Elementary watched cartoons and read Spider-Man comics, I followed politics and current events in the *Des Moines Register*, the *Iowa City Press-Citizen*, and the *Daily Iowan*. Our proximity to a politically progressive campus meant that anti-war protests and the social-justice movement became part of my daily life.

My dad's family had been in Iowa City since the 1840s, when

they opened a small grocery that became a well-known department store—Strub's Store for Everybody—in subsequent generations. After World War II, my grandfather sold the store but kept the appliance and bottled gas divisions, starting a propane gas company to service the postwar growth in suburban residential developments, which was the business my dad ran.

My mother's father was a shanty Irish entrepreneur, operating a pool hall and cigar store in Fort Dodge, Iowa, and promoting boxing matches in northwest Iowa and the Dakota territories early in the twentieth century. He died of lung cancer in 1931, right before she was born. Her mother, from a prominent lace-curtain Irish family in Cedar Rapids, died of breast cancer when my mother was two years old, so her childhood was nomadic; she bounced from one boarding school or convent to another, raised mostly by nuns. As a teenager, she came to Iowa City to live with an aunt and uncle and attend high school, where she met my father.

My parents weren't especially political; their Catholicism was vastly more defining than any political ideology. They never knew quite what to make of my obsession with politics, let alone the increasingly radical views I embraced in later years. I was the third of six children. My older brother was named Carl, after my father and grandfather; when I was born, I was named for my mother's Irish heritage and given her maiden name, O'Brien, as my middle name. My three sisters all were given Mary as a first name, after my father's devotion to the Virgin Mother. My younger brother, Thomas Jerome, was named after my father's close friend, who was best man at my parents' wedding.

The thrill of being away from home and near the nexus of power and politics in Washington was dampened by a humiliating secret. While many teenage boys at the time had a poster of television star Farrah Fawcett, with her long legs and blond hair, I was obsessed with Mark Spitz, the muscular and handsome 1972 Olympic swimmer. Even though I hadn't acted on my desire for men, I lived in constant fear that exposure would demolish my life as I knew it.

Homosexuals had no chance of finding love or affection, according to the Catholic Church, my family, and Dr. David Reuben's 1972 best seller, *Everything You Always Wanted to Know About Sex (But Were Afraid to Ask)*, which my parents hid under their mattress. We were condemned to a life of misery and empty sexual encounters. I thought my same-sex attraction was inherently evil; all I could do was hope it was a phase that might pass, like my youthful infatuation with magic. To the world, I looked like a young person with bright prospects, but I was damaged on the inside, shame smothering any vision of my future. That sense of alienation gave me empathy for others similarly marginalized or maligned and I think helped spark my interest in politics.

At thirteen, I briefly thought I had a calling for the priesthood, a period I now recognize as a desperate attempt to escape others' oppressive expectation that I become interested in girls. When I didn't pursue a religious vocation, I thought marriage might extinguish my attraction to men. However, my concept of marriage had nothing to do with love or creating a family. It was something to acquire or achieve.

I had it all wrong, of course. Not just about myself and the suppression of hormonal desire but also about the country's direction at the time. What I thought was a national renewal was, in fact, a curtain closing on liberalism. The building blocks of the New Right, the right-wing conservative movement exemplified by Reverend Jerry Falwell's Moral Majority, were firmly in place. The stage was set for the rise of the Reagan revolution, radicalization of the Republican Party, and destruction of the expanding social contract that had defined American politics since World War II.

I arrived in Washington as a virgin. I had never admitted my attraction to men to anyone, except in a confessional at fifteen, to a creepy priest who then interrogated me, wanting highly specific details of my sinful thoughts. Though I knew there was a gay rights movement on the political fringe, I had met only a handful of openly gay men or lesbians in Iowa City. San Francisco's Castro neighborhood and New York's Christopher Street were then already known around the world as coming-out meccas, but Washington was fiercely closeted, more like Iowa City, with a gay scene that was mostly underground. Washington was full of gay men who had devised an elaborate system of secrecy—with its own language, codes, and customs—and attended hidden bars and parties.

During those first few months, I tried to dress like preppy congressional staffers on the Hill and even bought my first pair of denim jeans to blend in after-hours with my peers. It was an opportunity to reinvent myself for new acquaintances who didn't know I couldn't throw a ball, wasn't interested in girls, and had been taunted for years as a faggot. Since the onset of puberty, I had been repressing sexual thoughts, so by the time I got to Washington, I was pretty good at it.

I was also pretty good at a key requirement for the elevator job: the ability to recognize senators. Every elevator operator was given a face book (long before that term's contemporary meaning); I had already pored over the encyclopedic *Almanac of American Politics*, studying the pictures and collecting arcane minutiae about candidates and campaigns the way sports fanatics study athletes and game statistics. I knew that the voting records of Iowa's two senators at the time—Dick Clark, who sponsored me for the elevator position, and John Culver—gave them the highest average rating from Americans for Democratic Action, a liberal advocacy group, of any state in the country. I knew which senators won in landslides and which narrowly slid through their last election; I read brief biographies on all the senators, which revealed where they went to school, their careers prior to election to the Senate, and information about their wives and children.

I started out as an operator on a bank of eight Senate-side public elevators. As soon as I saw a senator getting off the underground tram that ran between the Capitol and the Dirksen and Russell Senate office buildings, I made sure an empty elevator was held, ready for his private use. This adolescent precocity soon got me promoted to elevator number one, hidden around the corner from the main bank of public elevators. The Capitol had many such private senatorial sanctums— washrooms, barbershops, dining rooms, and hideaway offices—behind unmarked doors. The promotion meant I no longer had tourists or staff on my elevator, only members of Congress, cabinet officials, and the occasional Supreme Court justice, with any staff or guests who might accompany them.

The other elevator operators were the first people I met in Washington, and we often hung out in our break room, which was like a secret clubhouse in the bowels of the Capitol. It was behind an inconspicuous door at the end of a long, poorly lit basement hallway painted battleship gray, with exposed pipes overhead. The hallway led to offices serving the more mundane needs of the Senate, including one we called Jack the Wrapper, because they wrapped bulky packages for shipping, and a room marked SERVICE CLOSET, which housed a small snack shop for staffers.

In the break room, we entertained ourselves by playing cards and games or snapping rubber bands at rats scurrying along the baseboard. The Capitol was full of rats—a shocking revelation, I know—but they were a concern only on the rare occasions when they ventured into brightly lit public areas, startling tourists.

The oldest elevator operator, a middle-aged man, spent many hours in the break room reading. When I met him on my first day on the job, he was introduced to me as "the Senator." He never spoke to me, so I asked Jon, another elevator operator, if he knew what was wrong. "It's just that he used to be a member of the Senate," Jon said. "When he was defeated, he didn't want to leave, so he took a job running the elevator. But he's really proud and usually won't talk to someone new until they ask about his service in the Senate. Do that and it'll be fine."

I was intimidated, but a little while later, I was in the break room with several other operators and tried to strike up a conversation. "Senator, how long did you serve upstairs?" I asked tentatively. He let out a long, weary sigh and said, "Three terms, until that bastard Domenici beat me." Pete Domenici was a senator from New Mexico, so I said, "Oh, you're from New Mexico?" During our conversation, Gisele Gravel, an elevator operator and niece of Alaska senator Mike Gravel, came into the break room. Overhearing our exchange, she said to me, "They're pulling your leg. He's not a senator, he's an asshole."

Every elevator operator heard and retold a story about Texas Republican senator John Tower, known to be sensitive about his short stature. He dressed meticulously—shiny cowboy boots with an extra-high heel, carefully tailored suits, and sometimes a cowboy hat. He was arrogant and rude, especially to service staff, and known for his explosive temper.

One day a new operator was in his cab on the first floor of the Russell Senate Office Building when a short man wearing a cowboy hat and shiny boots walked onto the elevator and commanded, "Third floor!" The elevator operator closed the door and put the elevator in gear. As he passed the second floor, the call buzzer sounded three times, the code that it was a senator making the request. A call from a senator always took priority, so the new operator stopped the car with a hard lurch and reversed it. His passenger, furious, berated the operator. The elevator operator, initially nonplussed, looked at his passenger sternly and said, "Hold on, cowboy, we got us a U.S. senator coming aboard!" Tower exploded in rage and later got the elevator operator reassigned.

On my elevator, I saw senators on days they were happy and days they were upset. I saw them in the middle of temper tantrums with colleagues. I got to know most of them well enough to understand how best to greet them and when to stay entirely silent. Several senators, including James Eastland, Russell Long, Herman Talmadge, John Culver, and Lowell Weicker, frequented a hideaway office on the third floor that was mostly a private drinking club. Some were undoubtedly heavy drinkers, but just as many used the hideaway to drink strategically, loosening up colleagues whose votes they sought. Alcohol has always been an effective lubricant of democracy. After the first time a senator asked if I had a breath mint, I made sure to keep a supply on hand.

I took my job seriously, believing I played a small but important role in the legislative process. Crossing the crucial threshold from witness to participant made me feel less like an outsider, less like the bullied kid at the playground. Like with my earlier stint as an altar boy at St. Mary's parish in Iowa City, or later as a frequenter of Studio 54 in New York, the elevator operator position bestowed insider status. The costumes— whether the suits and ties of politics, the Catholic liturgical garments, or the glittering disco garb of New York nightlife—and the corresponding rituals were all part of the fun. Each milieu required a respect for the sanctity of its inner workings, and in exchange, participants gained membership, even if only a junior one, in the insiders' club.

Power is the drug to which all of Washington is addicted, and simply being in the presence of the powerful was intoxicating. It was only an elevator, but proximity to senators was the first step to access and influence. In Washington, fresh anecdotes and gossip about members of the Senate formed a currency that guaranteed an attentive audience; stories from my elevator provided a never-ending supply.

That first summer in Washington, I rented a spare bedroom in my friend Bill Flannery's compact ivy-covered basement apartment on Capitol Hill. While in high school, I had taken a journalism course at the University of Iowa and helped out as a gofer at the student paper, *The Daily Iowan*, when Flannery was its editor. He subsequently moved to Washington to work for the Center for Defense Information, a left-leaning think tank that studied U.S. military and foreign policy. Flannery was almost a caricature of a flaming radical. He was all of twenty-five and had adopted the tweedy academic look of an Oxford don. He had a small bust of Lenin on his desk, and he sometimes called me "comrade" as he lectured me on the blood-soaked history of the leftist movement. He gave me a political education, explaining what was "really" happening according to his own radical analysis.

Living as his tenant and semi-ward, I was a captive and sympathetic audience. A year earlier, I published the first and only issue of *Radical Rites Press*, a project in the journalism course, but I had only a peripheral sense of leftist politics. It was a mimeographed zine containing three manifestos (all written by me) in support of abortion rights, the legalization of both marijuana and gay marriage—all positions I know would have shocked my parents, if I had told them—and an endorsement of Mo Udall's presidential candidacy. It felt daring to put those opinions in print, even though its circulation extended only as far as my teacher's desk and to a few friends in the *Daily Iowan* newsroom.

I was proud when Flannery read it and said, "You've got talent, kid!"

Flannery and I had long talks, and I came close to telling him about my attraction to men. But when I managed to steer our conversation toward gay rights or homosexuality, he was either dismissive or pejorative. He wasn't a bigot, just uninformed. He grew to respect LGBT activism and, in time, treasured his openly LGBT friends. But in 1976, his insensitivity felt to me like a hammer sealing tight the already closed door to my suffocating closet.

I had to be home by ten P.M. every night or face a grilling from Flannery, who acted like a surrogate parent. He admonished me to walk only to the right, toward East Capitol Street, as I left our Fifth Street NE apartment. To the left, toward Maryland Avenue and Stanton Park, was too dangerous, he said. I felt on edge on the streets, especially at night, but the streets were where I eventually went in search of other gay men. I was self-conscious about my virginity, and it was becoming more difficult to believe my same-sex attraction was just a phase. I needed to experience actual sex with another man to know for sure. Gay men recognized me as one of them—and as an object of desire—and I started to understand that there were homosexuals in the world beyond the flamboyant stereotypes I could identify easily. Working in the Senate, both running the elevator and as an intern in Senator Clark's office, brought me into contact with many closeted gay men. I grew attuned to the subtle clues they used to signal each other—the lingering glance, a style of dress, or conversational innuendo. I developed gaydar and took notice of those men who were groomed more carefully than others, whose ties were tied perfectly symmetrically with a dimple in the knot, and who exuded awareness or heightened sensitivity that I associated with being gay. I learned to distinguish among cordiality, friendliness, and flirtation.

Flannery's curfew and babysitting style kept my desires in check temporarily, but they didn't stop me from spending countless hours privately speculating about whether this or that man was gay. My awareness of bigoted comments also became more acute. Jokes or slurs that wouldn't have caused me a second thought a year or two earlier now felt unkind, ignorant, or hateful. When I thought all gay men were flamboyant and obvious, those comments didn't apply to me because I wasn't like that. But the more I privately identified as a gay person, the uglier those comments sounded, and the closer they hit to home.

During those first few months in Washington, I started to accept my sexual desire as a permanent part of who I was. I began to see the injustices that gay men endured and to recognize the consequences. Surprisingly, I didn't view lesbians the same way; I saw their struggle as part of the broader feminist movement. I didn't understand what gay men and lesbians had in common, but I already had a feminist consciousness and was quickly developing a gay one as well. To the extent that I recognized a binary movement, I thought of it in terms of gay men and feminists.

My earliest political mentors were Iowa state senator Minnette Doderer, one of Iowa's most important feminists in the 1970s, and Jean Lloyd-Jones, president of the Iowa chapter of the League of Women Voters and later a state legislator. Minnette often gave me rides back and forth to Des Moines from Iowa City, and I worked on Jean's first campaign. I spent hundreds of hours with them talking about the Equal Rights Amendment, abortion rights, and other feminist priorities, but I don't think homosexuality ever came up.

My sexuality throughout my teen years existed in a conflict zone boundaried by my church, my body, and my conscience. Coming out wasn't an option I even considered. Keeping my desire private—and fighting to suppress it—was a survival strategy. Once I began to accept my desire, I realized the closet was only a temporary refuge, one I could not inhabit forever.

One night Bill Flannery took me to meet colleagues of his at the Tune Inn, a popular burger and beer joint on Pennsylvania Avenue, a few blocks southeast of the Capitol. One of the guys who worked with Flannery started telling fag jokes. Everyone at the table was laughing boisterously, and I did, too. While I drank my beer and ate my cheeseburger, I felt disgusted with myself. I wanted to say something to get him to stop, but I was a coward, afraid that if I objected, it would cast suspicion on my own sexuality. Was this the way it was always going to be? Sitting in silent misery while others made jokes at my expense? I knew I couldn't live my life that way and privately started to question how others could.

Part of my self-acceptance came from recognizing others—especially well-known and well-respected people in public life or from history—who were gay or lesbian. I also heard rumors about politicians and others in positions of great power and privilege who were gay but denied it, even some who spoke disparagingly of gay people or exploited anti-gay prejudice to further their own political ambitions. I was shocked by their hypocrisy. Years later it was confirmed that several of the leading architects of the late-1970s evangelical and conservative movement—men who publicly promoted intolerance of gay people—were at the same time cruising gay bars and having sex with men in private.

As my identity as a gay man took root, I also had the chance to observe, close up, some of the most politically powerful men in the world. My brief conversations with senators, forgotten by them the moment they got off my elevator, have remained with me. I once heard MSNBC host Chris Matthews, who worked for House Speaker Tip O'Neill earlier in his career, refer to feeling a "thrill up the leg" when in the presence of inspirational elected officials. I know exactly what he means.

When not ferrying passengers, I rested my elevator on the Capitol's second floor, outside the majority leader's office and just a few steps from the Senate chamber's main entrance. The majority leader—red-vested, fiddle-playing Democratic senator Robert C. Byrd—was a West Virginian who, when he died in 2010, had served fifty-seven years in Congress, longer than anyone in U.S. history.

Byrd was often in his office late into the evening, and one night he and several other senators could be heard from the hallway. As they argued loudly over a procedural matter, I saw a reporter—one known to be hostile to the Democratic leadership—lingering nearby to eavesdrop outside the office door. I daringly left my elevator, which was forbidden while on duty, brushed by the reporter, and knocked on the door. When no one answered, I timidly opened it to the small reception area where his private secretary usually sat. She had left for the day, so I walked over to the open interior door into Byrd's private office. When I poked my head in, the senators, surprised by my interruption, stopped talking; Byrd gave me an irritated questioning look.

I knew this was risking my job and could result in dismissal. My voice cracked as I informed them of the reporter outside the office. Senator Byrd's face softened, and he graciously thanked me. Within minutes, a Capitol police officer shooed away the unwanted reporter.

After that incident, I was a favorite of the courtly Senator Byrd. Once he gave me a message—"Tell him 'It's all worked out' "—to deliver to my patron, Senator Clark. I never found out what it meant, but I conveyed that single sentence as if it were a national security secret.

I loved meeting every member of the Senate, especially three of the Democratic liberal "lions"—George McGovern, Hubert Humphrey, and Ted Kennedy—whose careers I had followed closely. When I told Senator McGovern that I was his campus coordinator at my boarding school in Wisconsin during his 1972 presidential campaign, he asked, "How'd I do?" and I was proud to tell him, "You won, sir!"

When Senator Kennedy saw a copy of Leon Uris's novel *Trinity* wedged between the collapsible elevator seat and the wall, he told me that his mother had given him a copy when he was hospitalized. Over the next several weeks, he would ask me where I was in the story, about specific characters and turns in the plot. When Senator Humphrey, a failed presidential candidate but enduring statesman, found out I was a native Iowan, he said, "We midwesterners need to stick together!" He had brought me a signed copy of his newly published book, *The Education of a Public Man*, which Senator Walter Mondale, Humphrey's Minnesota colleague, saw in my elevator; I told him that Senator Humphrey had given it to me. The next day Mondale brought me a signed copy of *his* book, *The Accountability of Power*.

Senators weren't my only prominent passengers. Celebrities visited frequently, and the 1976 bicentennial summer attracted more stars than usual. Elizabeth Taylor, Billy Graham, sex expert Dr. Ruth Westheimer, and others were passengers. When Senator Jacob Javits squired Taylor around the Capitol, he looked like the nerdy high school kid who had lucked into a date with the prom queen. Another famous Elizabeth, the Queen of England, visited the Capitol in July for a lunch in her honor in the National Statuary Hall. There wasn't much room in my elevator, but I loved how large the world became for me within its walls.

In the 1970s, seniority meant everything in the Senate. It dictated chairmanships of the most powerful committees and the assignment of office space and parking spots; it earned the prize of the last available space on an elevator. It wasn't ideology but perks (especially office assignments and parking spaces) that caused the greatest friction among members.

Though the seniority system had serious flaws, it enabled more nuanced and complicated cross-party alliances than the lockstep party discipline typical today. A spirit of collegiality could transcend party politics, and senators were more independent in their political views. For example, Washington's senator Henry "Scoop" Jackson was so hawkish that he was called the "Senator from Boeing," after the major military contractor then headquartered in his state, but he was also a leading environmentalist. Mississippian John Stennis, an ultra-conservative Dixiecrat who staunchly opposed every piece of civil rights legislation, was one of the first members to publicly criticize Senator Joseph McCarthy's demagogic red baiting in the 1950s. In the 1980s, he opposed Reagan's nomination of ultra-conservative Robert Bork to the Supreme Court. Arizona's Barry Goldwater, an icon of the far right, was prominently pro-choice.

Stennis was not the only famous segregationist in the Senate in the late 1970s; others included South Carolina's Strom Thurmond, who ran for president as a Dixiecrat in 1948, and North Carolina's Jesse Helms, labeled the "master obstructionist" for his ability to delay legislation that he opposed. Helms was famously racist; in 1983 he filibustered for sixteen days, trying to prevent the Senate from approving a federal holiday to honor Martin Luther King, Jr. In the AIDS-defined years to come, he relished every opportunity to show his homophobia, railing against "the homosexual agenda" and ranting to all who would listen about the immorality of the "homosexual lifestyle." When President Bill Clinton nominated Roberta Achtenberg, the accomplished former head of the National Center for Lesbian Rights, to a post requiring Senate confirmation, Helms condemned her from the Senate floor as "that damn lesbian."

In my elevator, Helms was always distracted and slightly formal, courtly but not warm. At the time, I could not have fathomed that my future would intersect with Helms and that our encounter would one day involve the use of an extra-large condom.

I was spending my days in constant motion—going up and down— yet always arriving back where I started. My future was in a holding pattern as well, with an illusion of movement masking the fact that I was on standby, waiting to see if I might shake the secret that stood in the way. On some days, I had a growing sense that would never happen.

I desperately wanted someone—or something—to ring a bell three times and whisk me to where I wanted or needed to be. My real desire was to run for office, but I was certain that was impossible as long as I was attracted to men. That fear caused me to withdraw from my parents and family back in Iowa. As I took Washington's elite from one floor to the next, I feared being permanently grounded by my sexual orientation.

■ ■ ■

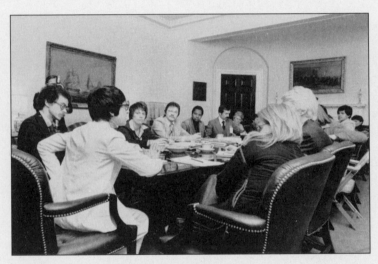

First meeting at the White House addressing gay and lesbian issues, hosted by Midge Costanza *(foreground, left)*, an assistant to President Jimmy Carter, in March 1977. Costanza ultimately was fired, in part because of her role in organizing this meeting. Jean O'Leary is the third person from the left.

CHAPTER 2

The Way Out

A few days after the country's bicentennial celebration, the 1976 Democratic National Convention was held at Madison Square Garden in New York. The week before it was to start, I was sorting mail in a large open room in Senator Clark's office, surrounded by desks where other several staff members worked, when the senator walked through and casually asked if anyone wanted floor passes for the convention. I don't think his offer was intended for the new intern, but I piped up anyway: "I'd love to, Senator!"

"Have you ever even been to New York?" he asked, smiling.

"Sure I have," I said, afraid he might think I was too young to go to New York on my own. It wasn't a lie, as I had driven through Manhattan once with a high school friend. Clark looked doubtful and asked, "Where would you stay?" I acted nonchalant and said, "Oh, I'm sure I can find a youth hostel." Clark ended up giving me his VIP floor pass (marked "U.S. Senator"), as well as the hotel room at the Statler Hilton provided to him by the Democratic National Committee.

Eighteen months before, when I applied to be a page in the Iowa legislature, I declined to declare whether I was a Democrat or a Republican, not wanting to limit my options. But I did know that my political beliefs were different than those of my conservative Republican parents.

Now here I was a short time later, a committed Democrat, with premium credentials and floor passes to the national convention. I had personally shaken hands with or spoken to eleven of the thirteen main candidates for the Democratic nomination. Not having met the two exceptions—Governor George Wallace, the Alabama segregationist, and Governor Milton Shapp of Pennsylvania—was, to me, like missing a couple of key players in a baseball-card collection. But of those I'd met, some I really felt I *knew*. I saw Senator Birch Bayh's humility when I got lost driving him to an event at the Izaak Walton League in Iowa City, and I was teased by Morris Udall, who wanted to see my driver's license before he got in my car because he thought I looked so young. I was awed by the fiery populist rhetoric of Fred Harris and thrilled to meet the genteel Kennedy-related Sargent Shriver. Former North Carolina governor Terry Sanford was president of Duke University; when he learned that I hadn't decided on a college, he encouraged me to apply to Duke. And months before Jimmy Carter became the presumptive Democratic nominee, I spent an afternoon making small talk while driving him and an aide around southeast Iowa. At the time, I found Carter sincere but his campaign quixotic; as a Southerner, he seemed foreign to me. I hoped to get close enough to him during the convention to remind him we had met.

With great anticipation, I hopped on the Amtrak train from Washington's Union Station to New York's Penn Station, underneath Madison Square Garden and across the street from my hotel.

For several years, New York City had been in a downward fiscal spiral, with exceptionally high crime, service cutbacks, and obvious neglect. With the city teetering on the edge of a financial abyss, President Ford's refusal to support a federal bailout prompted the famous headline in *The New York Daily News:* FORD TO CITY: DROP DEAD. But even as the Republican White House seemed to have written off the city, a miraculous turnaround was quietly under way. The Democratic

National Convention gave the city a chance to put forth its best face, focus national attention on its problems, and begin a dramatic turnaround.

That convention week would have been the perfect time for me to start to inch my way out of the closet and explore the city's gay scene. I was alone in the biggest and gayest city in the country. But I was determined to suppress my sexual desire and far too timid to consider entering a gay bar. Besides, nothing could compete with the excitement of my first national political convention.

I lived and breathed Democratic politics that week, practically sleeping with the credentials lanyard around my skinny neck. I never ventured more than a block from Madison Square Garden. I saved money by eating at free receptions hosted by state delegations, labor unions, and advocacy groups. I spent every possible waking moment on the convention floor, listening to Ohio senator John Glenn and Texas representative Barbara Jordan give the keynote speeches. Glenn was the first American to orbit the earth and a genuine hero, but it was Jordan's radiant oratory that brought tears to my eyes.

Jordan was the first Southern African-American woman elected to Congress, as well as the first woman and the first African-American to deliver the keynote speech at a national political convention. Her mesmerizing, stentorian voice became known nationally during her service on the Watergate Committee, where she once began her remarks by thanking the committee's chairman for "the glorious opportunity of sharing the pain of this inquiry" and then said her "faith in the Constitution is whole, it is complete, it is total."

At the end of her convention speech, she moved me when she quoted Abraham Lincoln: "As I would not be a slave, so I would not be a master. This expresses my idea of democracy. Whatever differs from this, to the extent of the difference, is no democracy." I didn't know then that Barbara Jordan was a lesbian and she never came out of the closet publicly. But when she died twenty years later, the press recognized Nancy Earl as her surviving partner of nearly three decades.

What I did know was that my secret sexual desire precluded any hope that I might speak at a convention. I had stopped attending Mass regularly when I was fifteen, but I prayed fervently that my sexual attraction to men would disappear. Still, I studied the faces, bodies, mannerisms, and style of dress of men I found attractive on the convention floor. Those I thought might be gay, I surreptitiously followed.

As I sleuthed my way around the convention and my own inner conflicts, I found a mention in *The New York Times* that Senator George McGovern, whom I admired, had advocated in favor of a gay-rights plank in the party platform. McGovern's support of gay rights justified my support as well.

Between the bicentennial and the convention, it was an exciting summer. But I was relieved when classes at Georgetown started that fall, because I could move out of Bill Flannery's apartment into a single dorm room. I grew up sharing a bedroom with my older brother, had roommates at boarding school, and moved in with Flannery when I arrived in Washington. At Georgetown, for the first time in my life, I had that prized possession of adolescence: total privacy behind a locked door.

Even though I had started school, my Washington life revolved around Capitol Hill, not the Georgetown campus, because I was still running the elevator and interning in Senator Clark's office. I was poorly prepared for college. I had left high school partway through the first semester of my junior year to become a page in the Iowa legislature. I attended Campion Jesuit High School, an elite Catholic boarding school in rural Wisconsin and the time I did spend there was atypical. The priests who ran it were divided between the old guard intending to "turn out fine Catholic gentlemen," as they had for decades, and a new generation of younger 1960s-era priests who espoused liberation theology and sought to produce "radical Christians" to oppose the war in Vietnam, fight for civil rights, and end poverty.

On the first day of class, the Jesuit scholastic (he wasn't yet ordained a priest) teaching my social studies course began the class by introducing himself. "Good morning, gentlemen," he said. "My name is Hal Dessel and I am a member of the Society of Jesus and I am your teacher. You may call me Mr. Dessel. I am also a Marxist and, if I am a good teacher, at the end of this course, some of you will be good Marxists." I figured out quickly that Campion wasn't going to provide me the education my politically conservative parents, who supported President Nixon and wouldn't let me grow my hair long, had in mind.

The rigorous discipline for which the Society of Jesus was famous had by the mid-'70s become a faint memory, and their internal battle resulted in a chaotic academic and living environment for students, with little structure, supervision, or guidance. Sexual abuse was rampant, scholastic oversight was virtually nonexistent, and both students and faculty members were openly dealing drugs.

Though high school gave me freedom from my parents' home, I wasn't stimulated academically. I wasn't any more focused at Georgetown, where my classroom education paled in comparison with my expanding political, professional, and, soon, sexual education on Capitol Hill. The only friends I made at Georgetown were residents of my dorm; I participated in no extracurricular activities and frequently skipped classes. Learning political science in a classroom couldn't compete with interacting with members of Congress, even in a service capacity.

The area around my Georgetown dorm was safer than where I had lived on Capitol Hill, but muggings and street crime were not uncommon. Despite the risks, I was drawn to the streets at night. I took long walks down Wisconsin Avenue, the main thoroughfare, passing slowly by the Georgetown Grill. Other boys in my dorm claimed it was a gay bar, so I sauntered by, trying to catch a glimpse inside without lingering enough to prompt suspicion. Other times I walked down the long and forbidding outdoor brick stairway featured in *The Exorcist*, leading to the Potomac River, silently searching for something I could not name.

Eventually I discovered "The Block," a popular cruising spot in a beautiful and expensive residential part of Georgetown. I don't remember how I came to know about it. Perhaps from a derogatory reference I overheard or even by instinct. The Block came alive late at night, after the elegant Georgetown dinner-party guests had gone home, with men appearing out of the darkness to claim several blocks, loitering along leafy streets lined with redbrick Georgian town houses. Some stopped to smoke a cigarette; others walked slowly or simply stood near the curb as if expecting a ride.

I joined their parade, scrutinizing them for clues, trying to figure out if they were like me. With each step, I felt guilt and vulnerability, as though my presence itself were a criminal act. Old-fashioned pedestrian streetlights lined the street, but long stretches were dark, shrouded by a thick canopy of stately oak and maple trees. Sometimes men strode past me purposefully, as if going somewhere, but after a block, they would do an about-face and walk toward me. Our eyes would meet briefly until I diverted mine, fearful of what they exposed.

Cars circled the block, the drivers inspecting the faces and bodies of those on the sidewalk. I first thought they were residents or undercover police trying to discourage men from cruising, but I soon realized they were cruising me, like the men on the sidewalk who asked, "Do you have a light?" or requested directions to a nearby and obvious destination.

An anxious hush hung over the Block; the brief conversations were low and soft. After several visits, I felt both familiar enough with the terrain and desperate enough to make a move. It wasn't so much that I wanted to have sex; I just wanted to stop being a virgin.

"Do you want to go for a drink?" a driver asked tentatively as he peered at me through the passenger-side window. He was older, maybe mid-thirties, seemed friendly and not too unattractive. The car was expensive.

I thought for a moment, my heart racing. "No. I have to get back to my dorm."

"Where do you go to school?" he asked.

"Georgetown," I answered.

"Good school," he said.

I didn't respond, but I didn't leave. After another moment he added: "Do you want a ride? It's lonely to be walking all that way at this hour." It was, at most, a fifteen-minute walk.

"No thanks, I'll walk," I said.

But he persisted. "It's getting nippy out, why don't you just sit in the car for a few minutes to warm up?" he said.

He did not seem like a serial killer. I was prepared to have sex with him or, more accurately, ready to let him have sex with me. I thought he might give me a blow job, which I had read about but never experienced. I had promised myself I would lie back and let him do it. I had no clue how we would get to that point. When I got in the car, the man was figuratively and literally in the driver's seat.

We small-talked. I asked what he did for a living, and he inquired about my classes at Georgetown. I didn't dare tell him I worked on the Hill. I can't recall any of my freshman-year classes or instructors, but I do remember his job: He was a lobbyist for the American Petroleum Institute.

"You're a good-looking guy," he said suddenly. "How old are you?"

I said I was eighteen.

"Eighteen." He let out a long, low whistle. "Wow, it's been a long time since I've had eighteen-year-old dick!"

The crudeness of his comment immediately turned me off. I made an excuse and got out of the car. When he offered me his business card with his home number scribbled on the back, I politely took it but then threw it away before I got back to my dorm, destroying the one scrap of evidence showing how close I had come to having sex.

A few days later, I ventured into an adult bookstore, intent on solving the mystery of how gay men had sex. The store was on the second floor of a building on a seedy block of Fourteenth Street and offered individual booths for watching pornographic films. It was foreign territory, and I was without a map. Nervously, I exchanged my dollar bills for quarters, trying to look casual, as if I did this all the time. I took the booth farthest from the clerk's desk and began watching the film in twenty-five cent increments.

The near-total absence of gay life in the world where I was raised left me, like a lot of young gay men, with many gaps in understanding. What I knew about gay sex was influenced by homophobic descriptions of gay life in sex manuals I found at the library as well as pejorative comments, jokes, and stories I had heard. I thought that men "fucking" referred to two men having sex of any kind. I knew some gay men fantasized about having sex "like a woman," though I wasn't sure it was possible for two men to have intercourse with each other. I once saw grainy pictures in a porn magazine of what seemed to be one man penetrating another, but I thought it was trick photography, an artful simulation of what heterosexuals do.

This misconception was confirmed when I was fourteen. After a night of drinking, a male faculty member at Campion, the Wisconsin boarding school I attended, tried to penetrate me. I blacked out, but horrible details—including blood in my undershorts the next day— have surfaced in bits and pieces of recovered memories over the years. Until I saw that porn film, I thought intercourse was something that some gay men fantasized about, but it wasn't *really* possible; indeed, when attempted on me, it resulted in injury.

Yet as I learned more about gay life, I heard of men who claimed to enjoy having sex this way. I wanted to know if that was possible. Standing in the small booth that night with a molded plastic seat affixed to the floor, watching the flickering writhing images up close, was confirmation and revelation. Not only was it possible; the men in the film looked like they were enjoying themselves painlessly. I watched their eyes and faces closely and became convinced that the pleasure depicted was genuine.

Not long after exploring the Block and making the research expedition to the adult bookstore, I had sex for the first time. I was relieved to

have finally "done it," even if the other guy had been drunk and afterward pretended nothing had happened. That was followed by several
fast and fumbling interactions with other guys that were little more
than exercises in mutual masturbation.

For a while, I also tried to have sex with women; my plan was to
alternate one for one, to be bisexual rather than gay. But the sex I had
with women, even if meaningful and enjoyable to me, was less satisfying than that with men.

One day I was buying a sweater at Britches, a fashionable men's
clothing store on Wisconsin Avenue. An attractive and friendly clerk
asked where I was from and how long I had been in Washington. He
was just getting off work, and when he suggested that we hang out, I
said, "Sure!" Right after leaving the store, he looked at me and said,
"So, are you gay or what?" I froze, as no one had ever asked me that
question directly. I assumed he was, and I wanted to spend time with
him, so I said, "Yeah," as though it were no big deal.

After that, I started to use the word "gay" as a descriptor, sometimes
of myself and sometimes of others, even if they vehemently rejected the
label. Having sex with a guy was one thing; being gay was something
else. My first gay friends were closeted. I don't think any expected they
would ever come out—we didn't use that phrase. Like me, most were
ashamed of their attraction to men, including the first man I thought
of, briefly, as my boyfriend.

Andy was a journalist, a decade older than I. He was intellectual, fun,
and led an exciting life, traveling frequently and forever at the center of
breaking news and political action. I was impressed with his British-
racing-green MG and emulated his style of dress, refined mannerisms,
and lifestyle. He was straight-acting, though that wasn't a phrase I was
familiar with either. If I could have become him, I would have.

We met through my elevator post; he would say hello as he passed
by on his way to the Senate's third-floor press gallery. If the Senate
wasn't in session, I let him ride in my elevator, and sometimes he gave
me a ride back to my dorm at Georgetown when my shift was over. He

teased me about my clothes, saying, "You look like you stepped out of a Sears Roebuck catalog." One day he offered to take me shopping at Tysons Corner, one of the first regional mega-malls, just outside D.C., in Virginia. I wrote down his address on a receipt from the Senate take-out restaurant and agreed to meet him at his apartment that Saturday afternoon.

His apartment, near the Capitol, was a small bachelor's pad, with contemporary furniture, bicycle and sports equipment strewn about, a large TV, and stacks of books on the floor. Driving to the mall in his sports car with the top down was like entering an exciting new realm where I was finally one of the cool kids. After our shopping expedition, we returned to his apartment. There still was no explicit indication that he was gay or interested in me sexually, but I didn't care; I was just glad to be with him. I was so conscious of my attraction to him that when I sat next to him on the couch, I worried I might sprout an erection.

As we ate pizza, he told me how great his girlfriend was and how much I would like her. It wasn't until later that evening, until the very moment he leaned over and gently kissed me, with a basketball game playing on the television, that I knew for certain. His kiss was electric, sending a tingling sensation to the end of every finger and toe, a sensation unlike anything I had felt before.

The sex we had then and later was limited to mutual masturbation. It happened silently and without any advance planning or discussion, almost as if it weren't happening at all. We would be sitting next to each other, talking, when Andy would lean over and kiss me.

Sometimes, after we finished and cleaned up, he would erase the meaning of what we had shared. "This stuff is just a phase guys go through," he told me once. "You'll get this part of your life out of your system and move on to girls. Just like me." I nodded, because I wasn't aware enough to recognize this as an attempt to compensate for his own shame by "setting me straight."

After a few weeks, we stopped hanging out together, but I didn't go straight. Instead, I started to explore Washington's gay nightlife.

*   *   *

Describing the Lost and Found as a gay discotheque made it sound more glamorous and potentially less stigmatizing than the gay bars I knew existed but hadn't yet visited. Going to the Lost and Found marked my first appearance in a public gay venue, and that felt irreversible, crossing a threshold from which I could not return.

The club was in a nameless warehouse district amid a small strip of sex-oriented businesses—including a gay strip club and an adult bookstore—several blocks southwest of the Capitol. The streets were poorly lit, and when clouds obscured the moon, they were dead dark. Prostitutes trolled the loading docks and parking lots, sometimes clustering under corner streetlights.

Going there was risky. Addicts in need of cash for a fix and young thugs preyed on men visiting the area, knowing that few would report the crime. For those who were extremely closeted, the biggest risk was being seen in or near a gay venue. One might just happen upon the Georgetown Grill or cruising areas in respectable neighborhoods; any number of reasons could excuse being there. But the Lost and Found was a singular destination; to be seen anywhere within a few blocks indicated guilt by proximity.

At the club's entrance, there were muscled doormen standing guard like sentries at a sanctuary. Once I passed them and entered, I was struck by the club's ultra-modern decor. The industrial design with clean lines and contemporary lighting contrasted sharply with the grittiness of the neighborhood, just as the safety and excitement inside contrasted with the danger and fear of exposure outside.

Meeting people at a gay bar or club meant they were as "guilty" as I was. On one of my first visits, I saw a Senate staffer whom I recognized. We had never spoken in the Capitol, but in the Lost and Found, he talked to me like we were old friends. A few days later, he was on my elevator with his boss, a senator. When our eyes met, he covertly held his finger to his mouth.

I learned that meeting gay men in a gay context—whether at a bar, private party, or other circumstance—invoked an unspoken omertà-like agreement not to share the secret life with others, even if it meant pretending we didn't know each other.

It was like graduating from a private closet to a semi-private one. By day, most of the men at the Lost and Found pretended to be heterosexual. At night, they lived a hidden culture. It reminded me of Marrano Jews during the Spanish Inquisition, who had been forced to publicly convert to Christianity but kept their traditions alive by practicing them in secret. By day I "converted" to heterosexuality, but my friends and I gathered as our true selves at night.

The friends I made at the Lost and Found were all white, like most of the club's clientele, and typically college students or young Hill staffers. It would be years before I knew many lesbians or gay men of color. I had no inkling of the breadth of gay culture beyond the men I saw in the Lost and Found and, soon, other gay bars. I had read about historic figures, such as Alexander the Great, Leonardo da Vinci, and Michelangelo, who were supposedly gay. But I thought they were stories, probably folklore made up by gay activists.

I was quickly adopted by a handful of gay men, an affectionate clique of barflies who campily called each other Mary. They hosted Sunday brunches and were regulars at the Wednesday gay night at a skating rink in Alexandria, Virginia. "Oh, just call me Mother," one of the older members said when I was introduced to him. They were shop clerks, bureaucrats, and a hairdresser, bound by love and caring rather than the politics or career ambition that united the guys I met on the Hill and at Georgetown.

They promised to corrupt me and pretended it was only a matter of time before I gave in to their seductions; in truth, they were fiercely protective and gave me a useful and cautionary education in gay life. They had opinions about every guy I found attractive. "Be careful of that one," Mother once said, "I heard he's got the clap." (Yes, I had to ask what that was.)

I was inching my way out of the closet, into a wider circle of friends and acquaintances met at the Lost and Found or at the parties and brunches I was starting to attend. I had never imagined the existence of such a vast underground. Every conversation with a gay man filled in details of a world that had, until then, been invisible to me.

It was not until I discovered the freedom of admiring men in a gay bar that I realized how much my appreciation of male beauty was tempered by fear. In junior high and high school, the tanned golden boys I wanted to look at ignored or taunted me. Now they were all around me. And some of them were looking at me.

In the months after my first visit to the Lost and Found, I had a lot of sex, but that wasn't primarily what I sought. I reveled in the attention and friendship, feeling for the first time that I belonged and was part of a group. I loved going out on a Saturday night, confident that I would meet someone with whom I could possibly have brunch and enjoy a movie with the following afternoon.

I was poorly prepared for sex, especially the casual kind. I knew little about my body and even less about my genitals or sexuality. I was ashamed of what my body looked like (skinny, no chest, and big ears) and its limitations. I wasn't any good at sports, couldn't dance, and was poorly coordinated.

I was neurotic and insecure, and my eagerness to be wanted left me vulnerable. I had little control over sexual contact. I thought of sex as managing someone else's desires—advances and aggression—rather than satisfying myself. I knew nothing about protecting my sexual health and believed condoms were exclusively for preventing pregnancy. In the eighth grade, several years before I hit puberty, my school separated boys and girls for an hour and imparted vague instructions about "family life." That was it. No one ever had the birds-and-bees conversation with me, let alone a birds-and-birds or bees-and-bees conversation.

Some of my early sexual experiences in Washington were painful. Today I see them as reminiscent of the sexual abuse I suffered as a child but didn't understand until years later. In both circumstances, I could not tell anyone without eliciting suspicion and shame, so I blamed myself. Eventually I recognized my self-hatred or understood its genesis in the sexual violence perpetrated against me.

*   *   *

In the spring of 1977, near the end of my freshman year at Georgetown and a few months after I started having sex, I was at Mr. P's, a gay bar on P Street near Dupont Circle. I was flattered when the muscular man on the stool next to me began talking to me. He was about ten years older and attractive—built like a football player, nicely dressed, a wide Slavic face, and narrow eyes.

His manner was abrupt, but when he introduced himself as Barry and told me about his job in marketing, he sounded important and interesting. When he found out I was looking for a place to live that summer—I had to move out of the dorm in a few days—he said he had an extra bedroom and needed a roommate.

At first it felt like kismet. When he showed me the apartment, he made a few sexually suggestive comments, though I thought he was joking. He was an older jock, confident and assertive; I couldn't imagine that he would be interested in me. I moved out of my dorm and into his extra room, agreeing to pay $256 per month, half the rent.

A few days after I moved in, I was lying on my mattress on the floor of my room, reading a book. Barry came in, wearing only gym shorts and white socks. When he lay down on the mattress and tried to make out with me, I could smell alcohol on his breath. I squirmed out of his arms and off the mattress, assuming he would take the hint. Instead, he grabbed me and, under the guise of playfulness, threw me back down on the mattress and began massaging my body.

"I'm reading, leave me alone," I said.

As I tried to get away, he threw me back on the mattress carelessly, as if I were a pillow. I froze, instinctively fearing that he would turn violent if I tried to get away again; he outweighed me by at least fifty pounds. I acted like it was a big joke and tried to wrestle my way off the mattress. When he stopped me, I said angrily, "Leave me alone!"

He laughed, saying, "Why do you think I rented you the room so cheap?" He pinned me facedown on the mattress with his body, one arm braced against my neck. With his other hand, he pulled down my pants, then wet his finger with spit and started to wiggle it in my anus, cooing about how tight it felt. I cried out in pain, unable to escape his grasp.

"Don't be a crybaby!" he said as he pulled down his gym shorts and penetrated me. I was on my stomach, defenseless. When I started to yell, he pushed my head face-first into the mattress. As I began to cry, he put one hand over my mouth and used the other to pull my head back up by the hair, saying, "Just relax, or you'll only make it worse." A few minutes later, he said, "Oh fuck, you're bleeding," as if that were my fault. Then he left the room.

I locked the door and stayed in my room until I heard him leave the apartment. In the bathroom, I inspected the damage with a small mirror while trying to avoid dripping blood on the floor mat. Over the next several days, while I looked for another place to live, I avoided him as much as possible. When I told him I was leaving, he said, "I was going to throw you out anyway; you're too much of a pussy."

It was a devastating blow to the sexual ownership of my body that I had just begun to acquire, reinforcing shame, self-hatred, and a sense of worthlessness. Intellectually, I knew what transpired was nonconsensual; he was violent, and I was injured. But emotionally, it damaged my already fragile sense of masculinity. I felt like I should have seen it coming or somehow avoided being in such a vulnerable circumstance. I blamed myself.

It was over twenty years before I could recognize and label this as rape.

My first positive experience of intercourse was with a gentle man named Eric, who was slow and careful. Eric was attractive—big-chested, with brown hair and a sturdy, confident air—but I was too newly out and too insecure to have an adult relationship with him. After two or three dates, I blurted out "I love you."

Eric castigated me, saying, "You don't know what you're talking about, and you shouldn't say that if you don't mean it." Though my feelings were hurt, I knew he was right. The truth was, at that point in my life, I didn't have *any* idea what romantic love felt like, and my feelings about myself would have made it impossible to recognize even if I found it. We stopped seeing each other after a few weeks but remained friends.

I kept looking for something I could not consciously identify, sometimes on weekend hitchhiking trips to New York, armed with an emergency hundred-dollar bill hidden in my sock. On one particularly charmed trip in April 1977, not only did I get a ride leaving D.C. that took me all the way to Manhattan—a stroke of luck in itself—I also met someone who was to become my first close friend in the city.

On previous trips to New York, I'd made a few friends who would let me crash on their couches. If these were unavailable, the West Side YMCA, on Sixty-third Street, was an acceptable backup plan. Most exciting was when I found someone attractive who invited me to his place. After arriving in the city, I had dinner at a Greek diner and then started touring the bars. Late that night I was in Uncle Charlie's South, a popular cruise bar on Third Avenue, when I noticed a cute guy standing against the far wall.

He was wearing a starched white button-down shirt. He occasionally glanced my way, reciprocating my attention with a shy smile. When another guy tried to strike up a conversation with me, I told him I was interested in someone else, expecting the guy to beat it. Instead he walked right over to the object of my attention and pointed at me. I was mortified. After a minute, they waved me over, and a little while later, the three of us left the bar together and headed to the apartment of the intermediary. The guy in that starched white shirt introduced himself as Jim Nall, originally from New Orleans. I was nervous, being in a strange apartment in a strange city with two strangers, including one I didn't particularly like, but the idea of a three-way was new and exciting to me.

After a few minutes of messing around, the host passed out. Jim asked if I wanted to leave and go to his place on Ninety-seventh Street. Relieved, I dressed silently, and we left without waking our spent host. We held hands in the backseat of the Checker cab; we had known each other only a few hours, but it already felt like we were friends.

Jim became my cultural mentor. On my subsequent visits to the city, he introduced me to opera, ballet, and museums, and he seemed interested in the political gossip and news from Washington that I shared with him. I wasn't conscious then of having a "type," but in retrospect, Jim had a manner and physicality that was similar to those of men I was to have important relationships with later. He was shorter than me, with straight brown hair and hazel eyes, and a tight, toned swimmer's build. He exuded a gentle spirit I found attractive, and his face was handsome, with a distinctive pockmarked patch on one cheek. I didn't think of him as a boyfriend, more like a close friend with whom I sometimes had sex. I always found myself relaxed in his presence, less conscious of the imperfections I saw in my body and less burdened by shame and guilt. It felt right to be with him.

Ultimately, what may have made the biggest impression was that Jim was neither closeted nor a gay activist. He just *was*—living as he chose. He didn't hide his sexuality, nor did he wear it on his sleeve. He had no fear of being outed and no impulse to out himself.

I had never met anyone like him.

Back in Washington, I picked up the *Washington Blade*, the weekly gay newspaper, at the Lambda Rising bookstore, and I started to read about lesbian and gay community activities and activism. The first "gay books" I bought were *One for the Gods* and *Forth into Light*, gay-romance novels by Gordon Merrick with sappy stories about gorgeous rich men tortured by their desires and struggling for self-acceptance. Despite the genre, they helped me envision a gay adulthood for myself.

I was struck by coverage in the *Blade* that used real names and photographs of openly gay and lesbian people. I wondered if their parents were dead or if they were so estranged from their families that they didn't care if they were identified publicly as homosexuals. In that first year or two, the thought never crossed my mind that any of the gay people featured in the *Blade* might have parents who were actually proud of them.

I followed closely the *Blade*'s coverage of NFL player Dave Kopay's 1977 coming-out memoir, which made *The New York Times* best-seller list. Many gay Washingtonians knew that Kopay had dated the Washington Redskins' star tight end, Jerry Smith. Even though Kopay didn't identify Smith by name in the book, his thinly veiled account of their relationship sold a lot of books and provided lively fodder for the insatiable Washington gossip mill.

I met Smith at a holiday party, around the time Kopay's book came out. I was nineteen, very slight, and hadn't yet reached my full height. I looked at least three or four years younger than I was. The party was packed with Washington's A-list gays. All the "better boys" wore pastel-colored sweaters; mine was an embarrassing dark brown. When I was introduced to Smith, he immediately treated me like a kid brother, picking me up and carrying me around on his powerfully muscled shoulders. It felt like I was wrapping my legs around a tree stump as we waded our way through the crowded party. He died of AIDS in 1986.

A *Blade* story that made a strong impression on me was about an historic meeting of gay and lesbian leaders at the White House in 1977. It was at the height of former beauty queen Anita Bryant's anti-gay crusade in Dade County, Florida, just weeks before the referendum that repealed the anti-discrimination statute. Never before had the White House even acknowledged the *existence* of a gay and lesbian community, let alone held a meeting for it. I was surprised and intrigued that Jean O'Leary, who led the meeting, was not only head of the National Gay Task Force but also a former nun. I wondered if any of her one-time religious colleagues still talked to her. Years later I learned that the meeting was arranged by Midge Costanza, a special assistant to President Jimmy Carter who ended up getting fired, in part because of that meeting. Costanza became quietly influential in national lesbian and gay politics, but she never publicly came out of the closet. Years later, when we became friends, I asked why she never came out. "I didn't need the complications, and now I'm too old," she said. "Who cares about an old lady's sex life, anyway?"

The *Blade* frequently featured Washington's leading gay activist, Frank Kameny, who organized U.S. Air Force Sergeant Leonard Matlovich's public coming out on the cover of *Time* magazine in 1975. That was the first time the gay rights movement had achieved such prominence in the national media. The *Blade* said Kameny had been looking for an exemplary gay service member willing to confront the military's ban on homosexuals. Matlovich, awarded the Purple Heart and Bronze Star during Vietnam, fit the bill.

A dozen years later, Matlovich and I were arrested together at an AIDS protest in front of the White House, and we ended up sharing a jail cell. A year after that, he died of AIDS and was buried at the congressional cemetery under a tombstone that does not bear his name but says simply: "A gay Vietnam Veteran" and "When I was in the military, they gave me a medal for killing two men and a discharge for loving one."

From the coverage in the *Blade*, Kameny, Kopay, Matlovich, and O'Leary became important role models for me. Before reading about these four, I knew of no one who was publicly homosexual and unashamed of it. As I began to accept that I was gay, I abandoned any hope of getting elected to office, though I did see new possibilities, exemplified by self-accepting gay men who had interesting careers or positions of political influence. Even if they remained deeply closeted, they gave me glimpses of a world where a man could be attracted to other men and still pursue a career, albeit with some limitations.

The key, it seemed, was to keep one's private life separate from one's career. Gay men who were out were then considered flamboyant or "flamers." Nothing in mainstream culture made it seem admirable or desirable to be honest about one's sexual orientation.

The loneliness I had struggled with since puberty had become my version of normal. But what I had thought was a tiny, hidden, and beleaguered population showed itself as a massive community hidden in plain sight. Beyond the bars, I discovered gay and lesbian bookstores, restaurants, and churches.

The idea of being publicly gay, however, remained beyond my comprehension. If I told my parents, I feared they might disown me; their feelings of anger and humiliation were certain. Trying to educate them did not feel like an option. I wasn't close to my older siblings, and I thought the younger ones would not understand. There was no one from my straight life I could trust with my secret.

On a visit home from Washington, my youngest sister, Megan, took me to her fifth-grade class at Lincoln Elementary for show-and-tell, to talk about my experience running an elevator in the U.S. Senate. When we were walking back home, I told her that I was gay. She didn't understand exactly what "gay" meant, only that it was an important secret. She didn't keep the secret from her friends, though, and later she told me they thought it was cool she had a gay brother. Intolerance is taught, and Megan's peers hadn't yet learned that lesson.

My homosexual "problem" had, in just a couple of years, evolved from something I prayed would magically go away to something I accepted as a secret and was able to share with those closest to me. I started to understand how it could be integrated into my otherwise "normal" life, and what had been a moral, religious, and existential crisis became more of a logistical obstacle for my career and life ambitions—one that could be managed with a proper strategy.

■   ■   ■

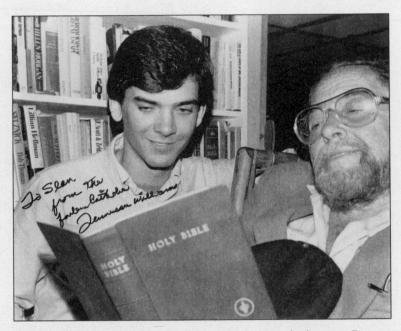

Tennessee Williams jokingly reading Bible verses to me, in his house on Duncan Street in Key West, December 1979, after dinner at the Pier House on Duval Street.

CHAPTER 3

Tennessee and Me

The first gay bar in Washington with a window to the sidewalk, Rascals, opened in 1978. This startling innovation helped make it popular with younger guys, the post-Stonewall generation, who were unconcerned with being seen in a gay bar.

One night at Rascals, a tall, impeccably dressed, and well-mannered gentleman came up to me and said, "Excuse me, but have you ever read *The Catcher in the Rye?*"

"Yes," I replied, amused at the pickup line.

"Well, you look just like I have always imagined Holden Caulfield might look. My name is Edmund Perret; that's spelled P-E-R-R-E-T. It's French, I'm from Louisiana, but no one here knows how to pronounce it," he said. He held out his hand in a regal manner.

At first I wasn't sure if he intended for me to shake it or kiss it. "I'm Sean," I said, extending my own hand.

Edmund was charming and, to my eyes, "old," meaning over thirty. A lobbyist for the American Psychiatric Association, he knew everything about gay life in Washington and relished tutoring me. During the next year, Edmund and I developed a platonic friendship, going to dinner or a party every few weeks.

One night when we had planned to get together for dinner, he told me to wear a jacket, code for a possible invitation to a party at an embassy, a congressional reception, or some other event. At dinner he asked if I wanted to meet his friend Tennessee Williams. My obsession was with politics; I knew nothing about literature. "Who is Tennessee Williams? Is he that singer?" I asked, confusing him with Tennessee Ernie Ford, a country music singer. Edmund looked shocked, and I'm sure in that moment I looked a lot less like Holden Caulfield.

He explained in a tone that made it clear I needed to pay attention: "Williams is the greatest writer in the English language alive today! He's world-famous and gay, and he lives in Key West, but he used to live in New Orleans." He added, "And we're old friends."

The party was in a mansion on ritzy Kalorama Circle, across the street from the French embassy. The hosts were a prominent gay couple, Bob Alfandre and Carroll Sledz. When a butler greeted us at the front door, we saw Tennessee and his entourage inside taking off their hats and coats. Tennessee and Edmund said hello with a grand and theatrical formality. They asked archly about mutual acquaintances, calling each other with exaggerated courtesy "Mr. Perret" and "Mr. Williams." Edmund had excellent posture and dressed beautifully, but Tennessee, beneath a scruffy growth of beard, was shapeless in a cardigan sweater with a hole at one elbow. Standing at Edmund's side, I could see Tennessee eyeing me even before Edmund got around to the introductions.

When Edmund introduced us, Tennessee's attention zeroed in. "How nice to meet you," he said, holding out a limp hand. "What's your name?" As I answered, his eyes twinkled with amusement. "Where, precious child, are you from?"

"Iowa City, Iowa," I said. "I go to school at Georgetown."

"Iowa City! Why, I went to school in Iowa City! In fact, I lost my virginity in Iowa City!" he said, taking my arm. "What's your name again? Let's go find a drink," steering me toward the living room.

"Sean Strub," I said slowly, enunciating clearly above the din of conversation and music.

"Did you say Strub? Are you perchance any relation to Strub's department store?" he asked, smiling, clearly proud that he had recalled something specific to his time in Iowa City nearly four decades earlier.

"Yeah, that was my grandfather's store."

"Baby, I'm going to have to buy you a drink sometime. I left town owing your grandpa's store some money! Is it still there? Right across from the campus?" I told him it had closed in the 1940s. "Extended too much credit to students, probably," he said, smiling, as we sat in a corner of the living room, where Edmund brought us drinks.

Tennessee reminisced about Iowa City and how E. C. Mabie, the head of the theater department when he was a student, was a terrible bigot who hated gay people. He described losing his virginity to a woman at a house on North Dubuque Street. "That was one thing Iowa City gave me," he noted wryly.

Tennessee had recently run into Paul Engle, the director of the renowned Iowa Writers' Workshop. I told him I knew the Engles because they kept horses in our field when I was very young, and Paul's daughter, Sarah, was our babysitter. When Paul and his first wife divorced, she gave me a box of his old *Playboy* magazines. I was twelve or thirteen at the time. When he asked, "Did they help?," I could only smile and blush.

I also told him how Paul Engle had brought me to his classes to participate in readings. I usually read the part of a child, but once I read the part of a young woman who was to scream at the top of her lungs. "My voice hadn't cracked yet, and Mr. Engle said my scream was better than what he could get from any of the girls in the class," I told Tennessee.

"Of course it was," Tennessee said, smiling. "Of course it was."

Other guests were edging closer, waiting for a moment to break in. Tennessee ignored them, talking to me like we were the only two people in the room. Edmund was beaming, proud that he had brought an attractive young guest who amused the Great One, but he finally broke in and said, "We mustn't monopolize."

As Edmund put his arm around my shoulder, moving me away, Tennessee said, "Wait, you've got to come collect that drink sometime, baby." Fumbling in his pocket, he extracted a small notepad and pencil and wrote down his name, Key West address, and phone number. When I told him I would take him up on his offer, he replied, "That would please me," smiling as he handed me the slip of paper. He then held my face in his hands and brought it close to his. He anointed me with a kiss on the forehead. During the next hour or so, until he left, I heard him telling funny stories, often with a ribald sexual reference or double entendre, though that wasn't how he had talked to me.

I had heard Key West was a gay Shangri-la, albeit expensive. However, after the humiliating experience with Barry, I had lucked out and found a housesitting arrangement with free rent, so I saved enough money to travel to Key West over the Christmas holidays.

I left a message with Tennessee's housekeeper to tell him the dates I would be staying at the Cypress House, a popular gay guesthouse in Key West's Old Town. When I checked in, there was no message for me, so I called again, and Tennessee answered the phone. He said he already had dinner plans that evening but asked me to meet him after dinner at the Monster, the big gay club. After we hung up, I wasn't certain he remembered me. After dinner, I went to the Monster with friends. Tennessee was with a group, sitting at a table littered with empty glasses. When I introduced him to my friends, his drunkenness was apparent and embarrassing. We didn't stay long. After I returned home to Washington, I didn't expect to see Tennessee Williams again.

CHAPTER 4

Sphere of Influence

Once Jim Nall and I became friends, I visited New York more often, usually staying at his apartment on Ninety-seventh Street. But learning my way around Manhattan and exploring gay vacation destinations such as Key West did not improve my comfort level back in Washington. I was still obsessed with politics, and collecting an expanding network of friends and contacts in congressional offices, consulting firms, and Democratic Party politics. I was also beginning to realize that my growing involvement in the gay world would be a permanent part of my life.

Fortunately, those realms came together through my friend Jim Prunty. Jim and I met over the pool table at the Lost and Found one night and started hanging out together. When he discovered I was from Iowa, he told me about his other friend from Iowa, Alan Baron. He said Baron wasn't very attractive but was a really smart political analyst and liked young guys. "He's harmless," Jim said, "but you might have to fend him off."

A few weeks later, Jim introduced us. Alan was from Sioux City, the opposite end of the state from Iowa City, and we talked for hours about

Iowa, politics, homosexuality, Washington, my future, and the political newsletter he had recently started.

Alan was one of the smartest people I had ever met, but he indulged his bad habits and eccentricities with devil-may-care devotion. He was morbidly obese—some unkindly referred to him as "The Sphere"— and had an ugly snatch of hair, appalling grooming habits, and the table manners of an infant. Yet Jim and I and many others were dazzled by his intelligence and generosity. Among his young friends, the utter disaster of his corporeality became merely a shared joke. His brazenness was an inspiration at a time when most of us strove to conform in appearance and dress.

Alan was a brilliant political strategist who might have toiled in relative obscurity if not for two fortuitous mishaps. When Jimmy Carter emerged as the likely Democratic nominee for president in the spring of 1976, the Democratic establishment went into panicked overdrive. The first time I ever heard of anyone being born again was when Alan warned me that it was part of Carter's religious faith. To me, it sounded fanatical and called to mind people speaking in tongues or handling snakes.

An "ABC" (Anybody But Carter) campaign was hastily organized, with Alan its ringleader. Leading Democrats denied their participation publicly while secretly trying to derail the evangelical outsider's candidacy in advance of the summer convention.

During a live television interview, George McGovern was asked if he supported the ABC effort. McGovern deflected the question, prompting the interviewer to read from a memo promoting the ABC campaign. He noted that a member of McGovern's staff, Alan Baron, had written it. McGovern, steely-eyed, looked directly at the interviewer and said, "Mr. Baron is no longer a member of my staff." Alan claimed that he had the pleasure of witnessing his firing on national television while sitting in McGovern's upholstered leather desk chair in the senator's office.

Out of a job and, after Carter was elected, virtually unemployable in a town scrambling to curry favor with the new president, Alan had the idea to start an insider's political newsletter. Every two weeks, *The Baron Report* arrived in the mail with insightful analyses of election returns, voter registration data, campaign news, and political trends, as well as gossip about important political players: media, lobbyists, labor-union officials, and senior staff. Much of what it reported was inside baseball, of little interest beyond the Beltway, and at $148 per year, subscribers were generally the political elite.

Printed biweekly on blue paper to thwart ready duplication by copy machines, *The Baron Report* gave Washington insiders smart conversational fodder. Subscriptions soared, and Alan was himself born again as a popular speaker and analyst, serving on *The Wall Street Journal*'s editorial advisory board and becoming a frequent guest on the highly respected *MacNeil/Lehrer NewsHour* on PBS.

The newsletter's biggest boost followed Alan's arrest on a cocaine charge. Alan rented the basement apartment in his town house to the owner of a male escort service. A young man who worked there was picked up for possession of cocaine. In exchange for leniency, he turned in Alan, a more significant arrest for the cops.

Alan wasn't a public person—his entire enterprise depended on access to sources that, in turn, depended on his own invisibility—and his arrest typically wouldn't warrant much attention, especially in those coked-out years. But human error intervened. *The Washington Post* police-beat reporter noticed that the publisher of *The Baron Report* had been arrested. Alan said the reporter confused his political newsletter with the venerable financial magazine *Barron's* and, thinking he had a hot scoop, called the *Post*'s business desk with the news that Alan Baron, publisher of *Barron's*, had been arrested on a cocaine charge. The business reporter laughed, according to Alan, and informed his police-beat colleague that Dow Jones & Company published *Barron's*, but neither Mr. Barron, Mr. Dow, nor Mr. Jones was alive to be using cocaine, let alone get arrested for it. He had heard about *The Baron Report*, however, so he told his colleague to call the *Post*'s political desk.

Every reporter at the *Post*'s political desk was, of course, a friend of Alan Baron. When the police-beat reporter asked, "Have you ever heard of something called *The Baron Report?*," the responses heightened Alan's importance: "Yeah, it's required reading for liberals *and* conservatives. It's the only publication that reaches the president's desk totally unedited."

The arrest of Alan Baron for cocaine possession thus made the front page of *The Washington Post* and was reported nationally on the *CBS Morning News*. Suddenly, Alan and his fledgling newsletter were having an improbable national media moment.

Almost immediately, Alan's phone started to ring. In a bizarre windfall, he took in tens of thousands of dollars within a few weeks, enough to not only secure the newsletter's viability but also to earn him some real money for the first time in his life.

After the arrest, Alan heard from many friends, including John Burton, a Democratic member of Congress from San Francisco. Alan said Burton called him the morning the *Post* piece was published and said, "A quarter of a gram! Goddammit, Alan, I spill more than that from the bathroom to the breakfast table!" Burton resigned from Congress in 1982, citing his addictions to cocaine and alcohol.

I met Alan after he started his newsletter and before the cocaine incident propelled him into national prominence. I was one of several people who helped him manage his life and business, especially after the newsletter became financially successful and he had more speaking engagements, bought a bigger town house, and began to entertain frequently.

Once Alan bought the new house, he needed more furniture than a desk, chair, and computer. Alan and I went on shopping excursions to department stores and suburban malls, breezing through and impulsively spending thousands of dollars on a big TV, living room furniture, dishes for the kitchen, whatever struck his fancy. Sometimes he wanted to buy clothes for me or other guys with us, and we would traipse into a men's store. "These are my nephews," Alan would assure the clerk.

Alan became the chief guide in my transformation from an observant politics-obsessed adolescent into a connected political operative. He was generous with introductions, allowing me to accompany him to meetings, listen in on his phone calls, and travel with him to speaking engagements. In the process, he taught me how to think about politics. When we discussed something in the morning paper, he would prompt me to think critically, like Bill Flannery before him. "Who was happy and who was unhappy reading this story?" he would ask. "Who is behind this story, and how are they spinning it? Who makes money from this news?"

My idealism was tempered by a heavy dose of reality as I learned that nothing passes Congress solely on its own merits; what passes is almost always the result of a complicated and sometimes years-long negotiation between competing economic interests.

Through Alan I met Roger Craver, who pioneered direct mail and telemarketing fund-raising techniques for progressive causes. Alan, who often consulted on these efforts, was well compensated for writing fund-raising appeals. A slight fraction-of-a-percent increase in the response to a mailing, or a fifty-cent difference in the average donation amount, could have an enormous impact on the success of a fund-raising effort that generated hundreds of thousands, millions, or even tens of millions of appeals each year.

One night at a party at Alan's house, Craver gave me a tutorial in direct marketing that was, to me, the equivalent of a Harvard MBA. We sat on the floor for hours—Alan's house was only partially furnished—and Craver explained response rates, average gifts, how to calculate the cost per thousand and revenue per thousand, and what made a fund-raising letter work.

He taught me the mechanics of database manipulation, response analysis, and innovative production techniques. He explained what type of celebrities worked best to sign fund-raising appeals; why some colors of paper and shapes, sizes, and types of envelopes pulled a better response than others; and why a stamp affixed to an envelope slightly crooked produced a better response than a straight one.

He told me that single-family homes with addresses ending in 0 or 1 were generally larger corner houses, likely to be slightly more affluent than their neighbors, and therefore better prospects. With large mailings, he warned me not to send all the letters out at once: "If there's a hurricane or the president gets shot, you're screwed, because no one's reading their mail; they're all watching TV."

Just as I thought no one understood politics better than Alan Baron, I concluded that no one understood direct mail better than Roger Craver. If Alan taught me how to translate focus group findings and survey research into persuasive messaging, Craver taught me how to take those messages and turn them into money for the causes I cared deeply about.

Most of the older gay men I met in Washington led carefully constructed double lives. They might manage a public social life with a wife and family, alongside a private gay life, sometimes under an alias. If unmarried, they might claim a mysterious girlfriend who lived in another city or was a flight attendant and traveled most of the time. They might be in a "white marriage," a nonsexual partnership with a woman who had her own Washington career or was a lesbian. If they didn't put up at least a pretense of dating women, they were considered confirmed bachelors, a code phrase for men who were unavailable to women.

The controlling power of the gay closet is difficult to comprehend by those who haven't lived in it. In the 1970s, many, if not most, gay men woke up every morning with the belief that they would rather kill themselves than be identified publicly as homosexual. During the "Lavender Scare" in the 1950s and '60s, a campaign instigated by the Eisenhower administration and Senator Joseph McCarthy resulted in a purge of homosexuals and suspected homosexuals from the State Department and other federal agencies. Some of them, upon learning they were under investigation or about to be arrested, took their own lives. For many gay men I met in Washington in the 1970s, those memories remained fresh and frightening.

The united front protecting the closeted gay world transcended party politics and ideology. Gay conservatives, including some of the most prominent anti-gay leaders and architects of what became known as the New Right, including White House aides, routinely socialized privately with Democrats, labor-union officials, and liberals. Ideological differences were irrelevant compared to the enormity of the secret they shared.

Gerry Studds, a gentle, down-to-earth patrician from Massachusetts who represented Cape Cod for many years, was the first member of Congress whom I heard was gay. He unintentionally became the first openly gay person to serve in Congress, after a scandal involving a consensual relationship with a seventeen-year-old page forced him out of the closet in 1983.

Studds was courageous and demonstrated exceptional integrity in the face of humiliating scandal resulting in censure by the House. He acknowledged that engaging in a relationship with a subordinate represented "a very serious error in judgment," but he refused to acknowledge any coercive element to the relationship, which the young man involved described as consensual. Eventually, Studds found lasting love with Dean Hara, whom he married in 2004.

Three years before he was outed, I met Studds and a friend of his at the 1980 Democratic National Convention in New York. I gave them a tour of New York's gay nightlife, including a stop at the infamous Anvil bar. Meeting a member of Congress socially felt like admission to a secret club.

When I was in Washington later that summer, Studds invited me to dinner. I met him at his condo in the Watergate complex. It was the first time I had a Cape Codder (cranberry juice and vodka), and I naively thought he had invented the drink, since he represented Cape Cod. We talked about politics, gay life in Washington, and why I'd moved to New York. I asked if he had considered coming out publicly, and he said, "I've thought about it a lot." But then he changed the subject: "Do you have a boyfriend?" he asked. "No, I don't," I said.

When he asked what kind of guys I was attracted to, I gave an answer that clearly didn't include him. "So I guess you probably aren't interested in an old guy like me," he said, smiling. I laughed and said, "Uh, no, probably not." There was no inappropriate grope, awkward pass, or guilt trip. We went to dinner, had a lively conversation, and he dropped me off where I was staying in Georgetown. We remained friendly until he died in 2006.

Several members of Congress were outed when they were arrested for public lewdness, solicitation, or hiring prostitutes. Jon Hinson, a Republican member of the House from Mississippi, was arrested in 1976 for exposing himself to an undercover police officer at the Iwo Jima memorial. Washingtonians were aware of Hinson's arrest, but in those pre-Internet days, it was successfully covered up and didn't become widely known in his district until his 1980 reelection campaign. He blamed the incident on alcoholism, denying that he was gay. An independent candidate entered the race and split the anti-Hinson vote, enabling his reelection, but he served only a few months before resigning and confirming that he was gay. Hinson died of AIDS in 1995.

I frequently heard rumors about Maryland Republican Bob Bauman, one of the rising ultra-conservative stars in the House of Representatives. A staunch Roman Catholic who often railed against the decline of morality in America, Bauman cofounded both the National Conservative Union and Young Americans for Freedom. In 1980 he was arrested for soliciting sex from a sixteen-year-old male escort. Like his colleague from Mississippi, he blamed alcohol. Bauman wasn't reelected, his marriage was annulled, and he then came out as a gay man, penning a thoughtful book, *The Gentleman from Maryland: The Conscience of a Gay Conservative*, in which he likened the clandestine world of gay politicians and government officials to that of closeted Catholic priests and Hollywood actors. In his book, he implied that the "confirmed bachelor" who defeated him, Roy Dyson, was also gay.

Deep closets are found in both major political parties, but an especially hypocritical anti-gay stripe has haunted right-wing politics for generations. Hinson and Bauman were two of a long list of conservative political leaders who were closeted homosexuals. Another was Terry Dolan, the founder and head of the National Conservative Political Action Committee (NCPAC), one of the most powerful right-wing organizations in the country. Dolan eventually died of AIDS, but not before AIDS activist Larry Kramer threw a drink in his face at a party, attacking him for viciously and repeatedly promoting anti-gay bigotry in direct-mail fund-raising appeals.

One of the other cofounders of NCPAC and a close Dolan ally was a peculiar man, Roger Stone, who called himself a "GOP hit man" and took pride in political dirty tricks. Stone wore a silver pinky ring in the shape of a horseshoe and tattooed his back with an image of Richard Nixon. He was a protégé of Roy Cohn, the craven, corrupt New York lawyer who was counsel to the anti-gay and anti-Communist Senator Joseph McCarthy in the 1950s. I always thought of Cohn as openly closeted—socially active and out among his circle of friends, but officially claimed heterosexuality. He denied he had AIDS to his last breath, claiming to *60 Minutes*'s Mike Wallace that it was liver cancer killing him.

After a *National Enquirer* exposé, Stone acknowledged that he enjoyed swingers' clubs but denied being gay. Once in the early '80s, I ran into him at the St. Mark's Baths, a gay bathhouse in New York City. Speaking to other patrons by name violated one of the unspoken bathhouse rules of that era. When recognizing someone, the proper protocol was to either ignore him or acknowledge his presence with a curt nod; however, when I saw Stone there, I said, "Hi, Roger," just to annoy him. In recent years, he was a consultant to the New York state senate Republican majority leader Joseph Bruno, who blocked marriage equality legislation in New York for many years.

Some of the most virulently homophobic voting records in Congress belong to men who were deeply closeted. Idaho Republican senator Larry Craig was first elected to the House in 1980; though he was the subject of rumors soon after he arrived, he escaped public exposure for decades. It wasn't until 2007, when he was arrested for lewd conduct at a restroom in the Minneapolis airport, that his sexual interest in men became publicly known. Craig's "wide stance" defense, claiming that his foot under the bathroom stall divider wasn't a sexual overture to the man in the adjacent stall but simply his habit when sitting on the john, became a national punch line.

Connecticut's Stewart McKinney was a moderate Republican who was relatively supportive on gay issues (despite remaining deeply closeted). When he died of AIDS, his physician and office claimed that he'd acquired it through a blood transfusion. Later, *The New York Times* reported what many people in national politics already knew: that he had been sexually active with many men.

Democrat Peter Kostmayer, who represented Pennsylvania's Bucks County, was openly closeted. From the time Barney Frank was elected and arrived in Washington in 1980, he was semi-out within a small social circle but didn't publicly acknowledge his sexual orientation until 1987. Studds, Kostmayer, and Frank were the first gay members of Congress to establish friendships and strategize with some of the early gay rights activists in D.C.

In the summer of 1978, right after my second year at Georgetown, I had left the elevator post and was working part-time for Alan Baron while I sought permanent employment. He took me to the Democratic Midterm Convention in Memphis and introduced me to Joseph Crangle, an important player in national party politics who had chaired the powerful Erie County, New York, Democratic machine for over two decades. Crangle was married with a large family, although some in the gay Democratic demimonde had seen him in gay bars.

When Crangle proposed hiring me to work in the Washington office of the Albany-based speaker of the New York state assembly, Stanley Fink, I was excited at the possibility. He talked as though the job was a done deal and when he made a pass at me, my brief protests were pro forma. There was no explicit quid pro quo, but we both knew what was going on. I needed the job, and using flirtation and sex to secure it seemed like part of a game played by everyone in Washington. I might have argued at the time that it was an "empowered" choice. Today I don't see my actions in quite the same light, but I do see how leveraging my body was an attempt to exercise a control over and ownership of it that had eluded me for years.

During the convention, Alan, Crangle, and I had dinner with five or six others, including the venerable *Washington Post* political columnist David Broder, then considered one of the deans of political analysis and reporting. Broder was straight, but most of the other men at the table were closeted homosexuals, including the Democratic chair of a western state, the head of a trade association, another journalist, a lobbyist for a labor union, and a prominent Republican public relations consultant.

Most knew each other professionally, but only Alan and I knew everyone's story. Table talk was replete with the mannerisms of the closet, double entendres and pointed references, raised eyebrows, and even some footsie playing, as the closeted gay men tried to suss each other out without tipping their cards to anyone else. As more alcohol was consumed, the comments grew racier and cattier. Broder, the odd man out, looked on in bafflement before excusing himself.

In a celebratory mood after dinner, the rest of us talked about where we might go for a drink. It was obvious to me that they wanted to go to a gay bar, but no one would suggest it explicitly; indeed, the word "gay" had not come up all evening. When I suggested a bar called David's Front Page, the others readily agreed to go. If I had described it as a gay bar, or said that I had found it listed in the *Damron Guide* (a gay men's guide to bars and meeting places), they couldn't have feigned ignorance and visited the bar "innocently."

This was typical of the era—as long as you cooperated with even an illusory closet, not forcing an explicit admission or recognition of anyone's homosexuality, the party could continue. Anyone too out was labeled a "militant homosexual" and sent to the sidelines, uninvited to insiders' parties—and unemployable in mainstream politics.

At dinner, I wanted to bring up the McDonald Amendment, a measure banning federal legal assistance in cases about homosexuality or gay rights. I was shocked that all 435 members of the House— every single one—had voted for the measure. But I was afraid, because I knew that if I did, it would silently brand me. Suggesting that we go to a bar where I knew it would be almost entirely gay men was fine, as long as I didn't use the word "gay" at the dinner table.

It was country-western night at David's Front Page, or maybe every night was country-western night. The place was packed with mustachioed gay men wearing plaid shirts, cowboy hats, and boots, dancing the two-step on a sawdust-strewn dance floor. Eddie Rabbitt's "I Just Want to Love You" blasted from the jukebox. "Where are all the girls?" Crangle asked, while winking at me.

A cute guy at the bar with poufy hair, tight jeans, and green-striped Adidas sneakers flirted with me. He spoke with a Tennessee twang, and I was surprised when he said he was a minister in the Church of God, a Pentecostal evangelical sect. "What if your congregation finds out you come here?" I asked.

"Once you learn to preach, you can preach anywhere," he said. "There are always people looking for a preacher. But if my family found out, they would kill me. You can always find a new congregation. But you can't just get a new family!"

When the bar closed, I managed to shake Crangle and took my new minister friend back to the hotel room I was sharing with Alan. An hour or so later, one of the other closeted dinner partners knocked on the door. He used the excuse that he was locked out of his hotel room and needed somewhere to stay. We let him in, and the preacher and I ended up going at it again, with the late-night visitor as an uninvited observer. Alan was snoring in the next bed the entire time.

The following morning, I saw several of the previous evening's dinner guests, including the one who crashed in our room, at breakfast. They discussed how much they'd drunk the night before as a preemptive strike, acknowledging the wild night without explicitly acknowledging that they had been with gay men in a gay bar. That was a pattern with closeted men I met in those years. They could be married to women, have large families, be prominent in their churches and even advocates of anti-gay measures. When the circumstances were right, they could also be campy, sing show tunes, and be sexually adventurous—that is, as long as they could deny it the next morning and blame "whatever happened" on the alcohol.

At the time, it was important for me and some of Alan's other young friends to make a clear distinction between being an escort—who was paid for sex—and being "above" selling our bodies. My gay world was about sophisticated people, trendy discos, and guppy (gay urban professional) bars, seemingly a world apart from street hustlers and denizens of seedier establishments notorious for prostitution. However, I and other guppies were not above sleeping with older men; though I would have been offended if they had offered cash, I was always alert to the opportunities these friendships presented. In Washington, knowing powerful people, no matter the context, was and still is a valuable currency.

Later that summer, after the trip to Memphis, I visited my family in Iowa. My mother and I were having dinner one evening when, out of the blue, she asked me if I was gay. The question was unexpected, but I didn't hesitate to tell her the truth, since I had known for some time that such a conversation was inevitable. We both proceeded to cry, and she made me promise not to tell my father. At some point, she told him, and a few months later, we had a conversation in which he awkwardly inquired as to whether I was "the man" or "the woman." I turned red and told him "It wasn't like that," and avoided answering the question. That was the last time my father and I discussed my sex life, which I'm sure he would agree is just as well for both of us.

Once my parents knew I was gay, I felt like I could come out to anyone. Infused with a new self-righteousness, I thought everyone else should take the same risk as well. I saw everything through the lens of my sexuality and was obsessed with who was or might be gay. Years later, my mother joked that there were two certain clues that someone was homosexual: "The first is when you find yourself having sex with members of your own sex," she said. "The second is when you suspect everyone else is doing the same thing."

At the time, my parents didn't find anything funny about it. They labeled it my "lifestyle," as though it were a pattern of behavior that I had adopted voluntarily. They didn't understand that what was important wasn't what they thought I had *embraced* but what I had *rejected*: shame, guilt, and constant fear of exposure. After coming out, I was immediately happier, and my social support network strengthened, even as my relationship with my parents frayed. That fall I didn't return to classes at Georgetown.

Instead, the job Crangle had offered finally materialized, so I went to work in the five-person Washington office of New York State Assembly Speaker Stanley Fink. The office was ostensibly set up to monitor federal legislation and support lobbying efforts for New York, but appeared to me that its main purpose was to entertain visiting VIPs and provide a few patronage jobs. I don't know if anyone—anyone at all—ever read the reports I prepared there.

I'd thought that sleeping with Crangle would be a one-time deal, but he seemed to expect it would be ongoing. That realization added to my private shame. He was annoyed when I deflected his advances during his visit to Washington that fall. When I was called to Albany for a meeting about an environmental issue, I was excited at the prospect of engaging in something substantive. But when I arrived, I discovered Crangle wanted another chance to get me in bed. I left Albany and quit the job a few weeks later.

The elaborate closet charades and the divergence between private behavior and public advocacy left me increasingly unsettled as my gay political consciousness took root. As the elation of having found a group where I fit in faded, I began to feel alienated from the closeted political class. This was around the same time I became an avid follower of gay and lesbian politics, although that felt like a hobby or a guilty pleasure. I didn't consider it a calling or career opportunity, like I considered the possibilities of mainstream Democratic politics.

That changed when San Francisco City Supervisor Dan White killed Mayor George Moscone and fellow supervisor Harvey Milk in November 1978. I knew little about Milk other than that he had been elected as an openly gay man. I was conscious that the media's primary focus was Moscone, a nationally known mayor; Milk's death was treated as secondary, collateral damage rather than a primary target. Milk's sexual orientation was initially mentioned incidentally, as a curiosity, an "only in San Francisco" aside, with no recognition of the historic importance of his election or what he meant to gay people. The discrepancy between how his murder was covered in the mainstream media and the *Washington Blade* was striking to me.

After his assassination, the compartmentalization of my life—between friendships forged on Capitol Hill and my increasing participation in the gay social scene—started to become more difficult. Career-oriented Washington gays distanced themselves from me as I talked about Harvey Milk and became more politically outspoken. Their reaction was more consistent with the media coverage than my sense of outrage; some were truly indifferent. To them, Milk was a local elected official at the other end of the country who had nothing to do with their world.

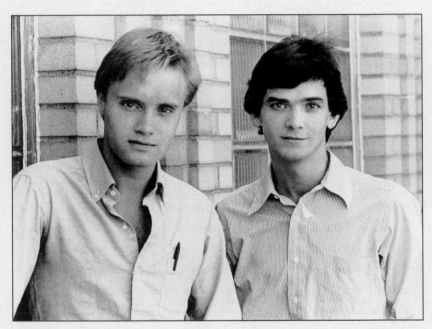

Max Westerman was a Dutch journalism student at New York University and became one of my first friends in New York. Here we are in Iowa City, July 1981. (Photo courtesy of the *Iowa City Press-Citizen*.)

CHAPTER 5

Making Movement

In the fall of 1978, my trips to New York on weekends became more frequent. I was attracted to a gay and lesbian community that had left their closets and adopted a strategically confrontational political stance.

Washington, ultimately, is a company town where almost everyone is connected to the political industry and its intrigues and machinations. New York felt so much bigger, not just in geography and population but in how it sparked my imagination and vision. If Washington was a staging area for my life, New York was the destination. I came to that realization during one enchanted night early in 1979.

I was visiting Jim Nall. We had gone to see a Broadway show with some friends; after dinner at Joe Allen's on Forty-sixth Street, we toured the bars. Sometime after midnight, we ended up at Studio 54, then the most famous nightclub in the world. I had never tried to get in, as admission was famously difficult.

We got out of the cab on Eighth Avenue, and as we walked east on Fifty-fourth Street toward the entrance, we saw a crowd of a hundred or more spilled from the sidewalk into the street, clamoring to be allowed in. "Marc!" they cried, trying to attract the attention of a trim blond man with fine, angular facial features who was the maestro conducting the admission orchestra on the sidewalk.

As we neared the edge of the crowd, Marc pointed our way and waved us over as though he had been expecting us. One of Marc's burly assistants lifted a red velvet rope, and the crowd parted to let us pass through. Why Marc chose us was a mystery; we were attractive but not model-handsome, nicely dressed but not especially impressive or stylish. Later I learned that there was artistry to creating the right crowd and ambience each night; there was no set formula. Sometimes it was about adding more young men, or more outrageously dressed people, or more couples, and sometimes it was about whoever was new and walking down the sidewalk, simply to rebuff those dressed to the nines who had been waiting for hours. Gaining admission to the sanctum sanctorum of New York's glamorous nightlife made me feel like I had won the lottery. I was conscious of every detail, hyper-observant, trying to experience and remember it all.

The dance floor was a stage left over from the building's former use as a theater. One could explore backstage in the wings, behind the curtain and scrim, the mezzanines, and if invited to the VIP room, the basement. I wasn't surprised to smell marijuana, but seeing people brazenly smoking it in public was startling. Around the necks of some dancers hung small plastic inhalers that held poppers (amyl nitrite). Others inhaled poppers directly from small bottles labeled Rush, Bolt, or Locker Room. In the bathrooms, the sound of cocaine being snorted behind the stall doors was commonplace; people occasionally snorted on the dance floor from small coke spoons.

The most physically beautiful people in the world, gay and straight, celebrities and drag queens, models and European jetsetters and muscle boys—many dressed wildly or hardly dressed at all—mixed on the dance floor. I was fascinated but self-conscious because I don't dance, a legacy of the sexual-abuse experiences that caused intense body shame. Even so, that night I was entranced by the pounding beat and cluster of humanity joined in extended rhythmic convulsion, with no beginning or end, melding into a single writhing mass of joy. It was like a pop-up utopian community, a ceremony re-created fresh every night, and it felt good to be near and experience it, even if I wasn't a direct participant.

When the music and evening reached a crescendo, a sense of euphoria enveloped the club. A giant grinning papier-mâché quarter-moon, covered with silver glitter, descended slowly from the ceiling above the stage. The crowd—on and off the dance floor—roared approval. A mechanical lever raised a gigantic silver coke spoon to the nose of the "Man in the Moon."

By three A.M., the crowd started to thin. By four or five, it was a small, dedicated, mostly drug-driven group of gay men pounding to the rhythm on the dance floor and in the dark corners of the club. The balcony seats doubled as a sexual playground, sprinkled with couplings of every variety and knots of three, four, or more engaged in orgiastic pleasures. When Jim and I staggered out the back door onto Fifty-third Street, it wasn't quite the crack of dawn. The dreamlike alternate reality inside the club gave way to what felt like an alien planet, with cold air, dirty streets, honking horns, and sidewalks filled with huge piles of smelly bagged garbage.

We went to the Brasserie, a twenty-four-hour restaurant in the Seagram's building on Fifty-third Street. Its sleek contemporary interior was where New York's nighttime club crawlers ended up after thrashing around on the dance floors at Studio 54, Xenon, and Bond's or writhing with others at the Mineshaft, Anvil, and other downtown sex clubs. In the bright restaurant light, costumes were gone, makeup was smeared, wigs were askance, and everyone was drenched in drugs and alcohol.

As we left the Brasserie, Jim suggested we walk through Central Park on the way back to his apartment on East Ninety-seventh Street. The serene beauty of the park at dawn was unexpected and magnificent. We strolled through meandering, misty paths alongside the earliest morning joggers. As we passed Bethesda Fountain, Jim pointed out the Ramble, a gay cruising area in a dense patch of underbrush, but he admonished me to avoid it because it was dangerous. We approached the Metropolitan Museum of Art, and when I said I had never been there, he promised to take me later in the day, after we had slept. In no hurry, we walked the long way around the reservoir and saw the sun rising in the east, its earliest rays reflecting on the still surface of the water. That's when I felt something transcendent, as if New York's vastness had become inviting and manageable, rather than intimidating or threatening. The previous few years had been a search for something I had now found. The dirt, grime, and sense of decay I felt on my first trips to New York faded away, replaced by the city's excitement, promise, and beauty. I realized I had to move to New York, and that the city would be a part of me for the rest of my life. Jim and I held hands as we crossed Fifth Avenue and approached his apartment, a daring move suited to the daring new life ahead of me.

In that Central Park dawn, I realized I could have a life in New York of my own invention that wasn't possible in Washington. Making a decision to leave Washington, and the political career I thought I wanted, for a city where I knew almost no one was monumental. It marked the moment I began to take true responsibility for and ownership of my body and life.

My years in Washington, bracketed by Nixon's resignation in 1974 and the election of Ronald Reagan in 1980, were optimistic and idealistic. Later, I recognized them as a brief interval before the stark turn to the right that dominated the nation's political climate for the next three decades. Even the most cynical observers in the 1970s couldn't have predicted the extent to which corporatism and the influence of money would come to define American politics.

Just as unimaginable was that a virus, then unknown, was already spreading secretly within my closest circles of friends, from one gay man to another, and that it would soon obliterate entire communities.

A few weeks later I heard that a friend of a friend, Scott, whom I had met briefly, was looking for a roommate in his studio apartment in Greenwich Village. It was serendipitous, so I packed my Washington life into two suitcases and a knapsack and hopped on a train to New York, planning to enroll at Columbia University after my credits from Georgetown transferred. My part of the rent on Scott's apartment was $153 per month, and we had to share a double bed, but I thought it was perfect.

The close living quarters precluded me from bringing anyone home, so my inaugural New York trysts took place mostly at the apartments of guys I met at the gay bars. I got to know my way around New York by waking up in various parts of the city and having to find my way back to Scott's studio. I also went to the New St. Mark's Baths, where young gay men re-created elements of a gentleman's social club and an orgiastic bacchanal.

New York was large and anonymous enough to permit sexual exploration that was not possible for me in Washington. It also cost more than Washington, so I found one job waiting tables at a restaurant on West Seventy-second Street and another at a retail boutique. I also started cleaning apartments—the pay per hour was better than any job I'd ever had—advertising on flyers I taped up on lampposts and phone booths.

Scott showed me his neighborhood haunts, including Julius's, a former speakeasy known as the oldest gay bar in New York, and the Ninth Circle, which catered to a younger crowd of NYU students. It was there, through Scott's boyfriend, that I met Max Westerman, who became one of my closest lifelong friends. He was my first friend in New York who was my age and shared my interests; that he was born and raised in the Netherlands only heightened my sense of having entered a more cosmopolitan realm.

I turned twenty-one soon after I moved in with Scott. I don't remember how I celebrated, because it wasn't a splashy coming-of-age moment or the threshold for accessing alcohol (the drinking age in New York at the time was eighteen). I do remember that a few days after my birthday, Harvey Milk's killer was convicted of murder but sentenced to the shortest possible term. I followed Dan White's trial on the evening news and, like many, was furious at the success of his "Twinkie defense," claiming "diminished capacity" because of the junk food he had eaten. There were riots that night in San Francisco. Thousands marched from the Castro to City Hall, clashing with the cops in hand-to-hand combat, smashing the windows and doors of the building and setting fire to a dozen police cars.

The "White Night Riots" remain the most violent and, in a certain sense, the most inspiring gay demonstration in American history.

Exacting a bloody revenge, White's former colleagues on the police force raided a popular Castro neighborhood gay bar—the Elephant Walk—and beat patrons, calling them "dirty cocksuckers" and "sick faggots." The next day San Francisco gay community leaders called for nonviolence, and the protests were muted, but despite pressure from Mayor Dianne Feinstein and others, they refused to apologize. Supervisor Harry Britt, who was later appointed to Milk's seat, told a press conference, "Harvey Milk's people do not have anything to apologize for. Now society is going to have to deal with us not as nice little fairies who have hairdressing salons, but as people capable of violence. We're not going to put up with Dan Whites anymore."

A decade later, ACT UP embraced a similar anti-fairy militancy, complete with a black-leather fashion statement, but the group favored civil disobedience over rioting and being arrested and jailed rather than setting fire to police cars.

The sentencing was protested in New York in Sheridan Square, near the Stonewall Inn, a five-minute walk from Scott's apartment. I stumbled upon the hundred or so demonstrators and stood frozen on the sidelines, feeling a queasy desire to join them; but I didn't, impeded by a reluctance I couldn't name. It wasn't a fear of exposure; I reveled in New York's vastness and went in and out of gay venues and events all the time.

The mood of the gathering made me uneasy. This was my first exposure to a group of *angry* gay people. My limited experience with gay politics had been built around the reigning mantra of earning access and a place at the table. Those furiously protesting the Dan White verdict were demanding something much bigger—justice—and were brave enough to put their bodies on the line. I was not.

My move to New York and the protests over the White verdict coincided with the peak of the gay male sexual revolution, a decade after the 1969 Stonewall riots ushered in an unprecedented era of sexual liberation and experimentation. Sexual expression was intertwined with political consciousness, and not just for gays and lesbians. The feminist rallying cry, "The personal is political" resonated powerfully with not only lesbians but also gay men fighting for sexual freedom. Political and sexual liberation, as I came to know them, were inseparable; one was achieved through the other. In those first months in New York, I met hundreds of people, made new friends, and had lots of sex.

In those days, there was no Internet, let alone Grindr or Manhunt, but in large cities, attractive men cruised the streets at all hours, and sex was available everywhere. I hadn't visited the baths, leather bars, hustler bars, or places with back rooms in Washington, but the anonymity and excitement of New York, coupled with a sense that I was playing catch-up sexually, made me curious about every venue and opportunity. Few places were more democratic or offered a more fluid social mobility than gay bathhouses.

Bathhouses have their own peculiar customs and rules, but when men strip naked or congregate with only a scrap of towel around their waists, a hierarchy emerges that isn't shaped by designer labels or expensive accessories. Bathhouses were an important part of life for most of the young gay men I got to know in those first years in New York. There we found a safe sanctuary to hang out, flirt, have sex, and make friends. Being naked or nearly naked with so many contemporaries created a bond that, in time, became a community. While it was agonizing for me to take off my shirt at the beach or swimming pool, I felt safe and comfortable doing so with other young gay men in a bathhouse.

My favorite was the New St. Marks, which opened in 1979, the same year I moved to New York. It occupied an old building in the East Village—James Fenimore Cooper lived there in the 1830s and later it became a public bathhouse for the local tenement dwellers—but inside, the decor was starkly contemporary. On weekends, a line often snaked down the front stoop and along the sidewalk. The line itself was cruisy; joints and poppers were passed back and forth, and sometimes guys left with each other before making it inside.

On the first floor was a brightly lit locker room with track lights illuminating a snack counter where activist Vito Russo sometimes worked. Small cubicles lined the perimeters of the upper floors with rows of them in the middle, creating a rectangular cruising track with a stairway at each end. Inside each cubicle was a foam mattress with a plastic or Naugahyde cover, a flimsy sheet, and a low-watt lightbulb with a dimmer switch.

The first floor pulsated with loud, thumping music, but the only sounds upstairs were the moans and grunts of sex, sometimes punctuated with ecstatic screams, laughter, or campy comments. Some guys rented cubicles where they would lounge on the mattress with the door partially open. Some circled the hallways while others stood in place, watching the parade. Regular patrons had favorite cubicles or preferred places to stand based on factors such as sight lines, lighting, or the blowing tempered air from the HVAC system. Though it wasn't unusual to spot celebrities, it was gauche to acknowledge recognition.

When I moved to New York, there were many gay bathhouses, fondly referred to as "the tubs." The most famous was the Everard (known as the "Ever-hard"), where a fire in 1977 killed nine patrons. A few years earlier, at the Continental Baths on the Upper West Side, a busty Bette Midler belted out songs to a crowd of men wearing towels, with a scrawny Barry Manilow playing the piano. I never visited either of those places, which I thought of as "sleazy" and catering to an "old" crowd.

The risks, as we perceived them in 1979, were crabs or gonorrhea; I had heard of syphilis and hepatitis but had not yet met anyone who admitted to having either. Though I had heard about "the clap," I didn't know the difference between syphilis and gonorrhea. I did know that the painful discharge soiling my underwear one morning meant I needed to see a doctor. I had seen a poster for a free VD clinic in Sheridan Square. The clinic promised anonymity, but I hadn't anticipated sitting in a waiting room crowded with other gay men. I was embarrassed, even though I knew we were all there for the same reason.

When it was my turn, I was ushered into a curtained cubicle with little privacy. The doctor was matter-of-fact, peppering me with questions no one had ever asked me: "When did you last have sex? What did you do? Where did you meet him? How often do you have sex?" He wrote out a prescription for tetracycline and said, "Don't have sex for about a week or ten days. Then you should be okay."

One of the doctors at the clinic was Joseph Sonnabend, a South African virologist, then in his late forties, who specialized in infectious diseases. Several years before, he had moved from London to New York to teach microbiology. He began working with the New York City Health Department, tracking sexually transmitted infections, and opened a private medical practice catering to the gay male sexual subculture of which he had become a part. I didn't meet Sonnabend then, but in a few years, our lives would intersect in ways I couldn't possibly have foreseen.

Soon after the clinic visit, I signed a lease for my own apartment on West Fifty-eighth Street, between Ninth and Tenth Avenues. I had just turned twenty-one, had come out to my parents, and felt I could do anything, go anywhere, and accomplish my heart's every desire.

That area on the West Side is trendy today, especially since the Time Warner Center was built at Columbus Circle. But in 1979 it was much different. There was a methadone clinic down the block, and the old Roosevelt Hospital emergency room was across the street. A walk to the corner bodega meant navigating panhandlers and addicts sprawled across the sidewalk. Burglars frequented the building where I lived, and muggings took place outside the front door. Once when I was in the shower, I heard someone in the apartment. I yelled, and the stranger angrily yelled back in Spanish. I locked the bathroom door, leaned out the window into a narrow airshaft, and knocked on my neighbor's window, asking him to call the police. By the time the police arrived, the burglar was gone, and I emerged from the bathroom wearing only a towel, facing cops with their guns drawn.

Nonetheless, I loved having a lease in my own name, and carefully refinished the floors and painted the walls. Most of the furnishings I found on the street; at the end of the month, when people were moving in and out of apartments, I went "shopping," rifling through discarded belongings piled on the sidewalk.

I moved in on the weekend of the 1979 Gay Pride March. I was in a state of ecstasy that day, surrounded by tens of thousands of celebrating LGBT people who shared the sense of pride and peace that comes from a feeling of acceptance—or at least self-acceptance. It bestowed on me a sense of normalcy I had never felt. Everywhere same-sex couples casually held hands. Many marchers wore outrageous costumes or carried signs that were not only political but descriptive ("Gay Realtors!") and clever ("Hey Mom, Guess What!").

Traversing the length of the parade, I realized how vast and diverse New York's gay community was. In comparison to Washington's hidden scene, New York's was an inseparable part of the culture of the city. The parade felt like a giant emotional sponge, wiping clean my angst. I began to think of gay people as a jubilant and protective "us" rather than a mysterious, alienating "them."

My involvement in gay activism was growing. When I heard about protests against the local filming of the movie *Cruising*, in which Al Pacino starred as a straight cop pursuing a gay serial killer on the loose in New York's underground S and M leather scene, I joined in. In our view, the film stigmatized the gay community and perpetuated the idea of gay people as deserving violence. We blew whistles, sounded air horns, carried signs, and tried to disrupt the filming in the narrow streets of the Village. (In typical gay-factional style, some leathermen mounted counterprotests because they believed that we were protesting against them and their sexual practices being used to represent the "mainstream gay community.") Although we didn't stop the production, I found the strength of our collective anger exhilarating.

*   *   *

My social life developed alongside and often intersected with my political activism. Although I didn't drink much, I frequented the Wildwood, a bar on Columbus Avenue near Seventy-third Street that was a ten-minute bicycle ride from my new apartment. Designed to look like a cowboy bunkhouse, the Wildwood had tall cocktail tables, long built-in benches and a bar made from exposed two-by-fours. Sawdust covered the floor, the lighting was dim, and a pool table in back was in perpetual use.

One night, as the jukebox incongruously blasted disco, a guy with a broad, open face and sandy hair cruised me. He was older than me but dressed like a college student in a crewneck, jeans, and loafers. I had just ordered a Heineken, at the time a new import from Holland.

"You like that beer?" he asked.

"Yeah," I said, "my Dutch friend told me about it." We continued talking and quickly discovered we had both attended Georgetown—though he had the benefit of a degree—and were both obsessed with politics. He put out his hand, announced, "I'm Tom Stoddard," and said he was a civil rights lawyer working for the New York Civil Liberties Union. I had met a lot of lawyers but never one who called himself a civil rights lawyer.

A few days later, Tom called to invite me to a meeting of the New York Political Action Committee (NYPAC), a gay political group that discussed political issues and local elections. It was at NYPAC meetings, held monthly at the Salmagundi Club on lower Fifth Avenue, where I met longtime New York gay activists who had been part of the Gay Activists Alliance, Gay Liberation Front, Mattachine Society, and other early gay rights groups.

Tom and I went out a few times. We would go to a movie or political event or fund-raiser, have dinner, and then head back to his prewar co-op in the West Eighties. One Sunday morning, I was snoozing in his bed while he read *The New York Times Book Review*. He let out a holler and poked me in the ribs: "John Boswell's book got reviewed in the *Times!*" Boswell was an openly gay historian at Yale, and his landmark study, *Christianity, Social Tolerance, and Homosexuality,* was a sensation; the imprimatur of *The New York Times*, in an exceptionally favorable review, took the book to a new level. Tom read me the beginning of the review with gusto, his delight evident while he enunciated each word as if reading the Constitution. "John Boswell restores one's faith in scholarship as the union of erudition, analysis, and moral vision," wrote reviewer Paul Robinson, a Stanford historian. "I would not hesitate to call his book revolutionary, for it tells of things heretofore unimagined . . . "

Tom excitedly called other friends to tell them. A review in the *Times* was the ultimate endorsement, especially to Tom. In later years, some of his friends teasingly called him "the *Times*'s favorite homosexual" because the paper quoted him so often on gay political matters, especially after he became head of Lambda Legal Defense and Education Fund.

At a NYPAC meeting, I met Paul Rapoport, a charming and funny man who sometimes invited me to dinner with other activists. When it was just the two of us, our conversations bordered on psychotherapy sessions. He queried me in detail about my family and growing up Catholic in Iowa. What did I think about being gay? About the LGBT movement? Paul talked to me a lot about shame, which he felt was a strong impediment to LGBT equality. When I denied feeling it, he said, "Shame is sneaky." It took me years to understand.

Paul was the first person to explicitly encourage me to consider a career in LGBT activism. At that point I was wrestling with how out I could be, but he depicted the burgeoning field of gay rights activism as full of opportunity: "We need people who can devote their lives to the movement." Hearing Tom and Paul refer to "the movement" evoked a mystical force uniting us all.

As I felt better about my place in the world and made friends who anchored me in the gay and lesbian rights movement, I came to regret aspects of my Washington life. I was embarrassed that I'd essentially traded sex for a job. That experience seemed emblematic of everything I had grown to dislike about Washington. Still, I had remained cordial with Joe Crangle, mostly because he was a powerful inside player in Democratic politics.

When he invited me to join him at a Yankees game with former

New York City Mayor John Lindsay, who was contemplating a U.S. Senate run, he made me an offer that he knew I wouldn't be able to resist. "Maybe there's a job for you there, helping with some of the early organizing," he said temptingly. That was an exciting prospect; Lindsay had a glamorous, independent, liberal veneer.

I met Crangle before the game at Lindsay's apartment in the elegant Café des Artistes building on West Sixty-seventh Street, just off Central Park West. I arrived with a fresh haircut and newly polished shoes. Mrs. Lindsay greeted me at the door and escorted me to a living room with a double-height ceiling, the nicest apartment I had seen in New York. Crangle and Lindsay had their jackets off and were talking over drinks.

We were picked up by a black Lincoln Town Car and driven to Yankee Stadium in the Bronx. George Steinbrenner, the mercurial owner of the team, greeted us personally, welcomed us into his luxurious skybox, and then disappeared. The Yankee team captain and star catcher, Thurman Munson, had died piloting a plane the day before, and the mood was somber. Terence Cardinal Cooke, who was at the game to say a prayer in Munson's memory, stopped by our box to greet Lindsay and Crangle. I was introduced to him by Crangle as "a fine Catholic lad from Iowa."

At one point, I picked up the phone in Steinbrenner's box—it was a WATS (wide area telephone service) line, which meant you could call long-distance without going through an operator—and dialed my parent's lake house in northwest Iowa. My dad answered the phone, and I breathlessly said, "Dad, you'll never guess where I am! I'm in George Steinbrenner's box, watching the Yankee game with Mayor Lindsay! Cardinal Cooke just stopped by and I shook his hand!" My Dad, without missing a beat, responded, "That's fine, Sean, how's school?"

After the game we left with two important Lindsay supporters in their chauffeured stretch limousine. It was late when we got back to Manhattan. Crangle and Lindsay had been drinking steadily since Lindsay's apartment, and the bars in Steinbrenner's box and the limousine had been put to good use. Lindsay directed the driver to stop by Herlihy's bar, on the Upper East Side, where he needed to "pick up something" from "a friend." We waited in the car while Lindsay went inside. He returned beaming and wiggled his eyebrows as he showed us a small glassine envelope in his palm.

I'm not sure who did or didn't snort cocaine that evening, only that I declined, saying I didn't feel well and needed to head home. I've never enjoyed being around people who are too drunk, and I knew Crangle, who was slurring his words, would get grabbier as the night wore on.

Crangle was annoyed and briefly argued with me, until he abruptly told the driver to pull over. "He can hop out at the corner," he said. "Okay, see ya, you're gonna miss a good time." No job with the Lindsay campaign ever materialized. And I never heard from Crangle again.

I did stay tuned in to the national political scene and frequently returned to Washington for weekends, usually staying with Alan Baron. Late in 1979, Ted Kennedy was considering a primary challenge to President Carter's renomination. Alan never warmed to Carter and had become close to Carl Wagner, who was one of Kennedy's closest political advisers. Alan hired me to call all ninety-nine Democratic county chairpersons in Iowa to get their thoughts about Kennedy's possible entry. From my West Fifty-eighth Street apartment, I was able to reach more than eighty of them, and the results of the poll—which showed broad dissatisfaction with Carter and enthusiasm for a Kennedy bid—were published in *The Baron Report*.

Despite his professional success, Alan's cocaine problem was getting progressively worse. He went on two- and three-day binges, sitting for many hours at a stretch at a boxy tan-colored Wang computer in his dining room.

Alan had become a well-paid speaker to corporate boards and had met An Wang, the computer manufacturer's cofounder. When the keys on his computer's keyboard started to stick, Alan had his secretary call Mr. Wang's office directly to complain. The next day, a repair service picked up the keyboard and, in a few days, returned it in perfect working order. The invoice showed no balance due, but it did note the repair: "Cleaned white powder caked around the keys, which caused keys to stick."

As Alan's addiction grew and his health declined, he began missing flights, appointments, and deadlines. He developed diabetes, and in one of those bizarre complications so common to addictive behavior, a simple nervous tic ended up costing him a leg. Sitting in his office chair for hours on end, he developed the habit of wedging his toes against one of the chair's casters to keep his foot from twitching. The friction caused a blister, which became an open sore, which ultimately became infected. Eventually, complicated by the diabetes, the foot turned gangrenous to the point where his leg had to be amputated.

In the fall, I started at Columbia. I had told my parents I moved to New York to transfer to Columbia, but I wasn't enthusiastic and skipped classes whenever I could get away with it. In October, I missed a week of school while attending the first National March on Washington for Lesbian and Gay Rights. I expected a gathering like that summer's jubilant pride parade, all festive, whimsical, and celebratory. The Washington march was different, with a more focused political energy and an undercurrent of urgency and anger. Until then, I had thought of drag queens as entertainers, almost like court jesters to the gay rights movement. At the march, they held the fiercest placards and led the chants, causing me to view them in political terms for the first time.

That day on the streets of the nation's capital, surrounded by so many energetic and determined people, I felt my horizons expand and my pride soar. New York's diverse LGBT community was sexy and full of promise, but the march in Washington cemented my political resolve. When I saw people I recognized along the route, I waved at them to join us. By the time Holly Near took the stage to sing the movement's anthem, "We Are a Gentle, Loving People," I felt completely in sync with the activists from around the country and both inspired and armored by their idealism.

My coming out wasn't a steady, linear process. It was more of a zig-zag, sometimes advancing in a surge and other times making a cautious retreat. That day was a giant leap forward.

When I returned to New York after the March on Washington, I wrote a long letter to my parents.

It's been one year since I told you about an important part of me and my life. Mom, the night I told you, we cried as though it were the end of something. I think you foresaw a very sad future. I hope in the year that has passed you've realized for me it's not a sad thing, but a very, very happy thing . . .

For the first time with them, I framed my sexual orientation in political terms and presented myself as part of the gay rights movement. My new boldness also came from a change in thinking about my career. I wrote:

If my lifestyle prevents me from running for political office, or from living without scandal in Iowa City, so be it. I've accepted that. No one can ever blackmail me, and I'll know I'm helping toward the day when there won't be 15-16-17-year-old gay men and women committing suicide or feeling self-hatred . . .

I began the letter as a greeting card, noting their wedding anniversary. Once I began, everything I needed to say kept spilling out of me and I ultimately sent them a fat envelope with the card and four or five additional handwritten pages.

It would be easy for us to get along for the rest of my life with your only acknowledgment of my gayness to be when you might occasionally meet a friend or lover. But I desperately want it to be more than that . . . The more of the world I see, the prouder I am of being an Iowan, Catholic, and your son . . .

I took a while to put this long, emotional letter in the mail. I unsealed the envelope and reread what I had written twice before taping it shut and dropping it in a mailbox.

Every day I hoped to find a message on my answering machine or a letter from them. Like my gayness itself, the letter was acknowledged only when I brought it up—which I did when I called them about ten days later—but it was not discussed. I was disappointed. Two decades later, I found this and other letters I'd sent my parents in a folder that my father had kept with my school records. The original was accompanied in the file by a typed version my father had his secretary transcribe, carefully replacing names of famous politicians I outed with "xxxxxxx." When I asked him why he had it typed up, he said, "Maybe I thought it was important."

Rereading the letter today, over thirty years later, I am struck by how resolute I was about my sexual identity during a period when other aspects of my life were chaotic and unfocused. I got by but did not excel at Georgetown and was repeating that pattern at Columbia. Any foundation I had established for a traditional political career was in jeopardy because of my growing gay activism. I had discovered sex and pursued it enthusiastically but sometimes in ways that were degrading, opportunistic, or self-destructive. I was a whirling dervish of activity, involved in many things, but without any structure or plan. I wanted to do something significant with my life, but I couldn't articulate what the possibilities were. Yet of the importance of LGBT liberation to my life, I had no doubt.

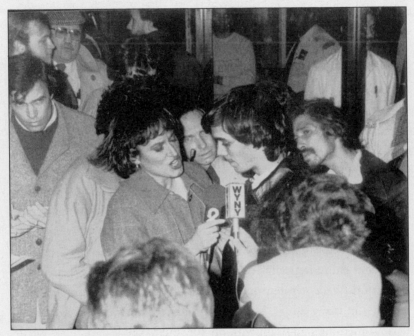

WCBS reporter Jeanne Downey interviewing me at the old Roosevelt Hospital emergency room, across the street from my apartment on West 58th Street, about an hour after John Lennon was shot. (Photo courtesy of Brent Lucik.)

CHAPTER 6

Virus and Violence

A few weeks after the march, I ran into Tennessee Williams at an after-theater event in a gay bar on the East Side. He talked about Edmund Perret—they'd had some disagreement—and I talked about the march and how exciting it was. He listened but didn't seem particularly interested in gay politics, a pattern typical of many gay men I knew then.

When I told him I had reservations to return to Key West for a week after Christmas, we made a dinner date. "Just come to my house, we'll figure out something then," he said. On the appointed day, I arrived by bicycle at Williams's clapboard Bahamian cottage at 1431 Duncan Street. He had two houseguests, and the four of us went to the Pier House for dinner. Gary Tucker was a theater director with the popular gay "clone" look: a short trimmed beard, tight T-shirt, and jeans hugging a muscular body. His boyfriend, Schuyler Wyatt, was a tanned and toned Adonis with blond ringlets. Neither of them had attended the march, but they were intrigued as we discussed it and gay rights activism in general throughout dinner. Tennessee seemed neither interested nor bored, more like he was observing us, gauging our excitement and enthusiasm.

During dinner, he was approached for his autograph several times and was gracious each time. He told us about a time he was with Truman Capote and a woman in a bikini asked Capote to autograph her stomach. As he did so, her drunken husband came over to their table, unbuckling his pants. "You want to autograph this?" he asked, exposing his penis. Tennessee, mimicking a nasal whine, said that Capote replied after a pause, "Well, I don't know if I can *autograph* it, but perhaps I could *initial* it!" Later I learned it was an oft-told story, but hearing it directly from Tennessee, over candlelight in the Pier House at the foot of Duval Street, felt like a privileged intimacy.

Back at the house after dinner, while Tucker rolled a joint and Wyatt made drinks, Tennessee showed me around the first floor, pointing out his painting studio. It was in the Florida room, an enclosed side porch with glass jalousies on three sides. There was a partially finished canvas on an easel with floral splashes of pink and green. I took some pictures of Tennessee with a brush in his hand. Then he took a picture of me standing in the doorway to his studio.

When we rejoined the others, Wyatt took my camera and snapped pictures while Gary and I discussed homosexuality and religion. Tennessee was sitting in an easy chair, sipping his drink, when he pointed to the bookcase and said, "Give me that Bible up there. You could all use a verse or two." He waved me over to his chair and said, "Come here and sit by my knee and look like you're learning something." He read a random verse in a loud, exaggerated fire-and-brimstone voice that sounded like the condemnation of hell while Wyatt snapped the shutter.

Later, he inscribed the photo of him reading the Bible to me: "To Sean from the Fallen Catholic, as ever, Tennessee." The photo he took of me standing in the doorway of his studio, he inscribed, "To my Gentleman Caller Sean, as ever, Tennessee."

When the Democratic National Convention returned to Madison Square Garden in the summer of 1980, I not only thought of myself as a political insider; I also felt like a true New Yorker. In 1976 I had been a naive eighteen-year-old too closeted to even visit a gay bar, but in 1980 I hosted out-of-towners, taking them to gay bars, nightclubs, discos, even Studio 54. I wasn't taking classes over the summer, but I had several part-time jobs—cleaning apartments, waiting tables, and freelance copyediting—and had made friends and contacts all over the city.

The Republicans had nominated former actor and California governor Ronald Reagan, an ultra-conservative whose views were considered so extreme that they were routine fodder for jokes on late-night talk shows. The Republicans' recent hard turn to the right was astonishing. Their support of the Equal Rights Amendment was one among a range of moderate positions to bite the dust. All of the Republicans I had known in Iowa supported the ERA, a simple effort to include women in the U.S. Constitution as equal to men. But the Republican party had changed.

Before the Democratic convention started, it was clear that President Carter had enough delegates to prevail over Ted Kennedy, who was invited to deliver the convention's keynote speech and encourage party unity to reelect the president. I was about fifty feet from the podium when Kennedy spoke. His closing words nearly knocked me over, at once so sad and so hopeful: "For me, a few hours ago, this campaign came to an end. For all those whose cares have been our concern, the work goes on, the cause endures, the hope still lives, and the dream shall never die." The crowd in the Garden leaped up with thunderous applause—many, including me, with tears in their eyes.

I wondered then if I had made a mistake by leaving Washington, by stepping off the electoral-politics track. I loved New York, and I was eager to forge a new activist path, but I wasn't progressing in a career. Seeing contemporaries in my adopted city with great political jobs made me feel unaccomplished. I was lagging behind, still in college, still scrambling at various pay-the-rent jobs.

Right after the convention, I met a trim, smooth-skinned man with warm brown eyes at St. Marks. When he saw me, he asked, "Are you

my birthday present?" He had just turned twenty-six. Despite the
cheesy pickup line, I was drawn to Robert Hayes's quiet demeanor.
We left St. Marks together that night and dated for a few months. He
lived on East Sixteenth Street, and I often bicycled the hundred blocks
from my classes at Columbia directly to his apartment. His mannerisms, interests, style of dress, and opinions intrigued me, and when he
declined to disclose where he worked, it gave him an air of mystery. He
wore Armani, so Armani became my favorite designer. He collected
photography, so I became interested in photography.

One night the phone rang while he was busy in the kitchen and I
answered it. An accented female voice asked for Robert. I asked who
was calling. "Just tell him it's Bianca," she replied. He spoke to her
briefly. The only Bianca I had ever heard of was Bianca Jagger, and from
hearing Robert's half of the conversation, I knew it was she.

It was then I learned that Robert was the managing editor of Andy
Warhol's *Interview* magazine. Warhol was to New York's downtown
cultural scene what the president of the United States was to Washing-
ton. When I hung out with Robert at his office, Warhol's Factory on
Broadway near Union Square, he told me not to speak to Warhol unless
I was spoken to first.

One day Gael Love, the magazine's executive editor, complained
that her IBM Selectric typewriter was broken and said she was calling
the repairman. Sensing an opportunity, I quickly offered to help. "Let
me take a look at it," I said, walking to her desk. I pulled the housing
off the typewriter, removed the round ball, and looked inside. A rogue
paper clip revealed itself and easily came loose; the typewriter was fixed
and an expensive service call avoided. Andy was pleased. "That's really
neat that you can fix things," he said. In an instant I knew my position
had changed from a Factory hanger-on to a useful presence, a higher
rung on the ladder to insider status.

Washington had taught me that proximity to power was an ana-
logue for power. In New York, glamour works the same way. The glamour headquarters—for Warhol and others—was Studio 54. Despite the

quick wave-in on my first visit with Jim Nall, gaining entry was typically tricky; the doorman unhooked that red velvet rope at his discre-
tion, ignoring the pleas of the unchosen. You needed a strategy to make
sure you could get in. For me, that was a shopkeeper named Barbara
Baxter who had a small clothing boutique right next door to the club.
The sidewalk frontage of her shop was located within the Studio 54
entrance zone, enclosed by the daunting ropes.

My roommate, Tito Hernandez, had become friendly with Barbara,
and we helped her out sometimes as handymen. As we loitered at her
shop in the evenings, the Studio 54 doormen occasionally began to
dispatch us to Thano's, a diner on Eighth Avenue, to pick up sodas and
sandwiches for them. These services won us and sometimes our friends
free admission to the club.

In New York, as at Georgetown, I found my off-campus education
far more interesting than classes. I was on my own, at loose in Sin City,
enthusiastically exploring the sexuality I had long denied myself.

My return to Columbia at the start of my junior year, in September 1980, was halfhearted, as I was more interested in volunteering
on Carter's reelection campaign. I abandoned both in October when
hepatitis B and a mysterious swelling of my lymph nodes landed me
at Memorial Sloan-Kettering Cancer Center for tests. By then I knew
people who had hepatitis and it didn't seem like that big of a deal, sort
of like an adult mononucleosis. I wasn't self-conscious or reluctant to
disclose I had contracted it. It did make me so sick and fatigued that my
mother came to New York for a few days to care for me. I spent all but
a few hours a day in bed for almost two months. The doctors couldn't
diagnose the lymph swelling and thought it might be some type of
lymphoma. Years later, flipping through medical records and a journal
I kept at the time, I realized the swelling of my glands probably signaled
the seroconversion sickness that accompanies acute HIV infection.

The last months of 1980 were a terrible time for me and many

others. I was depressed about being unable to work on the presidential campaign and was in bed recovering while I watched the election
returns on my twelve-inch black-and-white GE television. The race,
according to polls, was close in the weeks before the election, but I
was incredulous when Reagan was elected. Carter's landslide defeat was
demoralizing.

Two weeks after the election, a mentally ill gunman shot and killed
two gay men and wounded six others at the Ramrod, a gay leather bar
in the West Village. It wasn't a place I frequented regularly, but I had
been there enough to picture the carnage. The killer was later quoted as
saying that he believed gay men were agents of the devil trying to "steal
his soul."

I'd experienced Harvey Milk's murder two years before as a tragedy,
with the numbing distance of an outsider. The Ramrod shooting felt
personally threatening, almost an extension of the bullying and abuse
inflicted on me as a child. I wanted to attend the memorial vigil, but I
was too sick to leave my apartment.

A little over a month after the election, I was finally feeling better and
made plans to join Tom Stoddard for dinner. It was the first time I had
left my apartment in weeks. I brought along Rob Hershman, a friend
from Washington who had just moved to New York. The three of us
had dinner at Hisae's, a Japanese restaurant, and then took in the movie
Melvin and Howard. Afterward, I walked Tom and Rob uptown—they
lived close to each other—but when Tom invited us up for a nightcap,
I was too tired to accept.

I walked south along Central Park West, and as I passed Seventy-
third Street, I heard several loud cracks, like a car backfiring. I turned
onto Seventy-second Street, and a police car came speeding toward
me, lights flashing. I saw a commotion at the driveway entrance to the
Dakota, a dark and imposing nineteenth-century apartment building
made famous as the location for the filming of *Rosemary's Baby*.

Some people might have turned in the other direction, and given my illness, I should have. But my nature dictated that I find out what was going on. I reached the driveway entrance to the building's interior courtyard, a few steps from the corner, seconds after the arrival of the first police car. Two cops had jumped out of the car and grabbed a man standing just inside the entrance who looked calm, detached from the drama around him. Soon more squad cars arrived, and a small crowd formed.

That was when I noticed a man's body lying in the driveway a few steps behind the cops. A cop was leaning over him, urgently asking, "Are you John Lennon? Are you John Lennon?"

I didn't know much about music. I associated John Lennon with peace and kindness, progressive values, and opposition to the Vietnam War. I also thought of him as a family man. Just a few months earlier, I'd been having a picture framed at the You Frame It shop on Seventy-second Street when I saw John and his five-year-old son, Sean, at the next station, framing a picture Sean had made for his mother. "She's goin' ta like this," John said several times to Sean in his distinct accent.

Seeing him on the pavement with a dark wet spot on his vest growing as his life bled out of him, I felt faint. A moment later, two officers picked up Lennon, causing a little fountain of blood from the wound to geyser three or four inches from his chest. They immediately set him back down on the ground.

Another cop held Lennon's hand and said sharply, "We gotta go! NOW. We can't wait!" They picked him up again, gently, without a stretcher, and put him into the back of one of the squad cars. The clothes on his torso were glistening with blood, and a drip trail led to the curb from where he had lain on the ground. A handful of us watched in mute horror.

Yoko Ono appeared nearby, and when she saw the blood, she let out an eerie wail that lasted several seconds and hung in the air afterward. Yoko wanted to get in the squad car with him, but there was no room, so she climbed in a second car that followed the first, its siren already wailing as it took off toward Columbus Avenue, where it would turn left and go thirteen blocks to the Roosevelt Hospital emergency room.

A chaotic scene quickly formed in front of the Dakota. People in tears asked strangers what had happened and whether John Lennon had really been shot. I shared what I saw, as did several others, each of us dazed, barely absorbing what had happened.

A television crew arrived. Someone pointed at me and told them, "He saw the whole thing!" My explanation that I'd arrived after the shooting did not deter them. Their cameras were rolling while I answered questions as best I could.

Feeling faint again, I knew I needed to get home; by this time the crowd was growing rapidly. On my walk home, I called Tom Stoddard from a pay phone on the corner. My heart was racing, and I was barely coherent; the shock of what I had seen was starting to sink in. Tom told me to slow down, and he asked me to repeat several times what I had seen. He told me to take a cab home and call him when I got there. After we hung up, he called his friend Richard Meislin at *The New York Times*, which I later learned gave the *Times* about a fifteen-minute jump on the story.

The Roosevelt Hospital emergency room, where Lennon was taken, was across the street from my apartment on West Fifty-eighth Street. Alerted by the first radio and television coverage, a crowd had started to form by the time I got home. A neighbor rushed out of our building, camera in hand. "They've shot John Lennon!" he said. "I know, I know, I was just there!" I said, and told him what I had seen.

The phone was already ringing when I unlocked the door to my apartment. And it kept ringing; the news crew I talked to at the Dakota was from ABC, and within minutes, they had interrupted *Monday Night Football* with a special bulletin, including the interview with me. I was the only Strub in the Manhattan phone book; it wasn't difficult to find my number.

The neighbor I ran into at home asked if I would come downstairs to speak to his reporter friend. By then, many reporters had heard there was a "witness," and their flashbulbs popped as they shouted questions at me from all sides. Among the photographers was Annie Leibovitz, who had photographed John and Yoko earlier that very day.

Eventually, I tried to get away, but the crowd of reporters followed. I felt like a caged animal, alternating between answering questions and trying to extricate myself from the growing crowd. Jeanne Downey, a reporter with CBS, materialized and whispered in my ear: "You've got to get out of here. How about if I take you around the corner to my office, where it's quiet and you can use the phone and chill out." I nodded as she put her arm around my shoulder and took me away in a cab.

I spent most of the night at the CBS studio, just a couple of blocks away on West Fifty-seventh Street. They put me in a small office with a couch and a telephone, where a succession of CBS staffers interviewed me on camera for two hours. When a production assistant announced that Lennon had been pronounced dead, we all fell silent. The next day, Walter Cronkite's evening-news coverage of the Lennon story cut to footage of me, looking even more dazed than I remember being at the time, describing what I had seen outside the Dakota.

The media onslaught ratcheted up in the following days. Reporters were desperate to talk to me—some even offered money. There weren't any witnesses to the actual shooting, so a skinny kid who happened to walk by a few minutes later was the best they could do. I had to take the phone off the hook.

I declined most of the interview requests, except for one with *The Des Moines Register* and another with a radio station in Iowa City. To them I talked about what Lennon meant to me—as a symbol of peace and love—and how urgently we needed tighter gun control. It was an opportunity for me to stand on a soapbox and talk about my political views, and I took it.

For weeks afterward, curious strangers and Lennon fans who had seen me on TV pushed the buzzer for my apartment at all hours of the day and night. Some managed to get past the locked lobby entrance and knock directly on my door. One jittery guy offered to be my "protection," lifting his T-shirt to show me a gun he had stuck in his waistband.

After Lennon's death, I didn't return to Columbia. My teachers had accommodated my hepatitis, allowing me extra time to finish the coursework, but I never did. The incompletes turned to F's. My indifference made the decision for me; I was done with college.

Frustrated friends tried to reach me in the days following Lennon's murder only to get a busy signal. When Don DeBolt, a friend from Washington, got through to me, he said, "You need to get out of there. Why don't you join me this weekend at Andalusia?"

Andalusia is the magnificent Biddle family estate in Pennsylvania, about two hours from New York. I knew Don was very close to James Biddle, the family patriarch, who had lived in Washington when he headed the National Trust for Historic Preservation. In a little while, Don called back. "It's all set. Get on the five-forty train from Penn Station on Friday; Jimmy Biddle will be in the second car and expecting you to join him. You will recognize him by the beaver collar on his topcoat."

The Biddle family had been affluent for generations—Nicholas Biddle founded the Second Bank of the United States in 1816, and his father, Charles, was vice president of the Pennsylvania colony when Benjamin Franklin was its president. Don had told me that Jimmy was an extravagant and elegant host, a pioneer in historic preservation; in the early '60s, when Jacqueline Kennedy was renovating the White House, he was an adviser to the White House Fine Arts Committee. He said Jimmy's recent divorce from his wife, Louisa DuPont Copeland, had been difficult because Jimmy had "sort of" come out of the closet.

I easily found Biddle: He was sitting alone and looked precisely like the patrician he was. I sat across from him and, after some polite chitchat, endured an awkward ninety-minute ride in almost complete silence. I was intimidated and worried about saying or doing the wrong thing. I assumed this would be my one and only visit.

Andalusia was a bucolic three-hundred-acre patch of forest, pastures, and gardens with several mansions and a dozen meticulously restored barns, sheds, and outbuildings stretched along the banks of the Delaware River, just north of Philadelphia, surrounded by industrial parks and dilapidated residential areas.

The Big House, as the main mansion was called, was one of the earliest examples of Greek revival architecture in the country, fronted by a row of gigantic white columns facing the river. Biddle restored it with original Philadelphia furniture and family portraits. He lived a few hundred yards away in the Cottage, which was a little like calling St. Patrick's Cathedral a chapel. Biddle had restored it in Gothic Revival style, and with eight bedrooms, it was ideal for large weekend house parties.

Biddle managed Andalusia with precision. Gardening and housekeeping tasks and menus were planned well in advance and executed flawlessly by a loyal and efficient staff. Barbara, the Irish cook, took a shine to me but once admonished me, saying a "mickey" like me ought to be grateful to Mr. Biddle for "his kindnesses."

My fears during that first train ride were unfounded. After the awkward start, we hit it off over the weekend and became good friends. Jimmy welcomed me to Andalusia so often that it felt like my personal getaway. Throughout the 1980s I spent dozens of weekends at Andalusia, calling Jimmy on Thursday or Friday to let him know how many friends would be with me.

Jimmy became interested in and advised me about my career, friendships, and relationships. He taught me much about historic preservation, and in return I tried to raise his gay political consciousness. No one would have labeled Jimmy an activist on anything other than historic-preservation issues, but he was interested in passionate people and welcomed my activist friends to Andalusia. A few years after we met, Jimmy was working on an effort to subdivide and develop a part of Andalusia to create an endowment that would preserve the mansion in perpetuity as a public museum. There were local political obstacles, so Jimmy asked me for help. I organized a fund-raiser for the local candidates for county commissioner—whose support, if they won, could be crucial to approval of the zoning changes—and we held it in the Big House.

Jimmy's aristocratic mien set the tone. He greeted every guest, a mix of the county's Democratic Party activists, business leaders, and steelworkers from a nearby U.S. Steel mill. Jimmy spoke briefly to the group to introduce the candidates. At the end, he said, "I would like to remind everyone that the last time there was a political fund-raiser at Andalusia, it was in the 1770s and launched a revolution. So watch out!" The night was a huge success, and a few months later, when our candidates were elected and the rezoning request approved, I knew I had earned my keep at Andalusia.

■   ■   ■

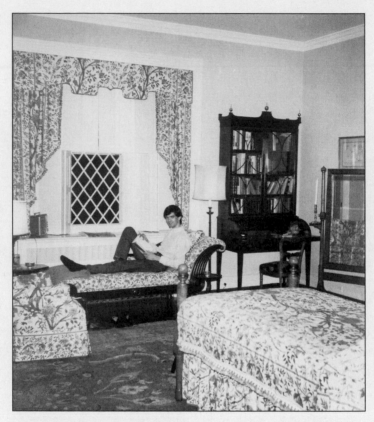

The opulent guest room where I usually stayed at Andalusia, the Biddle family estate outside of Philadelphia. Jimmy Biddle's guests weren't always interested in talking about AIDS, but he supported my work from the beginning. (Photo courtesy of Clifford Lefebvre.)

CHAPTER 7

Kentucky Fried Closet

I started 1981 in terrible shape. I had spent much of the previous fall tethered to my sickbed. I was disillusioned by Reagan's election, frightened by the Ramrod shooting, and traumatized by witnessing the gruesome aftermath of Lennon's murder. When I had been enrolled in school, my parents contributed toward my rent. Now I had dropped out of college, was on my own, and needed a real job.

Alan Baron told me that Matt Reese, a political consulting pioneer, was looking for an assistant. When I interviewed for the position, Reese said the job was already filled but asked if I would be interested in working in Kentucky as executive director of the state Democratic committee.

Reese's firm had been hired by Kentucky's new governor, John Y. Brown, to revitalize the state Democratic organization, converting it from a corrupt patronage mill into a genuine service center for local candidates and county Democratic organizations. Rich and ambitious, Brown was married to former Miss America Phyllis George and was the largest shareholder in Kentucky Fried Chicken. A newcomer to Democratic politics who was intent on making a splash, Brown spent freely of his own fortune on his campaign. When he was accused of trying to buy the election, Reese's firm created a TV ad featuring a blue-collar Kentuckian at a barbecue, holding a can of Budweiser, who declared, "I sure would rather have them rich going in [to office] than rich coming out!"

Brown promised to reform the state Democratic organization, which had been plagued with corruption scandals; several people involved with the state party had been sentenced to prison. It was rewarding to be offered a job because of my qualifications rather than my connections or my sexual partners, and I knew I could implement the training, fund-raising, get-out-the-vote, and voter-registration programs needed to create a modern political organization.

Even as I accepted the post, I was conscious that Reese never would have hired me for a job in conservative Kentucky had I been openly gay. I could feel my newly opened closet door closing a bit. I recognized that I was compromising my activist spirit, and I didn't feel good about it. But I wanted the job, and I told myself that while I wouldn't volunteer that I was gay, I wouldn't lie about it, either.

When I landed in Kentucky, I was met at Blue Grass Airport in Lexington and driven directly to the State Democratic Committee meeting underway at that moment in Frankfurt. I waited outside the meeting room with state troopers while Brown was addressing the group. When Brown was leaving, I was introduced and he shook my hand, and said, "God, you're just a kid! Reese didn't tell me you were a kid. How old are you, anyway?"

"I'll be twenty-three in a few days, sir."

"Not in Kentucky, you ain't. You're twenty-seven, do you understand that?"

It was to be the most substantive conversation I had with Governor Brown during my six-month stint. He named one of his business friends as the state chair, and we set about raising funds, recruiting candidates, and increasing Democratic voter registration.

I didn't know any major Democratic donors in Kentucky, and I couldn't raise funds for the party by selling lucrative state contracts, jobs with state agencies, or pardons, as had been a tradition in Kentucky politics. What I could do was create a direct-mail program; I had learned a lot from Alan Baron and Roger Craver.

The basement of the party headquarters was a wasteland of unused letterhead and envelopes from previous campaigns. I had the idea to use all that old mismatched stationery with a letter from the current party chair explaining how Governor Brown wanted the state party run more efficiently. By cobbling together various leftover components, I could send out eight thousand letters without having to buy new paper. The mismatched logos, colors, and paper underscored our thrift.

The appeal asked loyal Kentucky Democrats to donate $19.81 to our 1981 Victory Fund, and many did so. The letter carrier dropped off canvas bags bulging with responses to the appeal. The response rate was so high that the committee wanted to send out more letters. I had to print them up new, in the style of the old leftovers. In Kentucky, I was suddenly viewed as a direct-mail fund-raising expert.

I also experimented with database technology to improve voter registration. I took the newly computerized statewide voter-registration file and matched it against the statewide driver's license file to create a list of people who had a driver's license and were not registered to vote. Instead of giving precinct captains and county leaders a stack of blank registration cards, we gave them partially completed forms with the names of unregistered individuals whom we thought most likely to register as Democrats. The program was successful, and we reached a higher level of Democratic registration than any time in recent history.

When I analyzed the results county by county, I found the voter registration exceeded the population in some counties. In some counties, once someone was registered, he or she stayed registered even after he or she died. When I showed the analysis to one of the party leaders, his brow furrowed. "Let's not share this with anyone. I'm sure you've made some mistake here, Sean," he said, handing the report back to me. I got the message. Later I was meeting with party officials in eastern Kentucky and asked one county leader about the unusually high voter registration. "Weeeell," he drawled, "those are the graveyard precincts. We vote 'em the way they would've if they could've!"

While I was flexing my newfound political and fund-raising muscle in Kentucky, I was also secretly working on a project for Alan Baron and Steve Endean, a national gay rights leader I had gotten to know in Washington. Endean was also a politics-obsessed native Iowan, but unlike Alan and me, he'd arrived in Washington as an accomplished gay activist from his college days in Minnesota. He was also a member of the board of the National Gay Task Force, the most visible gay rights organization in the country, whose major success was in 1973, when they and other groups successfully petitioned the American Psychiatric Association to remove homosexuality from its list of mental disorders.

In the following decade, the gay rights movement morphed from a cultural and sexual liberation movement—encouraging coming out and self-realization—into a professionally managed civil rights movement focused on raising visibility, combating discrimination, and pursuing legislative, judicial, and political remedies. By 1978, there was an informal agreement among three national organizations: the Task Force focused on the executive branch of government; Lambda Legal Defense was responsible for the movement's advocacy in the courts; and Endean's newly launched Gay Rights National Lobby would exclusively lobby Congress.

One of Endean's first priorities was to try and persuade more members of the House to cosponsor the Equality Act of 1974, the first gay rights bill introduced in Congress, cosponsored by U.S. Representatives Bella Abzug and Ed Koch. He found that most members of Congress believed any public advocacy for gay rights was a political death knell; often he couldn't even get an appointment to discuss the legislation. The neighborhood activists and community groups who had such a powerful effect in municipal and statewide politics in Minnesota were meaningless in Washington.

Endean realized that to get access, he needed to be able to provide campaign contributions, so he decided to launch a gay and lesbian political action committee that would enable him to accompany his arguments to members of Congress with a check. Launching a PAC for a movement that few elected officials supported and whose constituents were mostly too frightened to identify themselves was uncharted territory, a far different scenario from other "identity politics" movements such as feminism and African-American civil rights, which already enjoyed champions on the Hill and tremendous public support.

But Endean's timing was right, because the threat of powerful new enemies—the Reagan administration, Reverend Jerry Falwell's Moral Majority, and a pushback from cultural conservatives opposing newly passed nondiscrimination ordinances—had alarmed the emerging gay and lesbian community.

Endean built relationships with powerful but closeted insiders, such as Alan Baron, who could give him entry to the capital's secret gay elite. He was an expert at identifying true believers who came to politics through a sincere and heartfelt commitment to progressive change. For his part, Alan felt pangs of responsibility toward the gay rights cause, and when Endean asked for his help with a direct-mail fund-raising program for the new PAC, Alan agreed. He had worked closely with television producer Norman Lear to create People for the American Way, and he helped create donor programs for the ACLU, Common Cause, and other progressive interest groups. He had an exceptional knack for translating complicated issues into emotion-laden messaging that brought in checks. Best of all, he could help Endean discreetly, without outing himself.

Endean and Alan quickly agreed the words "gay" and "lesbian" would not appear in the name of the new PAC. Many prospective donors wouldn't write a check to an organization whose very name disclosed the private truths of those supporting it. Many candidates would also refuse contributions from a group whose name contained those words. If a "closet name" was necessary, Endean and Alan felt it was a small price to pay for political power. Endean chose Human Rights Campaign Fund, believing that it provided a broader context for gay issues and created common purpose with other progressive movements.

Alan pointed out that the pro-choice movement was successful at getting Republican women to support it when the issue was framed in terms of "keeping the government's hands off my body" rather than as a right to abortion. He proposed a similar reframing for gay issues around the concept of privacy. "Conservatives love privacy; they love keeping the government out of where it doesn't belong. Let's call it the Privacy Project." The concept of privacy was one that donors could respond to in a personal way, regardless of sexual or political orientation.

It was too late. Endean had already registered the name Human Rights Campaign Fund, assembled a board of directors, and printed letterhead. When Alan pressed his case, Endean compromised, and the appeal to fifty thousand prospective donors raised funds for Privacy Project '82, referring to the following year's midterm congressional races. At the bottom of the letter, in mouse type, it noted that Privacy Project '82 was a project of the Human Rights Campaign Fund. The words "Human Rights Campaign Fund" didn't appear in the text until the fourth page; the phrase "gay rights" was only used twice, buried deep in the letter.

Jerry Falwell and his Moral Majority served as the letter's bête noire. Before Ronald Reagan's disheartening landslide victory, Falwell was considered a quaint, corny peculiarity of televangelism. Suddenly, his movement was identified in the news as the secret political weapon behind the Reagan election and a powerful defender of so-called traditional family values.

Alan began the letter with a chilling quote from a religious-right organizer: "After the Christian majority takes control, pluralism will be seen as immoral and evil, and the state will not permit anybody the right to practice evil." Alan focused on the threat that Falwell and "self-righteous moralists" posed to American values, privacy, and individual rights, the more broadly palatable euphemism for gay rights.

To lend additional credibility, Endean solicited a slew of endorsements from high-profile activists engaged in other causes, as well as respected elected officials. Feminist icon Gloria Steinem; the Republican president of the Los Angeles City Council, Joel Wachs (today an out gay man, then closeted); Endean's old friend Don Fraser, the Democratic mayor of Minneapolis; and Georgia state senator and civil rights hero Julian Bond were among the supporters.

I spent weekdays in Kentucky but frequently traveled to New York or Washington on weekends. One Saturday evening, I was at Alan's Capitol Hill town house, eating Chinese takeout with friends. We were discussing whom we could convince to sign the letter. Gregory King, another Alan protégé, and I pressed the idea that someone openly gay should sign the letter.

King suggested writer Gore Vidal, who was famous, politically active, and not ashamed of his attraction to men, even if he preferred the label "homophile" to "homosexual." (He felt that "homophile" described a person's sensibility and preference, whereas "homosexual" described a behavior.) Alan didn't think that Vidal would sign the letter, because he was rumored to be interested in running for the U.S. Senate from California in 1982. Moreover, none of us knew Vidal personally, though Alan's friend Warren Beatty knew him, and Beatty had spoken out in opposition to the 1978 Briggs Initiative in California, which tried to ban openly gay schoolteachers. But Alan wasn't out to Beatty, and he was afraid that if he asked him to ask Vidal, he would ask why Alan was so interested in the issue.

Greg's suggestion of Vidal got me thinking beyond political leaders and recognized activists. I said, "What about Tennessee Williams?" Williams had acknowledged in interviews that he was homosexual but had never discussed it at any length nor done anything, to our knowledge, for the gay rights movement. When I hear people talk about the importance of "role models," I think back to that dinner at Alan's house and the fact that none of us could name anyone else in the public eye who was openly homosexual and widely respected.

I was tasked with persuading Tennessee Williams to sign the letter, and in a few days Endean and Alan called me in Kentucky to follow up. "We're counting on you, Sean," Endean said.

"I'll send him a letter today," I said.

"Won't you have a better chance in person?"

"Yeah, but he lives in Key West," I protested.

"I'll pay for half your plane ticket," Endean offered.

Alan chimed in, "I'll pay for the other half, but *only* if you get the signature!"

By that point, I considered myself totally out in my private life, and I knew my commitment to the gay and lesbian movement would be lifelong, but I worried about my career. I was still certain that being identified as openly gay in Washington would destroy my future in politics.

So when I talked to Endean or Baron about the project from my office phone at the Kentucky Democratic headquarters, we spoke in code, never using the word "gay." I felt like an undercover agent secretly helping this subversive effort.

I wrote to Tennessee at his house in Key West, telling him I was planning a trip to discuss something with him. Within a week I got his reply by postcard, saying he was about to leave for New York and asking me to call on him the following week at the Elysée Hotel on Fifty-third Street.

A few days later I called him at the hotel and scheduled a meeting for the next day at two P.M. When I arrived, I went directly to the elevator, afraid that if I had the front desk call his room to announce me, he might postpone the appointment or not answer. When I knocked on the door to his room, there was no response. But I heard noise from inside, so I knocked again.

A grumpy, half-awake voice yelled, "Just a minute!" After three or four minutes, Tennessee opened the door wearing patterned cotton pajamas under the hotel's terry-cloth robe. He had a glass of wine in his hand. Though it was obvious he had just gotten up, he seemed pleased to see me. "Hello, baby, come on in, don't mind the mess," he said. He kissed me on the cheek and motioned for me to sit on a love seat covered with a stack of papers. "Just shove 'em to the side." He refilled his glass and poured me a glass of wine.

Within ten minutes, he had heard my entire spiel. When I mentioned Reverend Jerry Falwell and the Moral Majority, Tennessee leaned forward, listening intently. I told him how Falwell was mobilizing his faithful to support anti-gay referenda in various cities. I discussed the McDonald Amendment prohibiting gay men and lesbians from accessing the taxpayer-funded Legal Services program. I relayed how Steve Endean had said that every time the amendment came up in the House of Representatives, we won on a voice vote, but if it went to a recorded roll-call vote, we always lost.

I emphasized how influential the new PAC would be and how critical his signature on the letter would be to its success. I said he could set a powerful example to others. Getting him to sign the letter, I declared, would be the most important thing I had ever done in my life.

He looked at me thoughtfully. I couldn't tell if his eyes were smiling or dead serious when he said, "What would you do for it?" Tennessee had never made an overt pass at me; I thought that moment might have arrived. I took a deep breath and said softly, "Almost anything, but I hope I don't have to."

He laughed and stared at me for a moment. I was petrified, not sure what would happen next, so I changed the subject, telling him that his signature would single-handedly raise $250,000, a figure I made up on the spot. "The largest movement gift to date," I said.

I handed him the letter. He set it on the table and refilled our drinks. He put on his glasses and began reading. I sat in silence. It was excruciating. He finished and set the letter back on the coffee table without comment. Then he asked after Edmund Perret, our mutual friend. Then he asked when I was last in Iowa City. He wanted to know if the Jefferson Hotel and its café, the Huddle—which he claimed was a major cruising area prior to World War II—were still in operation.

He repeated the story he'd shared when we first met, about losing his virginity to a woman on North Dubuque Street in Iowa City in the late 1930s.

We talked for another ninety minutes about everything except the letter. Once or twice I tried to steer the conversation back, but he deflected those efforts, instead talking about plans for his new play, asking me about gay bars in New York, and making a phone call about some work he was having done to his house in Key West.

I smiled and tried to be charming, but I was focused on the letter sitting on the table between us. As our conversation rambled, I became convinced he was being nice to me to soften the letdown when he said no. When he mentioned his dinner plans for that evening, I realized his mind was drifting past the purpose of my visit. I felt sick to my stomach as I anticipated reporting my failure to Alan and Endean.

Finally, I stood up, said how nice it was to see him, and started making motions to leave. I felt dead inside, though I tried not to show my disappointment. Tennessee stood up to escort me to the door, pouring himself another drink. I put my coat on and was almost to the door when he said, as though he had just remembered something, "Wait a minute, baby, what about your letter?"

At first I thought he was reminding me not to leave it behind. When he said, "See if you can find a pen over there," gesturing to the telephone stand, I realized he intended to sign it. I retrieved a pen, and he scrawled his signature across the bottom half of the last page of the letter. "The lawyers are going to kill me," he said, chuckling. "The lawyers are going to kill me."

My heart was pounding; I thanked him profusely and hugged him, tears in my eyes. "It's good to believe in something important," he said.

I left the hotel exhilarated and a little tipsy. I called Alan collect from a pay phone at East Fifty-fourth Street and Madison Avenue. "I got it, I got it!" I shouted into the phone.

Through an initial test mailing to fifty thousand recipients and a subsequent rollout to hundreds of thousands more, the campaign generated more than ten thousand new donors to the gay and lesbian rights movement, more than had ever given before. HRCF's phenomenal fund-raising success over the years, relative to other national LGBT organizations, is due in significant part to its early focus on creating a massive small-dollar donor database.

About a year later, I ran into Tennessee at a restaurant in New York. He affected a tone of faux anger and said that HRCF had to stop using his name. "The lawyers are after me," he said. "You've got to stop it or they'll be after you, too!"

I told him we had another three hundred thousand pieces already printed and asked if we could send out the remaining inventory before retiring the letter. He agreed. A few months later, HRCF received a letter from an attorney representing Tennessee, demanding that they stop using his name. Despite the legal intervention, I know Tennessee was proud of his role. The last time I saw him before he died in 1983 was at a restaurant in Key West. He introduced me to his dinner guests and said that I was the person who got him to "help start the gay rights movement!"

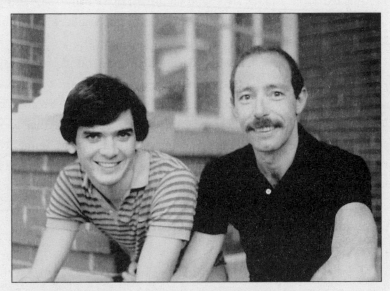

Vito Russo and me on the steps of Adam Reilly and Ev Engstrom's house at 1326 Emerson Street in Denver, Colorado, on June 5, 1981. That's the same day the Centers for Disease Control and Prevention announced that five gay men in Los Angeles were suffering from a rare pneumonia found in patients with weakened immune systems, making these the first recognized cases of what has come to be known as AIDS. Vito wrote in his diary that later that evening I told him, "If I were to die young, I wanted it to be after a day like this."

CHAPTER 8

The End of a Day Like This

The first media report that gay men were dying of a strange affliction was in the May 18, 1981, edition of the gay biweekly *New York Native*. The article wasn't prominently featured, and the headline read "Disease Rumors Largely Unfounded." The piece gave me the impression that the death of a handful of gay men from a rare pneumonia was a peculiar coincidence, more curiosity than threat.

Two weeks later, I flew to Denver for a meeting with the executive directors of the state Democratic committees and stayed with Adam Reilly and Ev Engstrom, two men I knew from Washington. Adam now ran the Denver Center for the Performing Arts, and Ev was a fellow native Iowan involved in Democratic politics. Gay activist and film historian Vito Russo was also a houseguest; he was in Denver to talk about his new book on lesbians and gay men in films, *The Celluloid Closet*.

I knew Vito slightly from the St. Marks Baths, where he sometimes sneaked me a free piece of carrot cake from his post at the snack counter. With his distinctive accent and attitude, Vito was, in my eyes, the quintessential New Yorker—and cute as well.

On my first morning in Denver, FedEx delivered a package for Vito. It contained the first two bound copies of his book. As Vito opened the package, the four of us were standing around Adam and Ev's kitchen counter. We were almost as excited about FedEx, then a new service—"Imagine, this was in New York just yesterday!"—as we were about seeing the book.

At the DNC meeting that afternoon, I ran into Ed Mezvinsky, who represented Iowa's First District in Congress from 1974 to 1978 and was on the Watergate Committee. He lived two doors from my grandmother and I knew his three daughters, but he made a strong impression on me when I was in the eighth grade and heard him speak passionately at a rally against the Vietnam War at the University of Iowa.

After Mezvinsky lost reelection in 1978, he moved to Philadelphia. When I saw him in Denver, he was on the verge of being elected to chair the Pennsylvania Democratic state committee. I was proud to tell him that I was working at the Kentucky Democratic state committee and thrilled when he asked if I would be interested in working in Harrisburg for six months to help him organize the committee. Pennsylvania was a much more important state politically than Kentucky, and more to the point, Harrisburg was a short drive from New York. We agreed to talk about it over breakfast the next morning at his hotel.

That evening back at the house, I mentioned my breakfast plans to Vito, who asked, "Does this guy know you're gay?" When I shook my head, Vito mockingly rolled his eyes and advised, "Ya gotta tell him! He'll find out anyway."

I thought I had come to the point where I didn't care who knew I was gay. But in accepting the Kentucky job, I had put my burgeoning identity as a gay activist on the back burner. Here I was, just a few months later, in the same fix: I didn't think Mezvinsky would care personally about my being gay, but I knew it would be sensitive politically. Still, I wanted to do the right thing; also, I wanted to make Vito proud of me.

Vito didn't totally nix the idea of my staying closeted if I took the Pennsylvania job—"That's a choice only you can make," he said—but he went full-tilt on the virtues of coming out, how being up-front about myself would make me happier, not to mention relieve my worry about being discovered. "You're right," I said, "I know you're right." I just didn't know how to do it.

Vito helped me practice. "Well, young Sean, how would you like to live in Harris*boig*?" he asked, doing his best imitation of a congressman and adding a Brooklyn twist at the end. I tried to respond in kind, but was laughing too hard to focus on the prospective job.

That night, the two of us squeezed into a single bed and snuggled. I loved how casually and comfortably Vito talked about the movement; I felt trusted as a partner in something bigger than myself, like when I met activist Doug Ireland and he began calling me "comrade," as Bill Flannery had. I was also more confident about my career after my success in Kentucky. I knew I had skills that were in demand. To others, my career still looked scattershot, but to my thinking, a sense of purpose had begun to emerge. I went to sleep in Vito's arms feeling mentored and protected, ready for my coming-out breakfast. Even if Mezvinsky reacted badly or I didn't get the job, I knew I had a new friend in Vito, and that was even better.

The conversation didn't go at all as planned. When Mezvinsky showed up at the hotel's restaurant, I was astonished to see he was carrying a small men's purse that matched his stylish new suit. Men's purses were enjoying a moment on runways and in magazines, but they were not found on the arms of U.S. politicians, especially those from culturally conservative states such as Pennsylvania.

At breakfast, all I could think was: This is ridiculous, I'm worrying about telling a man carrying a purse that I'm gay?

"Nice suit," I finally said.

"Yeah, I got it in London," he said. "But the weird thing is the pants don't have any back pockets, so they give you this." He held up the purse. "My wife, Marjorie, loves it."

We reminisced about Iowa City and talked inside baseball about politics in Pennsylvania and Kentucky and the logistics of my taking the job in Harrisburg. After about half an hour, Mezvinsky looked at his watch and said, "The DNC meeting starts pretty soon; we'd better get going."

He reached for his purse to pay the check, and all I could think was that he was about to walk into a Democratic National Committee meeting carrying a purse, accompanied by a guy whom some of the attendees knew was gay. He might as well be wearing a rainbow ribbon in his hair.

"Ed, you can't carry that into the meeting," I said.

"Oh, don't be so provincial," he said teasingly.

"Ed, I'm gay; if you and I go in there with you carrying that purse, they'll think we're boyfriends."

That stopped him. "Ohhhh," he said slowly. I could tell he was much more worried about the purse than about me. "Okay, let me run this back to my room."

When he came back and we headed toward the meeting, he said, "Do your folks know?" He asked a few questions about what it had been like being gay while I was in Kentucky, reassuring me, "If it's not a problem there, it shouldn't be a problem in Pennsylvania."

That was it. Ed knew I was gay and still wanted me to work for him. It was the first time I had come out to someone with something immediate and tangible at stake, a very real career risk rather than just an emotional one.

I was relieved and excited. So was Vito when I shared the purse story that afternoon. "You see?" he said. "Only good things come from coming out."

We spent the next day goofing off together around Denver. Late in the afternoon, we headed back to Adam and Ev's and smoked a joint, seated on the front steps of their wide arts and crafts–style porch. I began to hallucinate mildly.

"See that Volkswagen Bug at the bottom of the hill?" I asked him, pointing down Emerson Street. "It keeps turning into a frog. It's jumping up the street, hopping over the other cars!" Vito had me describe the frog in detail, and we laughed and laughed. We had become smitten with each other, and as our new friendship turned sexual, I felt comfortable and safe.

In 2010, writer Michael Schiavi was working on a biography of Vito and shared with me Vito's journal entries about meeting me: He wrote that meeting me was like "a patch of perfect weather," and at the end of the day we spent together in Denver, when we were cuddling in bed, I told him, "If I were to die young, I want it to be at the end of a day like this."

The next morning, before Vito left for San Francisco, the next stop on his *Celluloid Closet* tour, he gave me one of the two copies of his book that had been delivered by FedEx. The inscription reads, "I didn't see any frogs, but I know a prince when I see one!!! XXX Vito. June 6, 1981."

The day before, June 5, 1981, the Centers for Disease Control (CDC) first took note in their *Morbidity and Mortality Weekly Report* of a strange new disease killing gay men, the same story the *Native* had reported a month earlier. Vito would in fact die young, less than a decade later, at the age of forty-four. I treasure a photograph snapped that day of Vito and me on those front steps, laughing, carefree and feeling the liberating freedom of love and infatuation.

A few weeks after I returned to Kentucky from Denver, the *Native* ran a longer piece about a group of sexually linked gay men in Los Angeles who had died. The article listed three symptoms they shared. The first was a sudden or unexplained weight loss; even though that applied to me, it didn't especially concern me. I had dropped thirteen pounds since moving from Washington to New York, but I chalked it up to my fast-paced lifestyle—that and the hepatitis that had laid me so low the previous fall.

The second symptom, night sweats, hit closer to home. I wasn't sure what constituted a night sweat, but I noticed I perspired more than others, especially at night. When I came to the third symptom, persistently swollen lymph glands, I got queasy. "Lymphadenopathy," it was called. That was the word the doctors at Sloan-Kettering had used to describe my inexplicably bloated glands. I put my hand to my neck and felt them, still sensitive to the touch.

Recognizing that I had symptoms similar to the men who had died was troubling, but none of the doctors I saw about my lymph glands in those years suggested that whatever was causing the swelling might be transmissible to others. Even "gay cancer," as the disease was first labeled, implied that it was not transmitted from person to person. People got cancer by smoking, exposure to environmental toxins, or—ironically, given the profile of this new disease affecting young gay men—old age; they didn't give it to each other.

The reported deaths were frightening but considered rare and isolated incidents. No one I knew thought that swollen lymph glands meant we would get sick and die. Though the *Native* story got my attention, I wasn't yet frightened.

Vito and I corresponded while he was on his lecture tour. We hadn't left Denver with any commitment to each other, but I think we both expected to see each other again soon and explore our relationship further. Later that summer, he wrote that he had "fallen in love with a great guy from San Francisco who appears to love me, too, and my little apartment to which he may move soon!" That was Jeffrey Sevcik, who became the love of Vito's life.

I was both happy for Vito and a little jealous. But my focus was on making up for lost time in my career, which was starting to flourish. After I began working in Harrisburg, Vito encouraged me to do "something important" with my life. "This is not a dress rehearsal," he wrote to me in August 1981. "It's your one and only life, and you have to make it something right now, you do not have all the time in the world, it only seems that way. End of wise comment."

Vito may have been subtly telling me to stop playing around and get to work. Following decades of shame, the Stonewall riots had presaged an unprecedented explosion of gay male sexuality, which was the environment in which I came out as a gay man. Men who, only a few years earlier, might have committed suicide or stayed closeted in their hometowns had flocked to the safety and privacy of gay urban ghettos. Sex itself had become synonymous with liberation; it was the antidote to oppression, with some men seeking validation and pleasure in the arms of hundreds or thousands of partners.

By the time the first cases of disease were reported, we had elected a handful of openly gay and lesbian candidates to local offices and passed a few municipal nondiscrimination ordinances. We felt like we were on a path toward somewhere better, although there was no sense of inevitability to our struggle, particularly as the religious right emerged to push us back.

Despite the political gains, there were woefully few public venues for gay men to meet except those that were sex-oriented, such as bathhouses, bookstores, and backroom bars. These venues were defended fiercely; they were the only places where many closeted gay men could socialize safely. When public health authorities in some cities sought to have them closed as the epidemic grew, it drove numerous gay men to activism. They were protecting spaces they valued for themselves, as well as the only places where many gay men could be reached for education about HIV and safer sex.

While the post-Stonewall generation of gay men embraced their sexual liberation with gusto, most had been taught little or nothing about sexual health. The relationship between gay people and the medical profession, historically, had been contentious, mistrustful, and highly politicized. It was less than a decade before, that homosexuality was declassified as a mental disorder, yet many doctors clung to the idea that homosexuality required professional intervention to "cure."

Systematic oppression, a hostile culture, and self-hatred damaged gay men, and when the '70s presented a sexual liberation unimagined only a few years before, it resulted in sexual behaviors and environments that created the perfect storm for a sexually transmitted virus to spread rapidly. The lack of knowledge about gay men's sexual health and access to health care that respected gay sexuality compounded the problem.

When the Black Plague killed a third of the population in Asia and Europe in the middle of the fourteenth century, civilization gave way to barbarism. Societies were destabilized, families were destroyed, leaders abandoned their people, the rich fled, and Jews were blamed and burned.

AIDS did much the same thing in 1980s America. To say the Reagan administration abandoned people with AIDS implies that it was once at their side, however, and that was never the case, not for a single minute. Many of the rich and powerful turned a blind eye to the death and suffering, rationalizing AIDS in religious terms as God's punishment of homosexuals, even secretly welcoming AIDS as a eugenic societal cleansing. Instead of the Jews, it was the gays, intravenous drug users, and Haitians who bore the brunt of blame in the early years. They weren't burned, but they were left to die just as surely.

Broader society's neglect was only part of the problem; the gay community, while demonstrating profound love in caring for those who were sick and dying, made important mistakes of both omission and commission in those early years. Painful and politically unpalatable truths got in the way when a culture of unfettered sexual liberation was threatened by a terrifying struggle for survival.

Doctors treating sexually transmitted infections in gay men were the first to notice that something was happening to their patients. In New York, one of those doctors was Joseph Sonnabend.

Sonnabend was born to white Jewish parents in South Africa and raised in Rhodesia, now Zimbabwe. His mother and aunt were physicians, the first Western-trained women doctors in that part of Africa. They had a "white practice" and a "colored practice," and as a child, he has said, he saw servants treated like they were enslaved, imprinting him with a lifelong sensitivity to racial injustice.

Years later, Sonnabend observed that the "peculiar sexual ecosystem" among urban gay males in the late 1970s was, in some ways, reminiscent of tribal communities in southern Africa, similarly marginalized within the dominant power structure and repeatedly passing pathogens back and forth within a relatively closed sexual circle.

Sonnabend's father was a social scientist and propagandist who worked with the U.S. Army during the Italian campaign of World War II, following the Allied forces' march through Italy. He oversaw the replacement of fascist editors with supportive ones. He created literature drops informing German soldiers that their generals were living it up in whorehouses with fine food and wine while the troops were dying and struggling in the trenches. "I learned a lot about the power of the Big Lie; how if one says it often enough and loud enough, it can prevail," Sonnabend said.

Given all this, Sonnabend became an iconoclast, skeptical of self-appointed experts and strong on matters of principle.

Sonnabend reminded me of Dr. Rieux, the narrator of Camus's novel *The Plague,* who says, "When you see the suffering it brings, you have to be mad, blind, or a coward to resign yourself to the plague . . . It may seem a ridiculous idea, but the only way to fight the plague is with decency . . . Not doing it would have been incredible at the time." Rieux insists he's not a hero, just a decent man doing his job as a doctor, taking care of people, injecting serum, and lancing abscesses day after day. Sonnabend was like that, a decent man doing his job as a doctor. As a world-class scientist, with deep expertise in virology and sexually transmitted infections, he was also exceptionally well qualified.

In his practice, he treated gay men who were running extra laps on the sexual fast track, including many whose lives were defined by a sexual exploration and excess that was unimaginable to the general public. The waiting room in Sonnabend's office on West Twelfth Street often looked like a casting call for a Broadway show, filled with handsome young men in denim jeans waiting for their turn with "Dr. Joe." Sonnabend had become alarmed by how frequently his patients acquired sexually transmitted pathogens and how casual they were about such infections. Some thought having the clap was nothing more than a minor annoyance; they showed up for a shot of penicillin and then forgot about it, sometimes returning in weeks with a new infection.

Sonnabend compared the gay bathhouses and commercial sex establishments to a giant petri dish, cultivating and cross-pollinating sexually transmitted infections among their patrons. By 1980, he had patients going blind from cytomegalovirus, gasping for breath from strange lung infections, and developing resistance to antibiotics. Early in 1981, he treated a severely anemic patient suffering from parasites. While the patient was being intubated, purple lesions were found in his stomach. Sonnabend referred him to a specialist who contacted the National Cancer Institute and learned there were already a dozen cases of a rare cancer, Kaposi's sarcoma (KS), among young gay men in New York.

Within a few months, Sonnabend was urging other doctors to be alert to symptoms. However, when he asked one group of gay doctors to send out a warning flyer, they declined, believing Sonnabend's concerns were unwarranted and fearing that such a warning might reflect poorly on gay men or incite panic. He wasn't concerned with the morality of the sexual behaviors; he was focused on his patients' survival. He advised them—especially his regular visitors—to cool it and told them that subjecting their bodies to repeated immune-suppressing infections was dangerous.

I wouldn't meet Sonnabend until several years later, but in 1981 and 1982, he was quoted so frequently in the *Native* about the epidemic that I felt like I got to know him. Although reading about anal intercourse and "fist-fucking" and seeing words such as "rectum" and "sperm" in the media shocked me, as I'm sure it did many readers, Sonnabend's frankness engendered my trust in him long before I met him. There were few sources of reliable information.

The one source we trusted was the *Native*, where every two weeks, the story unfolded like a serial mystery. I usually bought the *Native* at the newsstand at the southeast corner of Ninth Avenue and Fifty-eighth Street, just down the block from my apartment, and read it over a grilled cheese sandwich and chocolate milk shake at the Flame diner on the corner. As I read about the sexual histories of those afflicted, I kept thinking back to my own sexual experiences over the previous several years or even the previous weekend.

As the first trickle of reports turned into a steady stream and then a tidal wave, and the obituary pages became one of the largest sections of some gay newspapers, any prospect for a simple explanation—not to mention a cure—faded further into the distance. Because of objections from gay rights groups and reports of the disease surfacing in people who were not gay, the label "gay cancer" was jettisoned at the end of 1982. When researchers dubbed the disease acquired immune deficiency syndrome (AIDS), the name took hold quickly, though it applied to what we now consider the end stages of the disease.

Meanwhile, swollen lymph nodes had become widespread among gay men, but the relationship to AIDS remained unclear. When I had a painful flare-up that lasted several weeks in 1982, I was working on a congressional race in Florida. The gay doctor I went to, recommended by a friend, diagnosed it as "persistent generalized lymphadenopathy" (PGL) but didn't mention any potential relationship to the epidemic or particular concern. I'm not sure he was aware of AIDS. I didn't mention to the Florida doctor my suspicion that what I was experiencing might be related to what was killing gay men. Another doctor told me that having PGL was a good thing, because it meant I *didn't* have AIDS. PGL "proved that my immune system was strong and responding," he said. The guys who were getting sick and dying had immune systems that were destroyed.

I'd read the feminist classic *Our Bodies, Ourselves* as a teenager and already viewed health care in political terms. I recognized that doctors who specialized in treating sexually transmitted infections in gay men, sometimes derisively labeled "clap doctors," had much in common with those who provided abortion services. Both worked in partial secrecy and were looked down upon by some of their colleagues and much of society.

The first time I did anything about AIDS other than read about it was early in 1982. I was settled into the state Democratic headquarters in Harrisburg, recruiting candidates, raising money, and organizing the state voter files. I often went back to New York on weekends. Walking through Greenwich Village one Saturday afternoon, I saw a group of cute guys standing around a table on the sidewalk. They were passing out pamphlets about AIDS from the newly formed Gay Men's Health Crisis (GMHC) and shook coffee cans at passersby to collect contributions.

I signed the sheet for GMHC's mailing list and stood at the table reading a brochure. I didn't want to take it with me; that would have betrayed too much interest. However, when one of the can shakers had to leave and asked if anyone could take over for him, I agreed. I don't remember much about reactions on the street that day, but I do remember worrying that some people might wonder if I had AIDS.

Most gay men were deep in denial about what was happening, refusing to discuss the emerging epidemic or, when they did, joking about it. A few of those who were the sickest had begun to find each other, often only weeks before death. Some already knew each other through sexual networks and friendships forged in bars, back rooms, and bathhouses; others met in doctors' waiting rooms, at the bedsides of dying friends in hospitals, or at the first community forums held by GMHC and other gay organizations.

In 1982, the first support group for people with AIDS began meeting in the East Village; similar groups sprouted up in San Francisco, Los Angeles, and other epicenters. A few people went public, including Phil Lanzaratta, Bobbi Campbell, and Dan Turner, becoming the first AIDS "poster boys." Media attention—especially as divergent views emerged about the disease's pathogenesis, prevention measures, bathhouse closures, and a whole host of other issues—led to internal community battles and sniping at those who were most public. Some even accused the new spokespersons of not really having AIDS, just claiming so in order to get attention.

For my own part, I worried that my symptoms were related to AIDS, but I thought the worst-case scenario was that I had a distant and weaker cousin to whatever it was that was killing people. I read the obituaries in the *Native* and other gay media, but for the first year or two, it was like reading about a foreign culture. I thought about those who had AIDS as luckless victims, a step removed from my own life. I had only just begun to experience sexual freedom, mentally as well as physically, and I resisted any scenario that would take that away from me.

CHAPTER 9

Of Mousetraps and Men

By the fall of 1982, I had finished my stint in Pennsylvania and was back living full-time in New York, trying to figure out what to do next with my life. Vito was pushing me to go back to school, saying, "If you don't do it now, you never will. You need that degree!" But I had been bored in high school, bored at Georgetown, and bored at Columbia. I didn't go back.

One night when I was at the Ninth Circle, the gay bar near New York University, I saw a guy I thought might be a young professor, wearing horn-rimmed glasses and a white button-down shirt with a rep tie and seersucker jacket. Though it was uncharacteristic attire for that bar, he looked entirely comfortable.

Pinned to the lapel of his jacket was a campaign badge for California governor Jerry Brown. I liked Brown, partly because he was a former Jesuit seminarian but mostly for his fresh, down-to-earth approach to politics. While Brown didn't get far in the presidential race in 1976, he had beaten Gore Vidal for the California Democratic nomination for the U.S. Senate in 1982.

I pointed to the pin and said, "I'm a Brown fan, too." The guy introduced himself as Tim Dlugos, flashing a big smile and extending his hand. It turned out Tim was a prominent poet, as well as having been a Christian Brother (a Catholic religious order) until he came out. Like me, he had lived in Washington; he had written an article about closeted politicians for *Christopher Street*, a gay literary magazine. His passions, he said, were "politics and poetry."

Also like me, he was involved in direct-mail fund-raising. He had created the first ever gay direct-mail campaign, for the National Gay Task Force, in 1978; his day job was as a fund-raising copywriter. I told him about Alan Baron, Tennessee Williams, and the Human Rights Campaign Fund. We bonded over a discussion of response rates, average gifts, "engagement devices," and the art of writing effective letters.

Tim was very social, often leaving upbeat messages on my answering machine: "Want to go with me on my rounds tonight? Meet me at seven." We would hit cocktail parties, theater openings, art exhibits, and political events, sometimes three or four in one evening.

In December, soon after Brown lost his campaign for the California Senate seat, I was brainstorming with Tim about a letter he needed to write for the American Friends Service Committee. He said, "Look, go home and write down what you just said—pretend you're writing the letter to me. Bring it to me tomorrow at my office, and I can pay you a hundred dollars." That night I scribbled a draft on a yellow legal pad, addressing the letter "Dear Tim," and dropped it off at his office the next morning. He liked it and immediately gave me another assignment, this time for the Gray Panthers, an activist group that advocated for seniors.

Suddenly I was a fund-raising copywriter. At first I thought copywriting would be just a way to earn a living between campaign assignments, but I became intrigued. I loved that, in calculating the average gift or the percentage response rate, I had a clear-cut measure of the success. I reveled in the figures and data that others found boring. Before I knew it, I had a copywriting practice, with a specialty in progressive social change organizations.

*   *   *

Even as I became more interested in politics, everyone who knew me as a child expected me to be in business when I grew up. My entrepreneurial nature was clear by the time I was five or six years old, when I started trapping mice for pay in our farmhouse not far from Iowa City. My father paid my older brother, Trip, and me half a cent for each mouse we caught.

Trip and I were competitive, and we each had a preferred recipe for bait, secret locations where we hid our traps, and traps that we believed were especially lucky. My bait recipe was a stringy piece of bacon threaded through the metal bait tab, then smeared with peanut butter and topped off with a sprinkling of sugar. Each trap cost nine cents, which Dad explained was a "capital cost." Once I had caught eighteen mice at half a cent each, the trap would be paid off, and I would start to make a profit. He explained that since I used my own labor and got bait free from Mom, I had no "operating expenses."

We set the traps before heading off to bed, sometimes hearing them snap in the middle of the night. In the morning, we raced to see whose traps had sprung and carry the dead mice to Dad, usually while he was having breakfast. He paid our bounties once a week.

One morning I brought my overnight haul to Dad, and he was suspicious, pointing out that one of the mice looked like it had been dead for a while. "Haven't I seen that one before?" he asked me. I told him it was from a trap I had placed underneath a cupboard in the pantry and then forgotten; the mouse had been dead for a while and desiccated. He wasn't convinced and imposed what, in business terms, would be called a "control," using a cigar cutter to clip the tail off each mouse.

Mice were my first childhood business, and that whetted my appetite for more. Before the age of fourteen, I had cut grass; shoveled snow; painted fences; pulled dandelions; sold greeting cards, magazines, and cookies door-to-door; organized yard sales; babysat; detasseled corn; cleaned houses; scraped propane tanks; scalped tickets; shined shoes;

collected bottle deposits; sold popcorn and soda at University of Iowa football games; and worked as a bag boy in a grocery store. From the second grade, I don't remember a time when I didn't "have a job" earning money, usually two or three at once. Making money made me eligible for loans and credit, which in turn enabled me to take financial risks: I bought a restaurant in Iowa City when I was nineteen; I bought a small apartment house in Harrisburg when I was twenty-two. Making money also earned me attention and respect and helped me avoid doing "normal" boy activities, such as sports or hunting. In time I would figure out that fund-raising gained me similar respect within a political movement.

Tim Dlugos became my first close friend as interested in AIDS as I was. We even kept a ghoulish roster of the dead, dying, and sick. We started it on a cocktail napkin, over drinks one evening, a list of everyone we knew of who was sick. Tim put it on his word processor and, every once in a while, updated it. "I think we'll eventually hit one hundred names," he told me one day. One column contained the names of people we heard or thought might be sick (usually because of how they looked), but for whom we'd had no confirmation, each name accompanied by a question mark. One by one, almost all were moved to either the "known sick" or "dead" columns.

But in most of my social circles, AIDS wasn't discussed. I heard about it from gay-activist friends, generally in the context of what the "gay cancer" might mean for our community's political agenda. I didn't have close friends who were sick and didn't personally know anyone who had died. It wasn't so much that we were avoiding the topic than that the disease hadn't yet hit us where we lived; we saw it as a political threat more than as a personal threat.

In November 1982 two men with AIDS, Michael Callen and Richard Berkowitz, published a shocking essay, "We Know Who We Are," in the *New York Native*. Speaking as self-proclaimed "sluts," Callen and

Berkowitz made a full-on assault on gay male promiscuity, which they viewed as responsible for AIDS. Callen and Berkowitz had met through Sonnabend, their mutual doctor, and under his mentorship, began urging gay men to modify their behavior and advocating "the end of urban gay male promiscuity as we know it today."

That was a terrifying prospect to young gay men like me who were recently out of the closet and enjoying a new-found sexual freedom. Callen and Berkowitz believed that repeated sexually transmitted infections had damaged the immune systems of highly promiscuous gay men and facilitated whatever it was that was killing them.

"We have been unable or unwilling to accept responsibility for the role that our own excessiveness has played in our present health crisis," they wrote. "But, deep down, we know who we are and we know why we're sick."

I felt uneasy when I read their essay because it publicly shared information about the gay-male sexual subculture that I had only recently learned myself. It felt like they were exposing the secret rituals of a private fraternity. It was, after all, our sexual behavior that others found abhorrent; to reveal details of that behavior and to suggest that it facilitated the spread of disease seemed dangerous, like it could put our world and community at risk, and even provoke violence against us.

When I read how they were encouraging gay men to support a search for "sexual alternatives" and a "difficult transition to new, medically safe lifestyles," I couldn't imagine what they meant other than no longer having sex. That didn't seem possible to me and I couldn't relate to much of what they wrote. Sure, I had been treated for STDs, but I hadn't heard of some of those cited in their essay. Sure, I'd had a lot of sex, but nothing like the astonishing 1,160 partners they quoted as the median for gay men. It felt like they were writing about some other gays, because I was focused on how I was different from the men they described, not the similarities.

Callen and Berkowitz seemed an unlikely pair to wag their fingers at gay men telling them to stop being promiscuous and getting so many

STDs. Berkowitz, a sexy New Jersey native with thick hair, dark eyes, and a compact, muscular body, had been a gay rights activist as a student at Rutgers in the mid-'70s. Now he worked part-time as an escort, specializing as an S and M top. Callen was tall and willowy, with brown hair. He was an Ohio native, among legions of Midwestern gay song-and-dance boys who migrated to New York with dreams of stardom on Broadway. He earned a living through clerical work, though his passion was singing and songwriting.

One paragraph in their essay did seem to address me specifically and it gave me an odd feeling as I read it: "The new kid in town, stepping off that proverbial plane from Iowa, might conceivably enjoy a couple of years on the circuit before he accumulates sufficient risk to develop AIDS . . ."

I had flown on that proverbial plane from Iowa and ever since I started having sex, I had made—and then broken—a series of rules that I believed distinguished me from guys who were "promiscuous." I didn't go to bathhouses . . . until I did. Then I didn't go to a bathhouse more than once a month . . . until I did. I didn't have anal sex, take drugs, or do threesomes . . . until I did.

I wanted to put their essay out of my mind, but I couldn't. My swollen lymph nodes wouldn't let me. The essay nagged at me, as I struggled between denial and recognition. It felt as if their harsh language was calling me out, trying to force me to be honest with myself and shed the excuses and qualifications.

The essay ended with a warning and admonition: "The motto of promiscuous gay men has been 'So many men, so little time.' In the 1970s, we worried about so many men; in the '80s, we will have to worry about so little time. For us, the party that was the 1970s is over. For some, perhaps, homosexuality will always mean promiscuity. They may very well die for that belief. The 13 years since Stonewall have demonstrated tremendous change. So must the next 13 years."

In the same issue of the *Native,* an article by the head of New York's gay doctors group titled "Good Luck, Bad Luck: The Role of Chance in

Acquiring AIDS" was easier to embrace. "A man could go out and have sex with several hundred others and happen to pick only those who do not harbor the AIDS agent. This is known as good luck. Another person could go out and meet only one person, who happens to have the AIDS agent. This is known as bad luck . . . Luck cannot be controlled . . . A person could be a model of health . . . he could decide to have sex with only one person each year and still be unlucky and catch AIDS." That article also advised gay men to reduce the number of their partners, but the message that fate played the biggest role in deciding who would get sick was what registered most strongly with me. We can't be responsible for fate, so it justified a sense that there was little we could do about AIDS.

The "luck" doctor, as well as GMHC and much of the gay leadership, had concluded that the disease was probably caused by a new viral agent that was transmitted by having sex with an infected person, which supported the idea of a "fatal fuck," sleeping with the wrong person. Sonnabend, Callen, and Berkowitz proposed that one's cumulative sexual behaviors—and subsequent infections—played the central role. Sonnabend, Callen, and Berkowitz didn't believe a single sexual contact would lead to AIDS. They didn't rule out a new single-agent cause, but they weren't prepared to wait until that question was answered before advising gay men to reduce their acquisition of sexually transmitted infections, by stopping the specific behaviors that transmitted them.

It was a matter of emphasis, Sonnabend et al. urging gay men to protect and strengthen their immune systems by modifying their behavior so they wouldn't get sexually transmitted diseases versus GMHC and the gay establishment's "fewer partners" message, which was undefined (fewer than what?).

Sometimes the "fewer partners" message was positioned as necessary only for a limited period, "until this thing passes." Even GMHC's full name, Gay Men's Health Crisis, suggested that AIDS was serious and important—a "crisis"—but implied it was temporary, as crises ultimately either pass or become a new normal, a prospect we could not imagine. Many of my friends expected that a cure would be announced any day and that this would all turn out to be an unhappy chapter in the onward march of gay liberation.

The gay and lesbian movement's first major victories, like the American Psychiatric Association's declassification of homosexuality as a mental disorder (1973), the first nondiscrimination ordinances in St. Paul (1974), Miami (1977), and a handful of other cities, the introduction of the first gay rights bill in Congress (1974, by Bella Abzug and Ed Koch), as well as the earliest self-proclaimed public homosexuals in the nation, were all fresh milestones achieved in the years immediately prior to the discovery of the AIDS epidemic in 1981.

But they felt fragile and were under assault, factors that influenced the gay and lesbian activist community's initial response to the mysterious new disease. The four years immediately preceding the awareness of AIDS were especially fraught with threats to the few victories we had achieved.

Anita Bryant's "Save Our Children" campaign in Dade County in 1977 had vilified us as child molesters in the national media, resulting in a referendum repealing Miami's landmark nondiscrimination ordinance. Voters in St. Paul, Wichita, and Eugene followed suit over the next several years.

Then, in 1978, Harvey Milk's assassination traumatized the community, even more so when his killer was let off with a light sentence in May 1979. Televangelist Jerry Falwell and his Moral Majority began to exert a new-found political influence, seemingly out of nowhere, while demonizing us and inspiring religious leaders across the country to rail against gay and lesbian "activists," sometimes equating us with the anti-Christ, as perverts destroying the soul of America.

The election of Reagan in 1980 was a shock—a prospect many considered far-fetched when he first ran in 1976—and it confirmed the sense that the gains we had earned were but tender green shoots, poking their way through a thick and nearly impenetrable cover of intolerance and hatred.

The Ramrod shootings were just two weeks later, when a deranged man sprayed gunfire from an Uzi, killing two gay men and shooting six others at the West Village gay bar. The cumulative effect of the rhetorical and physical violence perpetrated against us, combined with the repeal of the nondiscrimination ordinances at the polls, left some of us secretly wondering if our movement could grow further, or if it might not be but a blip, a political idiosyncrasy, one soon to disappear?

If AIDS led to a public awareness of what gay men did sexually, many feared it would cause a devastating backlash, almost certainly inciting greater intolerance and violence. That's a big part of the reason why there was an effort to downplay gay men's sexuality and promote the myth that gay men's sexual behaviors had nothing to do with AIDS and it was "only a coincidence" that AIDS surfaced first in the gay community.

Some of the community's leadership were reluctant to talk openly and honestly about gay men's sexuality in those early years, especially about anal intercourse and commercial sex venues. The sexual freedom we were enjoying was new and exhilarating, yet it didn't feel secure. It felt like something that we needed to protect at any cost. And to many, the epidemic wasn't important until they or someone they loved got sick.

In addition, the gay and lesbian movement was already drifting away from its foundation as a sexual liberation movement toward a focus on rights and assimilation. "We're just like everyone else" was the mantra as we began to focus on legal reform and mainstream acceptance. Alternative gender roles, open relationships, promiscuity, fetish subcultures, and other aspects of lesbian and gay life differing from social norms were downplayed by the movement's leadership.

No one wanted to associate gay politics with this horrifying new disease except our enemies. Sonnabend, Callen, and Berkowitz were widely attacked when they urged gay men to change their sexual behaviors and stop frequenting the baths and commercial sex establishments that so greatly facilitated the spread of sexually transmitted infections. People wrote furious letters to the *Native* and yelled at them in public. They were called "sex-negative" and "self-hating" and accused of "blaming" gay liberation for the epidemic.

A few weeks after Berkowitz and Callen's essay appeared they organized a group to pay for a large ad in the *Native* headlined "A Warning to Gay Men with AIDS." It started out like this: "We are a group of gay men with AIDS. We believe it is crucial for us to begin to share with others like ourselves our personal experiences in getting treatment."

The ad listed various treatment strategies with comments and citations. The closing paragraph read: "To date, there is not even one support group or health crisis center in our New York City gay community that is providing support to immuno-suppressed gay men who want to break the habit of promiscuous behavior, nor does the community itself encourage such a change. We must care enough about ourselves; obviously, others—particularly those who advise mere moderation of promiscuous behavior—do not care about us."

Sonnabend was telling people that the greatest AIDS risk for gay men was to be the receptive partner in anal sex. That is widely understood today, but at the time, it felt to me like he was making a minor distinction. Sexual contact was sexual contact, your partner might have AIDS or not, but why would it matter what one did in bed? In any case, neither I nor many of my friends would admit to being a passive partner in anal sex.

In a letter to *The Village Voice* in December 1982, Berkowitz wrote, "The reason for so much confusion about which gay men are getting AIDS is that most AIDS victims, like myself, are not honest about our sexual behavior—let alone our sexual excess. Most of us continue to lie . . ." Indeed, in the early years of the epidemic, it was common to hear about men with AIDS who claimed they never bottomed, never visited sex clubs, and weren't promiscuous. AIDS forced a mass exodus from the closet. Acknowledging being penetrated by other men was an even deeper level of closet to transcend.

*   *   *

In early 1983, I had no desire to dwell on the new disease. What began as a part-time gig writing fund-raising letters for Tim Dlugos had grown into a full-time enterprise providing fund-raising and marketing consulting services. I incorporated as Sean O. Strub, Inc., and with the arrival of my business cards, I felt like my future was settled.

I also had my first steady boyfriend, André Ledoux, and the relationship felt secure enough that we bought a small weekend home in Bucks County, Pennsylvania, a favorite weekend getaway for gay New Yorkers. Jim Nall and a cousin loaned me part of my $6,500 share of the down payment. André was a decade older than I, and though we cared deeply for each other, after a year, our relationship became more of a partnership than a romance. My outness was very different from his closeted life. He ran a mineral and mining ore-testing laboratory founded by his great-grandfather, and several times a year, he attended high-profile charity balls, always with an attractive woman on his arm. His membership at the Saint, the legendary gay dance palace in the East Village, was under a fake name and a P.O. box address. (When I started *POZ* years later, André was very ill, but he sent me a sweet note and subscribed, still using his fake name for his P.O. box.)

With the boyfriend, career, and country house boxes all checked off, I believed I was in a good place. My night sweats were intermittent but manageable. When our sheets were wet in the morning, André teased me that I had "gone swimming" the night before. As for my lymph glands, they had been mildly swollen for so long that I'd stopped paying attention to them except when they hurt to the touch. I thought of them as an early warning system; as long as they were manageable, I didn't have AIDS and wasn't sick. A doctor told me that my relative good health would continue: "If you were going to get sick, you would have already done so by now." Yet my social circle was no longer insulated from AIDS. André and I were hearing about friends of friends and acquaintances who became suspiciously scarce and then disappeared; later we would learn that they had died. AIDS was only rarely blamed—it was pneumonia, an unusual cancer, or, as

André claimed when he got sick, a rare virus acquired from traveling in an exotic locale.

The first AIDS death to hit particularly close to home was that of Joe McDonald in early 1983. Joe was one of the first male supermodels, and it seemed like every gay man in New York knew who he was. I didn't know him personally, but Tito Hernandez, my roommate at the time, had dated him. Tito and I also sometimes had sex with each other. When Joe died, Tito and I speculated about what we might do if we got sick. "I'd kill myself," Tito said. "I couldn't ever tell my family. But maybe I'd go out and get really drunk first!" My plan: "I would get rid of everything I own and just travel for as long as I could." We didn't dwell on our sexual connection to Joe. At that time, AIDS was a label for when someone got sick, looked horribly ill, and then died a fast and awful death. Tito and I were fine.

Despite disquiet about the Callen/Berkowitz essay, I resisted connecting my sexual behavior to my risk of acquiring AIDS until a few months later, when another powerful essay, this one by GMHC cofounder Larry Kramer, "1,112 and Counting," was published in the *Native* in March 1983.

While Callen and Berkowitz had directed their blast to fellow "sluts," Kramer's call to action was addressed to the gay everyman: "When we first became worried, there were only 41," he wrote. "In only 28 days, from January 13th to February 9th [1983], there were 164 new cases—and 73 more dead. The total death tally is now 418 . . ." One sentence was especially chilling: "These numbers do not include the thousands of us walking around with what is also being called AIDS: various forms of swollen lymph glands and fatigues that doctors don't know what to label or what they might portend."

I read the essay while sitting in Joe Jr.'s, my favorite diner, in the West Village. Reading the sentence about swollen lymph glands, I disassociated for a few moments, my mind in another place. When the waiter approached my booth to clear my dinner plate, I folded the *Native* shut so he wouldn't see the article.

Kramer was saying *I had AIDS* as surely as if he had used my name. That article snapped me out of denial and I became the guy who invariably brought up the epidemic in conversation with other gay men. That was often not welcomed. Many of the closeted, rich, and elegant bachelors I met at Andalusia found any reference to gay politics or AIDS distasteful. When I brought up those topics, I would be gently admonished, "Oh, let's talk about something more cheerful!" and the conversation would move on.

During one especially grand dinner party at the Biddles'—three tables of eight set with sparkling crystal and elegant china, the family's colonial-era silver, and fresh flowers from the estate's cutting gardens—I was the youngest guest, seated directly opposite Jimmy at the head table. To my right was a Philadelphia grand dame, heiress to the Tastykake baking company and one of few women at the party.

The conversation turned to the death of Angelo Donghia, a prominent interior designer known personally to several of the guests. When someone said he had died of pneumonia, I spoke up: "No, he died of AIDS." One of the men at the table—who had arrived that evening wearing a floor-length mink coat—chastised me, "What a terrible thing to say!" I replied, "But it is the truth. And lying about it makes things worse."

A heated discussion erupted, with one man saying Angelo wasn't "careful," another saying it wasn't the government's job to stop AIDS, and a third poking fun at AIDS activists. My protests were disputed or dismissed. Then the man with the mink pronounced, with an air of finality, "Well, that's enough of that dreary topic. Now, who's going to the garden show this weekend?"

Though Jimmy had been paying attention, he hadn't contributed to the conversation. For a minute or two, the talk turned to the upcoming Philadelphia flower show and other topics. I fumed silently.

When there was a brief lull in the conversation about the azaleas, lilies, and petunias, Jimmy asked, "Sean, what can we do to try and find a cure for AIDS?" He looked at me expectantly, as though he had passed me the baton. We had a back-and-forth across the table that drew others into the discussion. It was a sign of Jimmy's approval of my work. I never again felt hesitant to discuss AIDS at Andalusia.

If there was reluctance to discuss AIDS in some quarters, elsewhere it was discussed constantly, especially with speculation about its cause.

Some of the focus was on sex clubs, such as the infamous Mineshaft in New York's Meatpacking District. The basement dungeons in the Mineshaft were packed, sometimes with more than a hundred men in a night, from hard-core leather aficionados to curious boys just coming out. A sign at the entrance spelled out the rules for entry, including a "leather and Levi's" dress code and prohibitions on polo shirts, sneakers, and cologne. Inside, however, any semblance of rules disappeared. Men wandered around naked, played bondage games, and had sex through glory holes, in bathtubs, and in slings hanging from the ceiling. Some of the earliest AIDS deaths in New York were among Mineshaft regulars. Before HIV was identified, rumors spread that the club's walls and floor were encrusted with bacterial and fungal growths that might have a connection to the disease.

Drugs were also suspect, particularly amyl nitrite or "poppers," the Studio 54 dance-floor favorite, available at sex shops, gay bars, even convenience stores and bodegas. I was among those who used them for an extra rush during sex; when inhaled, they dilate blood vessels and make one light-headed. The health effects of poppers had been debated before AIDS hit, but they were a big source of advertising for gay publications, which rarely referenced, let alone examined, their risks.

In March 1983, Larry Kramer wrote in frustration, "For two years, we've heard a different theory every few weeks. We grasped at the straws of possible cause: promiscuity, poppers, back rooms, the baths, rimming, fisting, anal intercourse, urine, semen, shit, saliva, sweat, blood, blacks, a single virus, a new virus, repeated exposure to a virus, amoebas carrying a virus, drugs, Haiti, voodoo, Flagyl, constant bouts of amoebiasis, hepatitis A and B, syphilis, gonorrhea."

In the fall of 1983, I even thought that I might be on the trail of the cause, as absurd as that sounds. One of my clients was the Council on Economic Priorities, a corporate social-responsibility think tank that studied nuclear disarmament and environmental issues. I became friends with a physicist working at CEP, Dr. Ernest Sternglass, who was an expert on the long-term health risks of low-level radioactive fallout.

One day we discussed the epidemic over sandwiches at our office near Union Square in New York City. I was telling him about the many different theories when he said, "I'll bet it's the immune system, it has to be!" He explained how exposure to low levels of radiation in utero or during the first years of a child's life could permanently damage the immune system, leaving a person vulnerable to several types of cancer. In the 1950s, he said, there had been more than a hundred above-ground nuclear-bomb tests in Nevada. The fallout had spread lethal particles infused with Strontium-90, a radioactive isotope, across the continent. It had settled on the ground and ended up in cows' milk, he said, eventually damaging fetuses and young children whose immune systems weren't fully developed.

The long-term health effects of Strontium-90 were only starting to be understood, as children who had been exposed to the fallout reached adulthood. "If only I could get information on where and when AIDS victims were born," Sternglass said. "We could compare that to the levels of Strontium-90 in the milk supply in various cities at various times and see if there's a correlation."

I brought him copies of the *New York Native* and other gay publications that carried obituaries of men who had (presumably) died of AIDS.

Sternglass put a map of the United States on a bulletin board next to his office cubicle. We stuck colored pushpins in every city we knew to be the birthplace of someone who had died of AIDS, and we noted the date of birth. Most of the deaths were in New York, San Francisco, Los Angeles, and other big cities, but finding out where the deceased were born proved difficult. We didn't collect enough data to prove a correlation.

Sternglass's theory was no more outlandish than many others, and his explanation of the gradations in the strength of one's immune system made sense to me. His theory might explain why some of us "sluts" got sick while others remained healthy. Sternglass was also the first straight person I'd met whose interest in homosexuality wasn't framed in a moral context; he was interested simply by the science. Sternglass was a famous expert and helping him felt important; I secretly thought about what it would be like if I helped him find the cause of AIDS.

Mainstream scientific inquiry had begun to diverge between those looking for an as yet undiscovered virus responsible for making people sick and those who pursued the medical consequences of—like it or not—the so-called "gay lifestyle," like Sonnabend's "multi-factorial" hypothesis.

The idea that a singular cause was out there, hidden from us, just waiting to be discovered was seductive to many of us, partly because it put the focus on something other than on our sexual subculture and behaviors. I had no understanding of the psychological and political factors that were shaping how the gay community viewed the epidemic. That came later.

Many of the gay leaders who were angry with Callen and Berkowitz also reviled Sonnabend. But he was beloved by his patients and by many people with AIDS. When he walked with the People With AIDS Coalition in New York's annual Gay and Lesbian Pride Parade in 1983 and 1984, he was cheered with many waving their hands and shouting out, "Dr. Joe! Dr. Joe!"

Yet his multi-factorial hypothesis put him at odds with GMHC, which had quickly become the community's dominant voice on AIDS. As the first and largest AIDS service agency, GMHC also had started to gain cachet when socially prominent New Yorkers became supporters. The agency's main HIV-prevention message that I heard in those early years was that we must have fewer partners, not that we needed to stop specific sexual behaviors (like unprotected receptive anal intercourse) that put people at greatest risk. Berkowitz described GMHC's "fewer partners" advice while they also advocated the single theory of causation "like telling someone to play Russian roulette less often."

The difference in approach was so contentious that GMHC's doctor-referral hotline wouldn't recommend Sonnabend, even though he was one of the most knowledgeable AIDS clinicians. If callers to GMHC's hotline asked about Sonnabend specifically, they were sometimes told he was "crazy."

The split became more pronounced when condoms came into the picture. One day early in 1983, Berkowitz had an especially hot S and M session with a client. When Berkowitz realized they had great sex, without any exchange of body fluids, it was a revelation. That led him, along with Callen and Sonnabend, to write a pamphlet called *How to Have Sex in an Epidemic: One Approach*. It was a straightforward consumer's guide promoting risk-reduction and the use of condoms to stop the transmission of pathogens during sex.

Not long before, Sonnabend had asked Mathilde Krim, whom he knew from interferon work, for help raising money for a study of his patients. Krim was affluent, socially prominent, and a skilled fundraiser; soon she, Sonnabend, and several of his patients formed the AIDS Medical Foundation (AMF). Krim became its largest donor and board chair.

But when Callen and Berkowitz proposed that AMF publish their safe sex pamphlet, Krim balked, fearing the frank language about anal sex was too risqué and would turn off potential donors.

She did agree to let the foundation serve as a fiscal pass-through, so donations to print it would be tax-deductible. Randy Klose, a gay Texas Dairy Queen franchise heir, donated $10,000 to be used at the discretion of Sonnabend, who earmarked it for printing the booklet. Callen had just gotten a tax refund, which he also donated toward the printing cost.

The pamphlet was a sensation because it was specific and nonjudgmental, written in laymen's terms, and provided information not readily available. Its main idea, to use condoms for the foreseeable future when having intercourse, at first seemed inconceivable, a hysterical overreaction to a threat that still felt largely abstract. The fact that the main condom promoters and the authors of the booklet were two men with AIDS who were at odds with GMHC and vilified by gay community leaders as "sex-negative" and "self-hating" diminished the idea's legitimacy.

Yet in the months that followed and as I heard people discuss it, condom usage began to sound plausible. But the first time someone suggested a condom to me, I was torn between being offended (does he think I have AIDS?) and being scared (does he have AIDS?).

Eventually, GMHC did embrace condoms, paying to reprint and distribute the booklet through their growing network, both in New York and nationally. First, though, they required deletion of any reference to Sonnabend's multi-factorial hypothesis and his suggestion that cytomegalovirus (CMV) might play a key role in the development of AIDS.

Not long before he died in 2009, Rodger McFarlane, the tall, plain-speaking Alabaman who was GMHC's first executive director, and in whose kitchen rang the first AIDS information hotline, wrote Richard Berkowitz after seeing *Sex Positive*, the film detailing the history of safer sex and GMHC's initial reluctance to support the work of Berkowitz, Callen, and Sonnabend:

"I know exactly what you and Joe and Michael accomplished—and many thousands, yea millions, of us live on only because of what you gave us. And you did all that with little help from people like me. I have spent many years contemplating my complicity in several of our worst lapses over the years. I tell myself I was a kid, an ignorant hick, too inexperienced to inherit such epic responsibilities—like all of us.

*   *   *

Late in 1983, I saw two emaciated gay men at the grocery store in my neighborhood. One was in a wheelchair, his face and hands covered in KS lesions and his feet grotesquely swollen. The other was visually impaired and stooped over, walking with a cane in one hand and his other hand on the wheelchair, guided by his partner's verbal direction. They looked like they were in their fifties or sixties but could have been two decades younger. I was moved by their devotion to each other and wanted to speak to them, but I didn't know what I would say.

It was the first time I really understood that AIDS was calling forth courage and care from those who had the disease. There already was a groundswell of support from those of us who were not (yet) ill. The casual networks created by neighbors, coworkers, "bar friends," twelve-step recovery groups, and gay softball and bowling leagues offered the care and love denied by many families of the stricken, the medical establishment, and society at large. The waiters at Joe Allen's, in the theater district, showed up early for work so they could deliver free meals provided by the restaurant to people with AIDS in the neighborhood. Lawyers volunteered to help write wills or fight to keep landlords from evicting tenants with AIDS. Schedules were planned around caring for sick neighbors or friends, many of whom were alone and in tremendous need, without support from or rejected by their families.

This unprecedented response unified the LGBT community in new ways. Until the epidemic hit, the "community" between gay men and lesbians was fraught with tension. Many lesbians couldn't understand gay male promiscuity and the anonymous or public sex that some gay men valued; many gay men didn't respect women's right to reproductive choice and were unwilling to address their own sexism.

AIDS brought them together, because of the massive loss and because the political indifference to and exploitation of AIDS was an attack on the entire gay and lesbian community. AIDS helped us cement the concept of a chosen family of friends as the foundation upon which we built a massive and heroic effort to tend to our sick and dying.

Volunteers, mostly gay men and lesbians, signed up for "buddy programs" at AIDS organizations to help those who were ill by cleaning apartments, walking dogs, watering plants, or cooking meals. Often there was nothing to do but offer one's presence, to listen and to care.

CHAPTER 10

Stigma and Solidarity

The small support groups and networks of people with AIDS that emerged in 1982 and early 1983 created a nascent sense of an AIDS "community," but it existed only at a local level and included few beyond those who were extremely ill with the disease. There was no national movement and little communication among groups of gay men with AIDS in New York, San Francisco, Los Angeles, and elsewhere.

That changed in June 1983, when eleven gay men with AIDS from around the country gathered to strategize politically at the fifth Annual Gay and Lesbian Health Conference, held in Denver. During the conference, which was attended by hundreds of LGBT health professionals and activists, the eleven men with AIDS who comprised the People With AIDS Caucus gathered in a hotel room.

It was an event that set in motion ideas and activism that would shape the trajectory of not only my life but the lives of countless other people with AIDS.

Both Michael Callen and Richard Berkowitz were part of that pioneering group. Nearly all of the participants had symptoms, such as KS lesions, thrush (a yeast infection in the throat), or visible wasting. Years later, Berkowitz, the group's sole survivor, would recall in *POZ* magazine how fraught yet funny their meeting turned out to be:

> The men from San Francisco kept hugging and holding one another—a far cry from our [New York] tendency to complain, yell, and curse. But our differences went deeper than style. We argued over treatment approaches . . . causes [of the disease], and, most fiercely, the connection between promiscuity [and AIDS] (the theory advocated by the New Yorkers but denounced as homophobic by the San Franciscans). One night at dinner, Michael Callen suddenly asked, "Who knows how to take two dicks at once?" a trick question intended to reveal what, other than AIDS, the 11 of us had in common: We were all sluts . . . By accepting the role of promiscuity . . . as personally painful and politically provocative as it was . . . we could lead the way in protecting the gay community by promoting safer sex. For 11 men made to feel like lepers while aching more than ever for affection, this was a revelation.

As they got to know one another and created a sense of shared purpose, they wrote a manifesto that became the founding document of the People with AIDS (PWA) empowerment movement and influenced virtually every patient-advocacy group that followed.

The iconic text, now known as the Denver Principles, began with a preamble rejecting the word "victim," the walking-dead descriptor most common at that time, noting it is "a term that implies defeat." They also objected to being called "patients," which they wrote, "implies passivity, helplessness, and dependence upon the care of others." "We are People With AIDS," they declared, staking claim to the right to control the language used to describe themselves.

They went on to outline a series of rights and responsibilities for people with AIDS, health care workers, and allies. It recognized people with AIDS as catalysts for social change and declared that they could and should be their own health experts, especially by discussing issues of sexuality with one another.

They asserted a right "to as full and satisfying sexual and emotional lives as anyone else" and the right "to be involved at every level of decision-making . . . [to serve] on the boards of directors of provider organizations . . ." and that people with AIDS should "substitute low-risk sexual behaviors for those which could endanger themselves or their partners; we feel people with AIDS have an ethical responsibility to inform their potential sexual partners of their health status." At that time, most people, including many in the gay community, thought that once someone was diagnosed with AIDS, he or she would never have sex again. Serving on the boards of directors of provider organizations was also controversial. There was no one publicly identified as a person with AIDS on the board of GMHC until several years later; even the first board chairman was closeted, not just about having AIDS but also about being a gay man.

As the conference was wrapping up, the eleven manifesto co-authors stormed the plenary stage behind a banner that read "Fighting for Our Lives." They took the microphone and read the manifesto to a stone-silent convention hall. According to media reports at the time, at the end of the presentation, "there wasn't a dry eye in the house," and the audience gave them a standing ovation that lasted nearly fifteen minutes.

The concepts expressed in the Denver Principles manifesto weren't new—to a large extent, they were an embodiment of feminist health principles—but it was radical for a group of people who shared a disease to organize politically to assert their right to a voice in the public-policy decision-making that would so profoundly affect their lives. Never in the history of humanity had this occurred; for people with AIDS, the Denver Principles document is the Declaration of Independence, Constitution, Bill of Rights, and Magna Carta all rolled into one.

The Denver Principles defined the philosophical underpinnings of the self-empowerment movement for the AIDS epidemic and the network of service providers we created. It also quickly became a model for organizing by those with other chronic health conditions in the U.S. and around the world.

As important as that meeting in Denver was, I wasn't thinking that much about AIDS in the summer of 1983. I was working on the ramshackle 1840s house on Old Windy Bush Road in rural Bucks County, Pennsylvania, that André and I bought in July. I wouldn't have thought so at the time, but looking back, I think the purchase was partly a reflection of my unconscious urge to flee New York, seeing the city itself as the most dangerous risk factor.

Regardless of whether someone was at risk of AIDS, fear of contagion infected almost everyone in those early years. During a dinner party at a friend's West Village town house, I saw the host discreetly change the hand towels after a guest rumored to have AIDS used the bathroom. After dinner, that guest's dishes were washed separately, with scalding water. "You can't be too careful!" the host told me. Gay men discovered that family members and straight friends they once comfortably kissed or hugged now avoided physical contact. It wasn't unusual for linens to be thrown away or burned after use by someone with AIDS.

Health officials and AIDS organizations undertook educational campaigns to explain that AIDS wasn't spread casually. But the science concerning transmission was frequently doubted or ignored; paranoia persisted.

The extreme disfigurement of people with AIDS at the end stages of the disease became the image of AIDS in the media. Thick patches of black and dark violet Kaposi's sarcoma lesions on the hands, face, and neck; eyelids so swollen from KS lesions that they couldn't open; skeletal, emaciated bodies, reminiscent of photographs from Auschwitz, terrified and frightened the public, including gay men.

Politicians used AIDS to energize anti-gay supporters and religious conservatives who heralded it as a consequence of immorality. Pat Buchanan, an adviser to President Reagan, declared, "The poor homosexuals—they have declared war upon nature, and now nature is exacting an awful retribution."

A *Newsweek* article in the summer of '83 traced the newest wave of AIDS hysteria to an alarmist editorial by Dr. Anthony Fauci from the National Institutes of Health, published earlier that year in the *Journal of the American Medical Association.* Fauci had already become an influential voice on AIDS in Washington.

Public health experts had determined that AIDS wasn't spread by casual contact, but Fauci's editorial, in response to the report of an infant diagnosed with HIV, revived "the possibility" that "routine close contact, as within a family household, can spread the disease." If routine close contact might spread the disease, he wrote, "AIDS takes on an entirely new dimension, [and if] the possibility that nonsexual, non-blood-borne transmission is possible, the scope of the syndrome is enormous."

Fauci's article fed deep-seated fears. "Mere Contact May Spread AIDS" blared a *New York Times* headline, prompting the CDC to calm things down, issuing a statement definitively ruling out transmission by casual contact, food, water, air, or environmental surfaces.

Whether or not Fauci had intended to stoke fear, the public hysteria pushed the government to "do something" about AIDS. Congress finally authorized $12 million for AIDS research and shortly thereafter, Fauci was appointed the head of the NIH's National Institute for Allergy and Infectious Diseases. He essentially became the CEO of AIDS in America, a position he still holds thirty years later.

On April 23, 1984, at a packed news conference in Washington, President Reagan's secretary of Health and Human Services, Margaret Heckler, announced that human lymphotropic virus-III (HTLV-III, later renamed HIV) was the "probable cause" of AIDS. At her side was Dr. Robert Gallo, of the National Cancer Institute, and Dr. Luc Montagnier, of the famed Pasteur Institute in Paris, credited as "co-discoverers" of the virus. Heckler foolishly predicted that a vaccine would be available in two years.

I watched the press conference on television in my apartment on West Fifty-eighth Street. Though I wasn't indifferent to the news, I wasn't inspired by it. The press conference seemed contrived, like it was held to assuage the public's fear. They might as well have been in a different universe, with no understanding of what it was like to live with the disease in and around your life every day.

Any comment or pronouncement about the epidemic from federal officials didn't hold much weight, as they'd been absent and uncaring for too long. In any case, if I already had AIDS, Heckler's two-year prediction was not of much help.

My worry over every cough, cold, mosquito bite, or bruise became an obsession. I was especially fearful of pneumocystis carinii pneumonia (PCP) and Kaposi's sarcoma, then the two leading killers of people with AIDS. Like so many others, I became fluent in the acronyms for all the strange and previously rare opportunistic infections flourishing in the bodies of gay men. In addition to PCP and KS, we would hear "He's got MAC" or "I think it's toxo" or "It was the CMV that took his eyesight."

The acronyms were shorthand for conveying sketchy associations. We were learning that people with MAC infections shouldn't be near birds, that guys who spent more time in the Southwest or desert climates were more likely to get histo, and that while CMV was endemic among gay men, it could make a person with AIDS lose his vision. I memorized the words, not just the acronyms; I wanted to be able to say "progressive multifocal leukoencephalopathy," "mycobacterium avium-intracellulare," "cytomegalovirus," "histoplasmosis," and "toxoplasmosis." It was a tiny measure of control over a terrifying syndrome against which I felt helpless. Learning everything I could about AIDS felt like I was preparing my brain for the assault on my body that I feared was on its way.

While I, like many other young gay men, had once thought those getting AIDS were older, more promiscuous, and into more extreme sex than I was, by 1984 it was clear that there was an inexplicable randomness to who was struck. At first I saw these "atypical" cases as quirky anomalies. Then it started to feel like every case was anomalous, especially as they came closer and closer to my own life. When I heard of someone who was sick, an instant Venn diagram appeared in my head, reflexively sketching out the sexual relationships that might connect me to that person. AIDS was now the main topic of conversation among my gay friends. Sometimes, though, we craved an AIDS-free conversation. At a friend's birthday party that year, the host said, "Let's not talk about AIDS or any sad things tonight," which made it impossible to think of anything else.

Some tried celibacy or moved out of New York or San Francisco or Los Angeles to more remote areas where it felt "safer"; some left the country. We used gallows humor to cope: "Hey, you know what 'GAY' stands for? 'Got AIDS yet?' " When the epidemic seemed confined to what was called the "Four H Club"—homosexuals, hemophiliacs, heroin users, and persons of Haitian origin—the line was "How am I going to tell Mom and Dad I'm Haitian?" We shared halfhearted denials that we knew weren't true: "It's just a lot of hype, they're trying to scare us" or "I'm not a slut, so I'm safe."

I first heard the suggestion to use condoms when *How to Have Sex in an Epidemic* was published mid-1983 but knowing and doing are two different things. At first I didn't use them, nor did anyone I had sex with suggest we use them. Once I realized I needed to use them, the subject was difficult for me to broach, because it was stigmatizing and embarrassing. Condoms couldn't be suggested without risking raising an unspoken accusation against one's self or one's partner. Sometimes I did wonder if I posed a risk to my partners, but more often I was worried about whether they were a risk to me. My swollen lymph glands were hardly unique—it seemed like many of my friends had similar symptoms—and we hoped our continued relatively good health might be a sign that we were "immune" to AIDS. It wasn't until late in 1984 or early in 1985 that I began to use condoms with any regularity and even then it was inconsistent. In retrospect, I'm ashamed that it took me so long to use them at all, but at the time it felt as if I was one of the first of my friends to do so, and I eventually raised the matter first more often than did my partners.

Even guys who worked at AIDS organizations and were responsible for HIV prevention programs were seen having sex without condoms in back rooms, bathhouses, and sex clubs. In hindsight, the main problem was that the message was to "use a condom every time," for every type of sex, without recognizing the risk differential between oral and anal sex or between "topping" and "bottoming." In any case, no one I knew used condoms for oral sex. We understood that oral sex was far less risky—otherwise virtually the entire community would have HIV or AIDS—and decided it was a risk we were willing to accept, even if it was "against the rules."

I also heard gay men refuse to use condoms, saying, "If I get it, I get it, there's nothing I can do about it." Some said they would rather die than refrain from having sex the way they wanted. Once I asked a gay doctor I knew what he thought about using condoms. He rolled his eyes and said to forget about them: "Just be a Boy Scout and wash up after you have sex, and you'll be fine."

The disconnect between what was being promoted as HIV prevention and what gay men were actually doing was part of the dichotomy between what we wanted the public to think about our sex lives and the sex lives we actually lived. Saying "Use a condom every time" was politically palatable. A more accurate and explicit message—"Being a bottom is the biggest risk"—would have required politicians who provided funding and the public health officials who controlled prevention programs to tacitly accept the aspect of gay male sexuality they found most abhorrent. Eventually, the Helms Amendment forbade any federal dollars for any HIV programs that were deemed to "promote" homosexuality, which killed the most effective prevention programs.

Some AIDS organizations raised private funding for prevention work with gay men, to get around the Helms Amendment prohibition. But when confronted by activists who wanted a more accurate and detailed risk assessment in prevention messaging, highlighting receptive anal sex as vastly greater risk than oral sex, for example, they were told there was little science to support this approach.

At the time of the 1984 Heckler press conference announcing the discovery of HIV, I didn't know anyone personally who had died of AIDS. My concern, in terms of AIDS, was mostly about myself. I ricocheted between fearing I was about to become sick and thinking I had narrowly escaped getting sick. My lymph gland swelling wasn't nearly as bad as it was a few years before.

Though Joe McDonald's death was a shock, it didn't feel like death rapping at my door until later that year, when two of my exes, Robert Hayes, the managing editor at *Interview* and Jim Nall, the neurologist who inspired my move to New York, got sick and died.

One Saturday I was having breakfast at a diner in New Hope with Rupert Smith and his boyfriend, Patrick McAllister. Rupert, an artist who also worked for Andy Warhol, as a screen printer, had a cool contemporary house built around the ruins of a nineteenth-century stone mill not far from my own.

Over scrambled eggs, Rupert casually said, "I guess you've heard about Robert."

I felt a chill. "No, what about Robert?" I asked. "I heard he's got it" was all Rupert needed to say. That led us to talk about Joe McDonald's death, and Patrick said that he was worried about a ménage à trois he and Rupert had with someone who had dated Joe. My mind was stuck on the news about Robert, worrying about him and myself, thinking back to all the times he and I had condomless sex.

Then my attention fixed on a small oblong purple spot near Patrick's left earlobe. It was about as wide as the tip of a pencil eraser and about the same color. I had seen guys on the street and at AIDS benefits with KS, but their lesions were bigger and darker than Patrick's. Did he know it was there? Should I say something? There was no etiquette in the situation.

Just then Rupert said, "But Patrick and I got checked out by our doctor, and we're okay."

I was flustered for a moment, then heard myself blurt out, "Did the doctor see that spot?" I pointed at Patrick's ear.

Rupert took a peek, and his face changed. "I don't think that was there a couple of days ago," he said. Patrick, who could be prickly, said belligerently, "What? Now you think *I* have AIDS? Thanks a lot!" He left the table to look in the bathroom mirror and returned with an ashen face. I felt guilty, like it was my fault for having noticed the spot.

Patrick died just a few months later. Rupert hosted a memorial service on a long stretch of lawn next to a creek in his backyard. He planted a tree over Patrick's ashes. It wasn't long before Rupert's ashes were there as well.

Another friend told me that Robert was denying that his sickness was AIDS. I wanted to call him, but I hadn't seen him in over six months and wasn't sure what I would say. Acknowledging that I knew he had been seriously ill was an accusation by itself, even if I never mentioned AIDS.

About a month after that breakfast with Rupert and Patrick, Robert called me, ostensibly to invite me to lunch and to see the newly renovated space that Warhol had bought for his Factory, an old Con Edison power plant substation at Thirty-third and Madison. I thought he might want to talk to me about AIDS; since I read the gay press and was reasonably informed, he thought of me as an expert.

The moment I entered Robert's new office, I noticed how thin he was. As he climbed a short flight of stairs to show me more of the building, his breathing was labored. Midway, I asked, "Do you mind if we go directly to lunch?" Robert looked relieved, and we headed to

Saltimbocca, a restaurant on Madison Avenue a block away, where he asked the maître d' for the quiet booth in the back corner.

Robert told me that his boyfriend, Cisco, was near death from AIDS. Robert wasn't feeling well, either, he said, but it was just from the stress of taking care of Cisco. He insisted he had been "checked out" and didn't have AIDS. He hoped I might help get Cisco into drug trials he'd heard were going on at the NIH. Fred Hughes, who also worked for Warhol, had told him that influential gay men, friends of President and Mrs. Reagan, were in these trials and doing well. "You know all those political people," he said. "Can you find out?"

I told Robert that I would ask Alan Baron if he had contacts at the NIH. Robert's brown eyes were never more soulful than on that afternoon when he said, "Thank you, I really appreciate it. I've got to get Cisco some help or he's going to die." Then he started coughing and took a sip of water.

I showed Robert a trick I had just learned for testing whether you had pneumonia, often the presenting symptom that led to an AIDS diagnosis. I made a fist and put it in the middle of my chest; he did the same. "Now take a really, really deep breath, as deep as you can, and hold it," I instructed. We both did that. "Do you feel any pain in your chest?" No, he did not. "Good!"

"I'm sure I don't have AIDS," he said. He repeated the coughing test several times before we left the restaurant. On the sidewalk, our goodbye was a little awkward; when we hugged, he held me longer than he might ordinarily. We both knew he was sicker than he let on.

That was the first time I said goodbye to someone I thought I might never see again. Later on, with others, I couldn't bring myself to go through the motion of saying "See you later." Those partings were usually silent, or I might whisper, "I love you" into a person's ear.

Before Alan could find out about the rumored trials, Robert was hospitalized. His sister said he didn't want visitors, but she gave me the phone number. His voice was so weak that I could catch only bits of what he said. He died soon after.

What Robert didn't tell me—and I hope he never knew—was how freaked out Andy Warhol was by AIDS. In the audio diaries published after his death, Warhol voiced anxieties about AIDS that were typical even among urbane Manhattanites. After seeing Joe McDonald at a party early in 1983, Warhol said, "I didn't want to talk to him because he just had gay cancer."

But Warhol's entries about Robert are devastating: "I didn't invite Robert Hayes to ride with me because he was with his sister and Cisco, and he has AIDS so I didn't want to be that close to him . . . I'm worried I could get it by drinking out of the same glass or just being around these kids who go to the baths . . ."

In the fall of 1984, Jim Nall invited me to visit him in Texas, where he had taken a job at the Kelsey-Seybold Clinic in Houston. At baggage claim, a man I hardly recognized, wearing a baseball cap, waved at me. As he drew closer, I saw that the hat was shading KS lesions on Jim's face. I tried to act like everything was normal, even though my heart was pounding with worry. The first gay man I'd met in New York, the man who had introduced me to the city, was sick.

That evening when we were getting ready for bed, Jim started to make up the couch with sheets and a beautiful antique quilt made by his grandmother. I was hurt. We had always slept in the same bed. I asked him, "Why can't we sleep together?"

He said, "I assumed you wouldn't want to because of this," gesturing toward his gaunt, KS-covered face.

"I don't care," I said. "I won't get it by sleeping in the same bed with you. Besides, it'll feel weird not to hold you in my arms like we used to."

We snuggled under the covers, spooning. I had been so focused on his KS lesions that I hadn't realized how much weight he had lost until I put my arm around him and felt his bony, wasted body. My nose was at his neck, and I was sure I could smell the disease. I was self-conscious about touching such an obviously ill body, but I responded by instinct, drawing him close to me. Then I felt tears on his cheek. "What's wrong?" I asked. "Does that hurt?"

He gave a small laugh. "No, it feels good. I'm glad you're here," he said. "I can't remember the last time someone held me. People won't even shake hands with me anymore." Every time I visit someone in the hospital or comfort an ill friend, I always make sure to touch them, remembering Jim's comment, as well as how it felt later, when I got sick, and people were afraid to touch me.

Jim died a few months later. His executor called me to say that he had left me "an old quilt." It was the one his grandmother had made. The one I did not use the last time I saw Jim.

CHAPTER 11

Testing and Telling

Despite the growing toll of AIDS among friends, my own health was fairly stable. I hadn't lost any more weight. The night sweats and lymph glands flared up occasionally, but I had gotten used to that. AIDS was just a background anxiety that had come to feel normal.

I was excited about my business, which was growing rapidly, with a roster of prestigious clients. One of my largest clients was a political survey research firm, Penn+Schoen. Early in 1985, their chief of staff, Todd Collins, and I went into business together. Todd's analytical and tech prowess complemented my political savvy and people skills. I liked that he had gone to Harvard; having a well-credentialed business partner made me less self-conscious about having no college degree. He was straight, but I think he considered it cool that I was gay.

We focused the firm on homelessness, children's issues, and gay and lesbian issues, three areas where we thought there was great need and opportunity. AIDS wasn't mentioned in our detailed business plan; it didn't cross our minds. I thought of myself as an activist, and was already participating in street demonstrations for passage of the gay rights bill in New York City, protesting AIDS stigma and other issues, but thinking of AIDS as a business opportunity was the furthest thing from my mind.

Todd and I named the firm Strub/Collins, and our initial clients ranged from Senior Action in a Gay Environment and the National Gay Task Force to New York's Municipal Arts Society, Partnership for the Homeless, and Holy Apostles Soup Kitchen. Within the first two years, AIDS efforts became the largest part of the business. It happened by accident: We found ourselves in a situation where our expertise was urgently needed—far beyond what we were able to undertake as volunteers.

I once heard Gloria Steinem speak at a fund-raising event for a congressional candidate in New York. She pointed out how the values people claim to hold dear and the values reflected in their actions are sometimes very different. She said, "If you want to know what someone's real values are, take a look at their checkbook."

As I immersed myself in fund-raising work, I found myself paraphrasing Steinem's observation in direct-mail appeals. I also looked at my checkbook, thinking about my own values. I realized that my support for GMHC was limited to buying tickets to attend fun events where I met interesting people. Not much of a sacrifice and something I did as much for myself as for the cause.

When Robert died, followed quickly by a friend of André's, I wrote out a check to GMHC for five hundred dollars, the largest charitable donation I had ever made. Pushing myself to donate beyond my comfort zone made it easier to push others to do the same.

I expected an acknowledgment from GMHC, but none was forthcoming. My ego was bruised—I wanted my generosity to be recognized—and as a fund-raising consultant, I knew that GMHC needed to thank donors, the first step to getting another gift.

At a GMHC reception, I met one of their board members, Ira Berger. I told him I was a fund-raising consultant as well as a GMHC donor and launched into a mini-lecture about how GMHC would never retain donors if they didn't acknowledge gifts.

"I agree," he said, beckoning a man nearby to join our conversation. "And may I introduce you to Bill Jones, our new development director?"

Bill apologized for not acknowledging my gift and then asked me to volunteer. "We're just setting up the development department and our systems," he said. "You sound like you know what you're talking about. Can you help us?"

A few days later, I volunteered to help create a fund-raising mailing for GMHC. Another volunteer, Time, Inc. copywriter Steve Petoniak, had written a rough draft. Steve was a brilliant copywriter, but more experienced at selling subscriptions than soliciting donations. His draft positioned people with AIDS as victims and based the "ask" on sympathy for their difficult plight. I rewrote his letter with a more personal approach from the perspective of GMHC's openly gay executive director, Richard Dunne, and added an advocacy edge highlighting empowerment rather than sympathy. GMHC's board liked the letter, and they hired my firm to find lists and print and mail it.

Finding a printer was tough. "We don't print pornography, either" one firm said, as though an AIDS fundraising appeal was comparable. After we got them printed, we shipped the printed components to a letter shop on Long Island to be folded, inserted, sealed, and mailed. I got a phone call from the owner: "Our workers won't touch the letters because they are afraid of getting AIDS." We had to pick up the printed pieces and take them to a letter shop in New Jersey.

Vendors weren't the only obstacles. Even though GMHC had been around for three years, they had never sent fund-raising letters, in part because the board didn't think direct mail would work for AIDS organizations. "People will think the envelopes or stamps were licked by volunteers with AIDS," one board member said. "They won't want to open the envelopes." Because of privacy concerns, we could not use the words "AIDS" or "gay" on teaser copy on the outside of the envelope; even the return address said only GMHC, not the organization's full name.

We sent it to fifty-four thousand New Yorkers, and it grossed over

$125,000 against a cost of about $22,000. During the next several years, we sent more than three million GMHC fund-raising letters, creating a huge base of small donors and raising a significant part of the agency's budget.

The space Todd Collins and I rented for the company was on Forty-fifth Street, just off Fifth Avenue. It had a large communal area for our growing staff—by the end of 1985, we had six people working for us—and two private offices for Todd and me. On July 25, 1985, the entire office was glued to a portable television, watching a real-life drama unfold as the Pasteur Institute in Paris announced that Rock Hudson had AIDS and had recently spent ten days there undergoing an experimental treatment.

The public reaction was explosive, mainly shock at the revelation. While the media fixated on Hudson's homosexuality, it also addressed AIDS in greater detail than ever. In the weeks that followed, half a century of secrets kept by friends, relatives, tricks, and Hollywood insiders flooded the pages of the tabloids and magazines. AIDS and the Hollywood closet were having a moment.

I called a friend in Los Angeles who was one of Hudson's friends. "It looks bad, Sean," he said of Hudson's health. "We're praying, but I don't think he has much time left." I asked about the treatment Hudson received at the Pasteur Institute, the esteemed hospital where Montagnier and his team first identified HIV. "It didn't really do anything. We thought it might have at first, but it didn't," my friend said.

Hudson was a longtime friend of the Reagans, and there was hope that his disclosure would inspire Reagan to finally say something publicly about the epidemic. Reagan issued only a brief statement after Hudson died a few months later, noting that the actor would be "remembered for his humanity" and making no reference to the epidemic. Reagan's political ally Charlton Heston said that any actor who was "a member of a high-risk group has an obligation to refuse to do a kissing scene."

The HIV antibody test had been introduced earlier in 1985, and news about Rock Hudson began prompting some gay men to get tested. I wasn't eager to join them, particularly since I was feeling good, excited about my business, and thought that my "symptoms" were under control.

Those I knew who had gotten tested usually did so because they showed up at their doctor's office with KS lesions or at an emergency room with PCP or some other infection. If I tested positive, there was nothing to do about it; it would only add more stress to my life. Questions about the test's accuracy nagged at me. On some level, I was afraid to find out for certain.

I also feared stigma. Some families were already refusing to allow gay male relatives to join family holidays or to hold young nieces and nephews. Those who tested positive were sometimes welcomed at holiday meals on the condition that they use disposable utensils. People known to have AIDS lost their jobs and apartments. Sonnabend's landlord tried to evict him because he treated people with AIDS at his office in the West Village. Funeral homes wouldn't take the bodies of those who died of AIDS or charged exorbitant extra fees to do so. There was serious talk of quarantine, and by the end of 1985, an effort was under way in California to put such a measure on the ballot.

Only with my closest gay friends could I share my fear that I might have "it." I disclosed my health concerns when I dated someone, but often not to one-time hookups. Among my friends and me, the assumption was that we had all been exposed many times over the years, and who got sick was as much a function of unknown factors as it might be having slept with the wrong person.

There was an emerging divide between those known to be sick and the rest of us, who worried about getting sick. The introduction of the HIV antibody test gradually gave rise to another viral divide, between those testing positive and those testing negative, but at the time there was a lot more discussion in the gay community about reasons not to take the test than people actually taking it.

*   *   *

By the summer of 1985, André Ledoux and I had drifted apart, and I was dating again. One night around closing time, I wandered into a popular gay bar in the West Village. Uncle Charlie's Downtown was one of New York's first "respectable" gay clubs, with a preppy vibe, pop music, and large windows that let passersby cruise without having to enter. The bar offered little golfer's pencils and "trick cards" reading "We met at Uncle Charlie's."

When I first saw Michael Misove, Madonna's "Like a Virgin" video was playing on the screens hung in every corner. The bar was thinning out; the guys remaining were determined not to go home alone. Michael was powerfully built, with bulging muscles visible through a tight T-shirt. He had tousled sandy-colored hair, an open, smooth face, and blue eyes. When he looked at me, I averted my eyes, afraid he was out of my league. After a while I realized he was interested, and I reciprocated his gaze. As the lights flashed to indicate last call, I worked up the nerve to say hello.

We went from the bar to an all-night diner, talking for hours about politics, gay culture, books, jobs, relationships and families, and, of course, AIDS. Michael declared that he had no interest in ever taking the HIV test.

When I caressed Michael's neck that first night, I could tell he had swollen lymph glands, just as I did. When I mentioned it, he said they had been that way for several years. "Mine, too," I said. We didn't discuss using condoms.

Michael was from Kingston, New York, in the upper Hudson River Valley, the youngest of three children. His family lived in a small house built on a landfill next to a Catholic cemetery. Michael's father was of Czech descent and managed the produce department in a neighborhood grocery; his mother was Irish and orphaned as a child, like my own mother.

Although Michael was close to his mother, he never felt like he fit in his family. As a little kid, he believed that he and another baby must have been switched at birth. Like so many gay men of his generation, he was fighting a sense of unbridgeable difference.

Michael got a scholarship to Wesleyan University and, after graduating, spent several years in the navy. Then he moved to New York for a master's program at Columbia but left after a falling-out with his father, who cut off tuition payments. The rift between them never healed.

We were different in many ways. He was thirty-eight and I was twenty-seven. He had few friends and wasn't especially interested in meeting new people; my circle was large and constantly expanding. He did love to cook for dinner parties, but our guests were usually my friends and business associates. If he wasn't cooking, he preferred time with me alone. And when he didn't care for someone, he didn't care if the person knew it.

Once we had a dinner party and included a neighbor, Darren, whom we didn't know well. He turned out to be boorish, and right before dessert, when I announced that Michael had made a pecan pie from scratch, Darren exclaimed, "Oh! I had the best pecan pie the other day," and proceeded to tell us about his exceptional pie experience. When I went to the kitchen to help Michael serve the pie, he had cut it into seven pieces. I said, "We're eight, Mike!" assuming he had miscounted the number of guests. He said, "I know, but Darren's already had the *best* pecan pie. I'm sure he won't want to taste mine."

I don't think the reclusive and prickly personality I got to know was natural to Michael; it was a defensive response to what the world had done to him. Like me, he had bitter feelings toward Catholicism, had suffered torment from other kids in school, and felt familial and social disapproval because he was gay. In contrast to my anger, engagement, and willingness to argue, Michael's response was withdrawal into a rich and complex inner world.

He immersed himself in classical music and great literature. He especially liked three Russians: Dostoevsky, Tolstoy, and Nabokov. He loved opera but preferred to go alone. He had a refined sense of color and could discern among and precisely label a dozen different shades, all of which I would have called "peach." Sometimes, while walking in the street, he would say to me, "Stop! Look at that," pointing to a narrow sliver of brilliant blue sky visible between two skyscrapers, say, or to the sidewalk, where a pale yellow wildflower had blossomed in a sidewalk crack.

Even if Michael didn't rant or obsess about politics the way I did, he had a quiet rage, like many gay men. That collective rage grew with the death toll and fueled the rise of LGBT and AIDS activism.

In addition to his love, his regular schedule and practiced habits created a routine in our partnership that enabled me to be more successful and effective in activism and businesses. The deaths of Jim Nall and Robert Hayes, breaking up with André, and managing a fast-growing business with a new partner had made my life chaotic. My love for and life with Michael was the antidote.

Michael taught English as a second language at a school in midtown, half a block from my office. He loved teaching, especially adults. "Kids go to school because they have to; adults because they want to," he said. We had lunch together several times a week. On nice days I would get us take-out and meet him at Bryant Park so we could spend his whole lunch hour together.

He got off work precisely at five-thirty; I always worked later. By the time I got to his apartment on East Twenty-fifth Street, he already would have gone to the gym, shopped for groceries, and tried a new recipe from the *Joy of Cooking*, carefully noting in the margin how a dish turned out. In the mornings, we walked up Third Avenue and then went west, giving each other a quick kiss at the corner of Fifth Avenue and Forty-fifth Street before going to our respective offices.

On weekends, we explored bed-and-breakfasts as far away as Vermont. We took back roads through small towns, delighted when we stumbled upon a festival, yard sale, or farmers' market. When either of us traveled without the other, we sent postcards. Once, during a week-long visit to Hawaii, he sent me nine cards.

My busier schedule dictated when we could get together. I was constantly attending political events or fund-raisers, making business contacts, and socializing. I had big ambitions for my life; he focused on his daily routine and quality of life. My schedule was fluid, and I frequently needed to change or reschedule our plans at the last minute.

But when it was Michael who began canceling dates in our budding relationship, I was afraid he was trying to ease out of it. I finally confronted him when he said he couldn't switch a dinner from Wednesday to Thursday; I knew he had no other plans. "Are you going out?" I asked. "None of your business," he replied. "Michael," I asked him, "what is going on?"

He explained, "You seem to think all these nights I'm not spending with you have no value, that they can be swapped around at your convenience. You shouldn't consider an appointment I make—even if it is just with myself—any more easily rearranged than a meeting or event on your schedule."

The thought of losing Michael scared me in a way I hadn't felt. That made me prioritize my time with him above all else and to accept an unstated assumption that we were together permanently. We didn't talk much about our future beyond a few months down the line or until the next holiday break. On some unspoken level, I think we assumed it unlikely that we would grow old together. The odds against it were too great.

Max Westerman, the Dutch guy I met at the Ninth Circle soon after I moved to New York, had become my closest friend. When I wasn't with Michael, I was often with Max, going to movies or parties or hitting the bars and clubs, sometimes staying out most of the night. Max didn't come to the U.S. until he was eighteen, but he knew more about U.S. politics than almost anyone I knew besides Alan Baron. We shared a fascination with Roy Cohn, the redbaiting right-wing legal counsel to Senator Joseph McCarthy in the 1950s.

Cohn was intensely homophobic and openly closeted; he vehemently denied being gay, sometimes threatening litigation against
those who suggested otherwise. He was a fixture at Studio 54 and other
quasi-gay glam nightclubs, often accompanied by at least one if not
several tall blond muscular men. He liked Quaaludes and cocaine and
lived a life as colorful as it was dastardly. Max had become friendly with
Cohn's private pilot, who shared stories about Cohn's exploits.

When Max and I learned that Cohn had AIDS, we knew it was a
great story and decided to write a biography of him. On the Saturday
after Labor Day in 1985, we had plans to get together at my friend
Doris O'Donnell's apartment to discuss the project. Doris and I met
when she volunteered at the Council on Economic Priorities, a think-
tank client of mine. She knew a lot about Cohn, in part because she
grew up in Washington in the 1950s, and her parents were both political columnists. Michael was out of town, and a friend of his was using
his apartment, so I was staying at Doris's apartment that weekend.

But when Max arrived on Saturday, I was in terrible pain. I had
woken up with eruptions of painful sores along the entire right side of my
torso. I could barely move, let alone sit and discuss a new project. Even
the fabric of my T-shirt brushing against the blisters caused sharp jolts of
pain. The previous weekend I had cleared brush at my house in Pennsylvania; I knew there was poison ivy nearby, but I thought I had avoided it.

Max called a doctor friend, Nathaniel Pier, who said he would meet
us in his office at Sixty-eighth and Broadway, even though it was Saturday. Pier took one look at the rash and said, "You've got shingles. Do
you know what that is?" When I told him I didn't, he said, "It's the
chicken pox virus that erupts in adults who have suppressed immune
systems." Hearing the phrase "immune system" made me forget the pain
and get right to the point. "Do I have AIDS?" I asked. "Not necessarily,"
Pier said, "but we can find out for sure with a test. The results will take
a couple of weeks to get back." When I didn't immediately respond, he
asked, "Do you want to do it?"

"Yes, let's go ahead," I replied.

In the intervening two weeks, I hoped desperately the test would come back negative. I tried reciting the Catholic prayers of my childhood, something I hadn't done in years. Michael knew I had taken the test, but our focus was on my recovery from the shingles, which took several weeks.

Another friend had recently gotten his positive result, and his doctor called him personally to deliver the news. When Pier's assistant called me to say the results were in and for me to make an appointment, I thought it was a good sign. I sat in the waiting room, flipping through the big *People* exposé on Rock Hudson's gay life. When the office assistant showed me in, Dr. Pier was organizing papers on his desk. He didn't look up. When I sat where I had sat on the previous visit, he suggested I move to the chair next to his desk.

He took a small intake of breath and then spoke briskly, businesslike, as though he had to get through something unpleasant. "Your test came back positive, Sean. I'm sorry to have to tell you that you have HIV." I froze, trying not to react as a rush of thoughts swirled in my head. He continued. "This doesn't mean you have AIDS. A mild case, like what you have, is what we call AIDS-related complex." When I tried to ask questions, my voice caught in my throat. Pier reached out with his hands and held one of mine. When I asked if he thought I should make a will, he looked at me with moist eyes and said, "Sean, these days you can have two good years left."

When I left Pier's office, I was in a daze. It was a warm, bright afternoon in late September. Walking down Broadway toward Lincoln Center, I passed people on their way to or from lunch, wandering in and out of shops, as if it were an ordinary day. My head felt like it was floating, and I found it impossible to concentrate. Everything was different, but I wasn't ready to face my new reality.

That night I told Michael the news in a matter-of-fact way, and he responded calmly, as I'd known he would. He gave me a long hug and said, "I probably have it, too, but I still don't want to know. If I've got it, I've got it. There's nothing different I would do." I didn't try to talk him into getting tested; it was his choice, and until I came down with shingles, skipping the test had been my choice as well. I never considered that Michael might reject me or that the test result would change our relationship. Having the comfort and security of knowing he would care for me, no matter how sick I became, made coping with the news much easier.

Telling others was more complicated, particularly making the distinction—which was so important to me—between my ARC diagnosis and AIDS. ARC was considered "AIDS lite," not AIDS, but plenty stigmatized. (Back then we didn't colloquially refer to it as being HIV-positive, as we do today.) Some who had tested negative didn't tell people because acknowledging you had been tested was stigmatizing. Sharing the news of a negative test among your gay friends could also feel unseemly, like it was a boast or taunt.

Not long after my positive test results came back, Michael and I tried using some flavored and brightly colored condoms from a gift bag I had brought home after a benefit gala. We ended up blowing them up as balloons. That was the only time we used condoms with each other. We did have a tacit agreement to use condoms if either of us had sex outside the relationship. We accepted that one of us might have sex with someone else on occasion; sometimes we shared that information with each other, sometimes not.

Over the next several years, I brought articles home about the science and the politics of AIDS, and Michael would read them. He didn't join me at demonstrations or other AIDS events. He was supportive, but AIDS was my arena, not his.

As I gradually told friends I was HIV-positive, some looked at me with a tragic expression or outright fear. Others became momentarily quiet and then offered support, saying, "You know you can count on me" or "We'll get through this together." Sometimes the first question was if I'd told my family. One relative's first comment was "I hope you've got good insurance." I never cried when telling people I had HIV unless they did first; my reaction frequently reflected theirs.

When I told my business partner, Todd Collins, I played down the drama of the news, saying it wasn't a surprise. But he was mad. "If you suspected it, you should have said so before we went into business together!" He wasn't concerned about the usual things—casual contagion and stigma—he was angry because he wouldn't have quit a good job and risked a new venture with me if he had thought I was terminally ill.

When I told Vito Russo, he said, "Oh, honey, I'm so sorry," and hugged me tightly for a long time. It was a hug that melted past the awkward moment when you expect the squeeze to end but then realize your hugging partner is holding on. I was nourished by Vito's hug, as if some energy or spirit had been transferred from his body to my own.

I hadn't fully grasped what a diagnosis would mean for me logistically, or for those around me, until it happened and I had to deal with the repercussions. In the months following my diagnosis, I wrote a will, naming Megan and my other younger sister, Gilbey, an attorney, as co-executors. I was psychologically preparing myself, and perhaps them, for what I believed was my inevitable sickness and painful death.

I wanted my estate to be as simple as possible, so I put my house in Bucks County on the market, intending to take the proceeds and live every day to the fullest even as I proclaimed my intention to "beat this thing." My life had become surreal. Upbeat clichés helped provide a framework for how I would make sense of complicated and contradictory emotions.

Despite losses, I hadn't lived through caring for someone up close, day in and day out, as they inched painfully toward death. The practical realities of dying remained a step removed. Now it seemed like my first experience through a decline to death was likely to be my own.

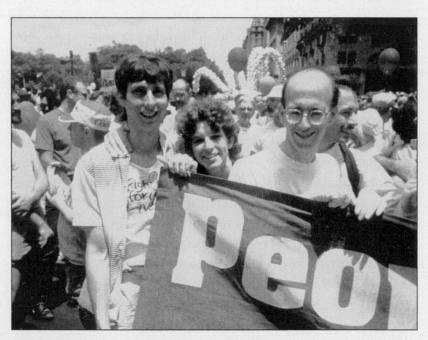

I took this picture of Denver Principles coauthor and cofounder of the People With AIDS Coalition, Michael Callen, photographer/activist Jane Rosett, and PWAC executive director Michael Hirsch at Gay Pride in New York City in 1986. "The Michaels" were important mentors to me; Jane Rosett documented photographically the early days of the epidemic in New York.

CHAPTER 12

The Living Room

In the fall of 1985, just a few weeks after I was diagnosed, a friend took me to the Public Theater to see Larry Kramer's powerful play, *The Normal Heart*, about how poorly and slowly Mayor Ed Koch and his administration were responding to the emerging epidemic. The play devastated me, and I began quietly sobbing, releasing emotions I had held tightly inside since the day Dr. Pier delivered the bad news. By the time I left the theater, I was inspired and angry but also ashamed. I had just turned in a freelance writing project, a fund-raising letter for Koch's reelection campaign. As closely as I thought I had followed the epidemic, I had been clueless about Koch's poor response.

Worrying about who knew or might find out I had HIV didn't seem nearly as important after I saw *The Normal Heart*. Its emotional impact made me focus on what I needed to do to stay healthy and survive as long as possible. In the months that followed, I surrounded myself with others who could encourage that purpose and understand what I was experiencing as a person with HIV.

A few days later, Vito called to ask if I would distribute flyers at the gay bars in Bucks County for an upcoming demonstration against the

New York Post's AIDS coverage. The *Post* had fueled hysteria since the first days of the epidemic. The *Post* routinely ran headlines such as "L.I. Grandma Died of AIDS" and "Junkie AIDS Victim was Housekeeper at Bellevue"; referred to gay clubs as "AIDS dens"; and ran cartoons depicting "AIDS dragons" threatening children. The headlines were so absurd that Pop artist Keith Haring made collages from them.

On a rainy Saturday night, I sloshed through the muddy parking lot of the Prelude, a large gay disco in New Hope, and put soggy flyers under the windshield wipers of every car. Most of the patrons were, like me, gay twentysomething or thirtysomething New Yorkers with weekend homes in the area, exactly the group we wanted to get involved in advocacy.

My sister Megan helped me that night. She'd graduated from high school in Iowa City the year before but wasn't getting along with our parents. I offered them advice once too often, and our frustrated mother finally said, "Well, why don't you take her?" When Megan moved east to live with me, it was intended to be for a month or two until she enrolled in college; instead, she became my ally in activism, my closest confidante, and my business partner. Over time, our lives, friends, finances, and aspirations became intertwined in ways that made our relationship markedly different than those we have with our other siblings. I told Megan about my diagnosis right away, but I delayed telling the rest of my family.

At Thanksgiving in Iowa that year, I realized that Megan was becoming an activist. It was not long after our sister Gilbey had come out as a lesbian. In discussing AIDS activism, Megan made a reference to the Stonewall riots. When Gilbey said, "What's Stonewall?" Megan was shocked. "I can't believe you don't know about Stonewall!" she said, and proceeded to explain the historical importance of the event.

There was another message from Vito on my answering machine later that fall, asking Megan and me to attend an upcoming meeting, again protesting the *New York Post*. "Bring everyone you can, we really need you!" More than seven hundred people jammed into the Methodist Church at

Seventh Avenue and Thirteenth Street to hear Vito's passionate speech. Feeling inspired and supported, I looked around the church at the huge showing and began to feel a part of a community working together.

I also saw an African American man who clearly had AIDS; even though my infection wasn't visible to others, I felt the stirring of a kinship with him that was new to me. Sharing the stigma of AIDS struck me as more relevant than the racial divide between us.

In November, when I read in the *Native* that the People With AIDS Coalition had opened the Living Room, a small office and drop-in center, I checked it out. The address was an old town house on a tree-lined street in the West Village. Several buzzers were positioned next to a wrought-iron gate at the side of the building. A handwritten label said "PWAC Living Room." I pushed it, and a raspy buzz unlocked the gate. I opened it and walked tentatively through a tunnel-like horse walk that ended in a garden area, where there once were stables. I stepped into bright sunlight, surrounded by lush plantings.

The garden was reflective of PWAC itself, vibrant and full of life. Inside there was a living room with a random collection of chairs and couches that looked like flea-market rejects. Every surface was piled high with gay newspapers, medical journals, and AIDS pamphlets. A balding man with glasses was talking on the phone at a makeshift desk near the back of the room. He put his hand over the receiver to welcome me with a mock whisper, mouthing, "Just a minute, I'll be right with you." When he got off the phone, he stood up and stuck out his hand. "Hi, I'm Michael Hirsch," he said, and proceeded to give a well-rehearsed spiel on PWAC and their work supporting people with AIDS. He was well into describing their newsletter, board structure, and fund-raising before I even asked a single question.

Hirsch was friendly and campy, but I could see how careful he was to avoid making assumptions about why I was there. He never asked my name; later, I found out that was the policy. Though Hirsch's warmth was disarming, I found it difficult to tell him that I had HIV, because I sensed that the information would have no effect on him. I had grown accustomed to handling deep concern and sometimes tears, but telling someone who might say "So what?" or "Yeah, me, too" was a new experience.

Before I left that day, I did tell Hirsch I had HIV but made it clear I had ARC, not AIDS—a distinction I clung to and that felt less stigmatizing. Lots of people had ARC—that was a big club—but only an unfortunate few had AIDS.

Hirsch filled my knapsack with a small stack of AIDS reading material. Until that day, I had read little about the epidemic from the perspective of those with the disease. As I read through the literature, I realized the voice of PWAC's membership wasn't desperate and despondent; nor was it strident or didactic. It was thoughtful, practical, and often funny. Members wrote about their lives and health without assuming death was imminent. They shared experiences of struggling through a difficult challenge together, recognizing its realities while finding and sharing the joys of living. They had no interest in pity, which was all too abundant in response to people with AIDS.

When I read the Denver Principles in a PWAC newsletter, they resonated deeply. More than a political manifesto, as I had thought of them when I first read about them in 1983, they were a guide to living in the shadow of a potentially fatal illness. The document was like a life preserver thrown my way by other people with AIDS.

At PWAC, my eyes were opened to a world of people with AIDS—mostly but not entirely gay men—who were living vibrant lives. Others, often including HIV-negative or untested gay men, sometimes didn't get it. I heard one sweet guy who was very thin and clearly ill talking about how he was opening a florist shop in Brooklyn. When he was out of earshot, a guy who didn't know I had HIV said, "He's delusional; he's not opening any shop, he's got AIDS!" I was shocked, because when I heard the florist-to-be's plans, I thought, "You go for it!"

Callen once told me, "An AIDS victim is sad and pitied, but a person with AIDS who tries not to be defined by the disease, or, God forbid, dares criticize anything about the gay community's response to AIDS, is considered to be in denial, a threat, or an ingrate."

I saw people with AIDS who retreated from their lives, giving up in the daunting face of death, while others struggled for survival. Some did so in private, in contrast to those whose path was gladiator-like and public. It sometimes seemed like the more powerful and influential a person's position in life was at diagnosis, the more poorly he handled the news. A "master of the universe" Wall Street investment banker might crumble in humiliation and defeat, while a struggling actor, waiter, or retail clerk often found new courage and emerged as a leader.

One day at PWAC, I ran into Joe Foulon, a friend I hadn't seen in four or five years. We had dated a few times around 1980 and seen each other occasionally at parties or nightclubs. Seeing him was a relief—he was alive—but it also had me worried: Being at the PWAC office meant he was probably sick. When I saw a postage stamp–size purple KS spot in the middle of his forehead, like a permanent tattoo of Lenten ashes, I had no doubt.

Joe was stunning to look at. He had thick, straight dark hair and perfect skin, with amazingly high cheekbones. His eyes at first seemed brooding and soulful, but once you got to know him, they were equally impish. He was one of those genetically blessed men who turned heads wherever he went. If he hadn't been so nice—Joe was modest and kind— he would have been easy to dislike. The KS lesion on his forehead was an imperfection that gave him an appealing touch of vulnerability.

Joe said he was on PWAC's board and two years earlier in 1983 had helped launch the National Association of People with AIDS. I was impressed. I knew Joe as a beguiling waiter/actor; I'd thought I was the political activist. Hearing how involved he was and how much time and effort he had given to fighting AIDS made me realize how little I had contributed. I felt like I had been asleep for several years while this horrific tragedy was unfolding around me.

Joe's boyfriend, Mark Senak, was one of the first employees at GMHC. He was a lawyer who helped people with AIDS prepare wills and fight for benefits and access to services. "Every day there's an RIP [Rest in Peace] list distributed to all the GMHC staff, listing the clients who had died," Joe told me. "Sometimes the list is more than a dozen names, filling a whole sheet."

On that somber note, Hirsch piped up from his desk, "Okay, tell me: Inquiring minds want to know. Did you guys do it?"

A few months later, I invited Joe to join me at a big party at my old boyfriend André Ledoux's loft on East Eleventh Street. It was crowded and noisy, and the loft had no air-conditioning. At one point, Joe and I climbed through a window and sat on the fire escape to cool off and talk quietly. We held hands, watched the night sky, and listened to the muffled sounds of music and laughter coming from inside. "Doesn't it seem like a really long time ago that we met?" he asked. "It's a whole different world now." We were quiet for a minute, and then I said, "It seems like everything has changed."

We were talking about AIDS but just as easily could have been talking about finding PWAC, which is where I learned how to live with the disease. Through PWAC, I met a large circle of guys like Joe who had been involved in AIDS work for several years. They weren't from the upwardly mobile circle of ambitious professionals and entrepreneurs I knew best, who served on the boards of GMHC and other community organizations. They were aspiring artists or actors working in restaurants or service jobs. They were members of the Gay Men's Chorus or played on gay softball or bowling teams. They shared holiday celebrations and most lived in New York's emerging "gayborhoods" such as Chelsea, the East Village, or Hell's Kitchen. They ate in gay restaurants, patronized gay stores, and when they went to Jones Beach on hot summer days (Fire Island was out of their price range), you were sure to find them in the gay section. They shared personal bonds far deeper than the political interests I shared with many of my first gay friends.

Joining these PWAC guys gave me a sense of belonging and purpose. I soon was wishing that I had started helping out at PWAC earlier. In retrospect, I realize that I viewed the first AIDS activists—who were PWAs—as professional homosexuals, highly promiscuous, and, as Callen and Berkowitz forthrightly put it, "sluts." From the time I had first come out, it was important to me not to see myself or to be seen by others as associated with this way of being gay. My fear of this association, coupled with my fear that others were likely to think I had AIDS, held me back. It did not, however, hold me back from fund-raising for, and volunteering at, GMHC, which was led by gay A-listers—the group that had become socially popular.

As I made friends with the PWAC men, my misconceptions fell away. I began dropping in at the Living Room regularly, to pick up new literature, lend a hand, or just to say hello to the two Michaels— Hirsch and Callen. The Michaels were fun, outgoing, and intent on keeping track of PWAC members' social and especially sexual lives. When Hirsch told Callen I had dated Joe Foulon, Callen declared Joe was the sexiest man with AIDS in New York. Hirsch then blurted out an unforgettable response: "He's so cute, I'd lick his lesions!"

With Callen at the helm, PWAC was a leading proponent of "safe sex"—shorthand for using condoms—and distributed thousands of copies of *How to Have Sex in an Epidemic* throughout the country. The group's strength was in its peer-to-peer philosophy and the bluntness of its mission. We didn't speak in euphemisms; indeed, getting diagnosed seemed to come with a heightened ability to detect BS. There was no time for dancing around the facts, cultivating social niceties, or worrying about political correctness.

Their medical advisor was Dr. Joseph Sonnabend, who by 1986 had been branded "controversial" for his hypotheses about AIDS, as mainstream research and treatment settled into an orthodoxy following the discovery of HIV. Once when a reporter was interviewing Callen and referred to his and Sonnabend's "camp," Callen replied that he, Sonnabend, Berkowitz, and their relatively few supporters hardly composed a camp. "It's more like a pup tent," he said. I remained wary about being identified as a member of any camp, even as my confidence in Sonnabend grew.

*   *   *

After my diagnosis, Michael and I settled into my first extended period of monogamy, or close to it. Spending fewer evenings prowling around the bars and clubs meant I got more rest and my health improved. Every three months, I returned to Dr. Pier's office. He would draw blood and feel my lymph glands before we spent fifteen or twenty minutes talking.

Pier shared some of Sonnabend's independence and kept up on the latest research and gave his patients copies of scientific papers. I had never read medical journals and sometimes couldn't understand them, but it was reassuring to know that someone, somewhere, was trying to find treatments. Pier's prognoses about the epidemic became increasingly optimistic. "There's definitely progress, but you're in a race against the clock," he said. "All my patients are."

Rumors spread about a drug known as Compound S—later known as AZT—that supposedly showed miraculous results in experimental trials. We started hearing about people with AIDS who went from being bedridden and near death to walking around and feeling great. Some suggested that AZT was the breakthrough that would turn the tide of the epidemic.

One day Pier asked if I was interested in taking AZT. "When did it get approved?" I asked, surprised that I hadn't heard the news. "It isn't," he said, "but I think I can get it for you through a compassionate-use program that makes it available to people who are extremely ill and likely to die otherwise. You're not that sick, but I'll say you are. What are they going to do, yank my license for trying to save my patients' lives?" I was flattered at Pier's willingness to lie to get me the drug. I felt lucky to have a doctor who had also become a friend.

What wasn't widely known at the time was that the benefits of AZT were short-term, lasting until the virus mutated and developed resistance to the drug. For those who were otherwise on their deathbed, it often provided a dramatic benefit, but for most people like me, who were largely asymptomatic, it ultimately would do more harm than good.

There were a few canaries in the AZT coal mine raising an alarm, but not many listened to their song. Sonnabend was suspicious of the drug from the start and highly critical of the research and political process that ultimately garnered its approval. For most people with HIV, he believed, its toxicity would outweigh its benefits. Callen minced no words, labeling AZT "Drano." He was disappointed when I started taking it. "Do. Not. Take. AZT," he said, reading aloud a list of potential side effects and explaining that the research behind it was flawed. "Plus, it will make your dick go soft, but they won't tell you that," he added.

I was to take two 100-mg pills every four hours, around the clock. The first dose sat on my kitchen counter for several hours before I took it. It felt almost ceremonial when I finally swallowed those first two pills. I wanted so badly to believe they would save me, not unlike the way I once felt about the consecrated host at Catholic Mass. AZT tasted nothing like the unleavened bread of a communion wafer, however; it left a metallic taste in my mouth, and in the days to come, it would upset my stomach and seem to drag down my body and mind.

My spell on AZT didn't last long. Getting up in the middle of the night to take it was so annoying that I missed doses almost from the beginning. Within a few weeks, I stopped taking it; as much as anything, it was because, despite my diagnosis, I felt healthier than I had in years and taking AZT made me feel like a sick person. Some of the guys I met through PWAC had lived three or four years and that gave me confidence that I could outlive Dr. Pier's two-year prognosis. Taking AZT felt like I was buying in to more sickness than I experienced, and I instinctively felt it wasn't helping me.

Discontinuing AZT was a turning point for me. It did take guts, because this first HIV drug was almost universally being hailed as the advance we had all been waiting for. Other than Callen, Sonnabend, and the *New York Native,* I heard few critics. I now believe that had I continued to take it, I very likely would have died, as did thousands of others.

Though Pier didn't agree with my decision to stop AZT, he respected it. At the time, I didn't realize Pier was also sick; he kept it a secret until not long before he died in 1989. He, too, took AZT.

Pier also connected me to another experimental treatment. Even though AZT was available under a compassionate-use program, there were no formally approved treatments. That didn't stop independent experimenters, armchair chemists, entrepreneurs, activists, and con artists from stirring up concoctions in their bathtubs, promoting products through an underground network, and sometimes exploiting desperation. I dismissed anything that was too expensive, promised miraculous results, or had a deadline to participate; I knew those characteristics as the hallmarks of scams.

But when Pier mentioned AL721, an experimental treatment made from egg lipids, I was intrigued. "Robert Gallo's written about it," Pier said. "He thinks AL721 inhibits the invasion of cells by HIV." It had not been through FDA-approved clinical trials, so the agency prohibited it from being marketed as a medical treatment, even though it was a nontoxic food product. Pier encouraged me to spend two hundred dollars to help the newly founded PWA Health Group have a supply privately manufactured.

AL721 seemed much less risky than other treatments, and Pier explained its mechanism persuasively. He said the fatty lipids coated the surface of white blood cells, which made the surface of the cells sort of slippery, so it is tougher for HIV to adhere and invade the cell. I was a science club dropout, but when Pier said the word "slippery" I got it, and signed up right away.

Thomas Hannan, Callen, Sonnabend, and others associated with PWAC formed the PWA Health Group in 1987, around the time ACT UP was formed. It was the first buyers' club for people with AIDS, pooling resources to investigate and procure experimental treatments that had not been stamped with FDA approval. I met Callen at the PWAC office and gave him the two hundred dollars in cash. It felt like a back-alley drug deal, and I was a little nervous. As an organic substance, AL721 was not technically a drug, but the government had cracked down on companies commercially marketing it. I didn't want to leave a paper trail, because it wasn't clear to me whether there could be repercussions from the police, the FDA, or some other agency.

The PWA Health Group had problems with that first batch; it needed testing to make sure the 7:2:1 ratio between its components was correct before Sonnabend would authorize its release. They found a lipid chemist at Brown University who agreed to help, but he dropped out after someone at the NIH advised him not to have anything to do with Sonnabend or the PWA Health Group. The delay only made me more eager to get my hands on AL721. Once I decided to participate, I wanted it right away; the tougher it was to access, the more magical properties I ascribed to it.

Eventually, the PWA Health Group perfected the formula and began providing over a ton of AL721 every month to about a thousand people. Whenever a supply arrived, people with AIDS and ARC lined up at the PWAC office and other distribution sites. Each customer picked up a quart-size plastic container holding a three-month supply of a yellowish-tan goopy paste.

I kept mine in the back of my refrigerator and, every night, spread a tablespoon or so on a few saltine crackers and ate them before I went to bed. Sometimes Michael would make them for me and stud them with raisins or nuts in the shape of a happy face. On a few occasions when I tried to get friends to taste it, they recoiled as if they might get AIDS from tasting the treatment. It sounds absurd, but I was careful to not put leftovers next to the AL721 jar in the refrigerator. AIDS stigma extended to irrational corners.

AL721 was one of many experimental treatments surrounded by intrigue—and hope. After a few months, when I didn't feel any benefit, I moved on to dextran sulfate. Available in Japan as a blood thinner, dextran sulfate came in shiny foil blister packs and commercial packaging, which made it seem more potent; this was a *real* drug. It wasn't approved for sale in the United States, so Jim Corti, a nurse in Los Angeles, had created an elaborate smuggling network. Flight attendants, traveling businesspeople, and tourists visiting Japan were enlisted to stuff their suitcases with the maximum amount allowed "for personal use."

Jim already had a network of smugglers making regular trips to Mexico for supplies of an anti-viral called Ribavirin. I knew about him through one of my direct-mail fund-raising clients, National Gay Rights Advocates. NGRA had wealthy board members with AIDS who funded the group to pursue litigation against the FDA and NIH to force faster action on drug development and approval, including for AL721, Ribavirin, and dextran sulfate.

NGRA's lawsuit accused the FDA of an insider arrangement, accelerating review and approval procedures only for AIDS drugs sponsored by the NIH; AL721, Ribavirin, and dextran sulfate were not on that list. The suit claimed: "NIH concentrated its research into NIH-sponsored drugs, or into drugs developed by companies with which NIH or its researchers had developed special relationships, such as Burroughs Wellcome or Hoffman-LaRoche . . . [They] ignored or seriously delayed consideration and testing of other promising drugs . . . NIH's decisions were affected by essential conflicts of interest, namely, royalty payments from manufacturers licensed to develop NIH-sponsored drugs."

Until the epidemic, I thought the FDA and NIH were agencies of professionals who were above politics and immune to the reach of special interests. I was idealistic, believing that they employed scientists working solely for the public good. I was shocked when I learned how pharmaceutical companies and government decision-makers manipulated the research and drug-approval process.

These official complications drove our efforts to experiment with unapproved or illegal treatments. What we viewed as necessary illegalities—ranging from drug smuggling to exaggerating one's condition to qualify for compassionate-use treatment or a drug trial—became regular aspects of AIDS culture in the '80s. People often lied to qualify for insurance; I knew of two men who obtained health care under an insurance plan that covered only one of them. They pretended to be the same person, alternating visits to have their blood drawn, and the clinic maintained a single medical chart for both.

It wasn't just that the established systems lacked urgency; it was also that the government, the pharmaceutical industry, and the entire health care establishment didn't care if we lived or died. To them, it seemed, the epidemic was an opportunity to profit politically or economically. If surviving required that we bend or break rules, it wasn't going to keep us up at night.

What did keep us up at night was fear of pneumocystis carinii pneumonia (PCP), a rare fungal infection that in the 1980s was the leading killer of people with AIDS. It also is a dramatic example of the ineptitude that marked the federal response to the epidemic.

As early as 1977, infectious disease specialists knew that an inexpensive sulfa drug, Bactrim, or another generic equivalent was effective at preventing PCP in immune-compromised patients, such as children with leukemia and organ transplant patients. It was in use as a treatment for people with AIDS who got PCP, but when a large number of Sonnabend's patients had recurrent bouts, he began using Bactrim prophylactically, as it was used with patients with other conditions who were at high-risk of PCP.

It worked well, so he and Callen tried to educate doctors and people with AIDS; they sought to enlist gay doctor groups, published articles in the *PWA Newsline* and elsewhere, and campaigned for the federal government to issue a recommendation to physicians treating people with AIDS. Some community physicians got the message, but many ignored it. In May 1987, Callen and several other activists met with Anthony Fauci at the NIH to, as Michael wrote, "beg" Fauci to issue guidelines recommending the preventive treatment.

Fauci was uncooperative. He dismissed previous research, saying he wanted data proving that prophylaxis helped prevent PCP specifically in patients with HIV. His colleague Dr. Samuel Broder, who was head of the National Cancer Institute, suggested it was justifiable to *discourage* the use of PCP prophylaxis on the grounds that the approval of AZT would make it redundant, even though there was no such evidence.

Ultimately a clinical trial was undertaken to test aerosolized dosing of pentamidine, another off-patent drug used to prevent PCP. A generic drug manufacturer, Lyphomed, sponsored the trial because they stood to make a fortune if they could demonstrate their aerosolized delivery system for pentamidine was effective. In 1981, an investor had purchased Lyphomed for $2.7 million; just before the pentamidine trial was finished, he sold the company for nearly $1 billion to Fujisawa, a Japanese company. In the end, generic Bactrim in a pill—the treatment Sonnabend had advocated—was more effective and vastly less costly than either form of aerosolized pentamidine.

Fauci's unwillingness to help when petitioned by Callen and other activists was typical of the lack of urgency at all levels of the federal government as well as of the disrespect community clinicians and people with HIV often faced when dealing with federal officials. In this case, a private company's potential to profit was protected at the cost of many lives.

By 1989, when the federal government finally recommended PCP prophylaxis, 30,534 people in the United States had died from a disease that was known to be preventable since at least 1977. Callen estimated 16,929 of them had died between the time he went to plead for Fauci's support and more than two years later, when the guidelines were finally issued. I had lost count of how many of them I knew.

CHAPTER 13

Rolo-dead File

My early experience with AZT was valuable in one way: It set me on a journey to understand and strengthen the strained connection between my mind and my body. Well into my twenties, I paid little attention to my body, a sense of shame at the failings I saw in it complicated any opportunity to take pride or find joy or pleasure in it. Catholicism had taught me that it was the "temple of my soul," but as I grappled with my attraction to men, I came to believe I had no soul, which weakened the temple metaphor. When I heard people say they listened to their body, I had no idea what they meant.

That changed after I was diagnosed, as I read about chemistry and biology and paid much more attention to my health. I learned to recognize how I reacted to different foods: Eating red meat made me feel sluggish, chocolate made me hyper, and onions and spices gave me vivid dreams, sometimes nightmares. At the same time, I learned to appreciate food more, partly because I was trying hard to gain weight. For most of my life, I had treated food like fuel; I was either hungry or not, and the food on my plate either tasted good or it didn't.

Michael tried to fatten me up with his cooking. His physique and encouragement inspired me to join a gym for the first time in my life. I also experimented with meditation, acupuncture, and a macrobiotic diet. Each venture delivered small revelations, and I began to bridge the gap between who I was and the body I inhabited.

Many people with AIDS turned to spirituality and self-actualization programs. New age gurus, most notably Louise Hay and Marianne Williamson, became popular nationwide draws as the epidemic grew. These events felt too much like organized religion to me, so I generally stayed away. One I did attend, at Town Hall in New York, was led by a woman who specialized in "visualization." I was with a friend who had been recently diagnosed, and I wanted to be a good sport, so I played along. The lights went down except for a gauzy pink spotlight on the guru at the front. "You may close your eyes now," she said slowly.

She asked us to think about our immune system and our CD4 cells—what they looked like, tasted like, and thought about. I created these mental pictures the best I could.

"Now think about the virus and what it looks like as it courses through your veins, seeking cells to attack. Is it angry? In a rush? Sly and devious, or just inconsiderate and reckless?" I envisioned something Darth Vader–like, ominous and threatening.

Then she asked, "Has anyone seen the commercial on TV for that toilet-bowl cleanser called Scrubbing Bubbles? You know how they show the little scrubbing bubbles as soldiers, marching around the toilet bowl, busily attacking grime? Think of your CD4 cells like that— like little Scrubbing Bubbles soldiers, marching through your body, cleaning up, and getting rid of the HIV."

This made me laugh, but it created an indelible image in my mind's eye. To this day, when I think about my immune system, I see a small army of cartoon bubbles in military uniforms efficiently patrolling my bloodstream for viruses to vanquish.

Visualizing those cartoon bubbles helped me picture my own survival; Michael even took to whistling the jingle from the TV commercial.

*   *   *

When I came out as a gay man, I gave up hope that I would ever hold elective office. After my diagnosis, I gave up hope of a career in politics in any capacity. My disillusionment with party politics—my youthful passion—came home to me with surprising force at the 1984 Democratic Convention, when I realized that gay and AIDS issues were driving me more than the "D" that remained the defining factor for the friends I saw there. Given the devastating effects of the AIDS crisis, Democrats behaved only slightly better than Republicans in meeting our needs, and my self-image as an AIDS activist increasingly trumped partisan preference.

For a long time, I resented the friends who drew away from me in the years after I disclosed my diagnosis. Some backed away when I became an activist. These people reminded me of Washington, where one could be good enough to sleep with or socialize with in private but not good enough to be seen with in public. Others were in denial about the epidemic, including their own risk, or were just frightened. As I revisit those years, I realize the divide was as much due to my withdrawal from them as it was their withdrawal from me. I needed the support of others with AIDS to create a protective cocoon to become the activist I needed to be.

I was already proud that my firm raised a lot of money for GMHC, but I was also proud that we provided necessary information to people with AIDS and those at risk. It elevated the fund-raising function by making our mailings more important and gave me satisfaction, knowing we were providing a useful service.

In early 1986, I pitched the idea of a direct-mail campaign to Michael Hirsch, PWAC's executive director. He was enthusiastic. I knew PWAC didn't have any money to put at risk, so I convinced Todd, my business partner, to allow our firm to advance the postage money. I personally guaranteed payment of all the expenses if the mailing wasn't successful.

PWAC's board chair, David Summers, was a Texas-born cabaret singer and actor who had made his New York debut in a groundbreaking play called *The Faggot*, where he sang "The New Boy in Town." He was also the first person in New York arrested for an AIDS-related act of civil disobedience, when he was refused the opportunity to testify at a 1985 New York City Council hearing. PWAC's fund-raising letter was from David, describing why PWAC was so important to him.

> I found . . . stifling solicitude from friends could be just as damaging as the vicious hostility of enemies . . . something important was missing. That "something" was self-determination, our own chance to meet our needs, and to affirm each other as "PWAs"— People With AIDS, not victims, patients, or outcasts . . . The PWA Coalition is America's only organization for people with AIDS run entirely by people with AIDS . . . we speak out to let the world know that we're not going to curl up and play dead. Nobody is going to quarantine, persecute, discriminate against, or otherwise make us the scapegoats for this terrible epidemic . . .

In the postscript, David wrote, "Very soon, if we can raise the money, we'll be starting our group for Women With AIDS/ARC." We included a "PWAC Family Album" brochure composed of black-and-white snapshots of David, Michael Hirsch, and other people with AIDS, showing them with friends, family, and one another and in public roles as educators and advocates.

The brochure was designed to resemble an old-fashioned photo album, with pictures set against a black background, picture-mounting corners, and text printed in gold. David and PWAC loved the mailing, and it was successful, but David told me not to make our next design so "funereal"; to him, the black-and-gold motif was reminiscent of mourning. "Our materials should be vibrant with life!" he said. Our next letter for PWAC, signed by Amy Sloan—one of the first women

with AIDS to speak to the media—embraced that philosophy and had
no morbid design elements.

Michael Misove frequently edited my fund-raising letters. Despite
attending excellent schools, I never learned formal grammar, took a
writing class, or studied literature. Michael, ever the English teacher,
was amused by the style and urgency of my fund-raising appeals. He
parodied them in notes he left for me:

> *Dear Sean,*
>
> *Quite frankly, the situation in the refrigerator is severe and getting
> worse. There is virtually nothing there; we are at risk of starving. I
> implore you to act today and go to the grocery store. Please, do not set
> this urgent appeal aside, or we will have nothing to eat.*
>
> *Love, Michael.*
>
> *P.S. To delay may mean to forget! Act now!*

Strub/Collins had quickly become more than a direct-mail fund-raising
consulting firm; we were an advocacy hub for lesbian and gay activism
and AIDS politics; our fund-raising projects closely tied what was happening in the media and with grassroots activism.

The tension in our community was palpable and growing. We were
under siege, we were dying, the country's leadership didn't care, and
our very right to be intimate came under assault in the courts. Atlanta
bartender Michael Hardwick was in his bedroom with another man
when a police officer entered his home and charged him under Georgia's sodomy statute, which prohibited gay sex.

The case had worked its way to the U.S. Supreme Court and in
June 1986, the *Bowers* v. *Hardwick* decision was handed down, uphold-
ing the Georgia sodomy statute. In the ruling, Chief Justice Warren
Burger quoted descriptions calling homosexual sex an "infamous crime
against nature," "worse than rape," and "a crime not fit to be named."

Within hours, angry crowds had gathered in cities across the country and at the Supreme Court Building in Washington. That night, I went to Sheridan Square—where we always spontaneously gathered when there was an important political development—and joined the outraged crowd. As the crowd swelled into the thousands, we marched and chanted our way to Sixth Avenue, where we sat down in the street and blocked traffic. With the death toll mounting all around us, the Hardwick decision was like putting a match to dry kindling; we were now as angry as we were scared.

A few weeks after the *Hardwick* decision, I was in Los Angeles visiting Jean O'Leary, an activist ex-nun who now ran National Gay Rights Advocates. She took me to a fund-raising event at a swanky house in Beverly Hills owned by a rich gay man. About forty gay men and lesbians sipped cocktails around a David Hockney–esque pool while activist David Mixner described Proposition 64, the radical measure on the California ballot that would quarantine people with HIV. The proposition was ahead in the polls, and Mixner, along with activists Torie Osborn and Bruce Decker, was running the "No on 64" campaign to defeat it.

Donors were put on the spot. The microphone was passed from one person to the next, so each could declare a pledge. I knew Jewish organizations had raised enormous amounts of money this way during the Six-Day War in 1967. The comparison was apt: In both situations, the threat was immediate and had grave and far-reaching consequences for a beleaguered minority.

The mood around the pool was somber. Many, perhaps most, of the men present had HIV or AIDS or had partners who were sick or had already died. Some took the microphone, spoke quickly, and sounded nervous. Others were slow and deliberate, remembering a deceased friend or offering an explanation for their generosity:

"Hal and I never give to politics, because we support the arts. But if they start locking us up, there won't be anyone left to create art or to support it. We'll give a thousand dollars now, and maybe we can do a bit more closer to the election."

"Vicky and I talked about this last night. We were going to renovate the kitchen at our restaurant, but this is more important. We'll donate five thousand dollars."

"I haven't closed Bobby's estate yet, so I'll donate a thousand dollars from it in his honor. He would have wanted me to. Tomorrow he would have turned thirty-two."

A soft clapping of hands followed each person's pledge. The prospect of quarantine was almost too horrific to contemplate, yet the measure had been leading in the polls. Jean and I were near the end of the line. She wasn't affluent, so no one expected a large pledge from her. I was a visitor from New York and one of the youngest people present; no one expected a pledge from me.

Jean whispered in my ear, "If I sign a letter and we use NGRA's list for an appeal, how much do you think we could raise?"

"Why just you and NGRA?" I said. "If the executive directors of NGLTF, HRCF, Lambda, and the other national groups declared this a national community emergency, and jointly signed a letter, I'll bet I could raise at least fifty thousand dollars." Jean's eyes widened. "For real?" she asked. I nodded.

When the microphone got to us, Jean put her hand over it and whispered in my ear, "You're sure you can do this? I don't want to be embarrassed." I told her I was certain, but my heart was pounding hard. I was about to make a very big public commitment.

"Sean Strub says he can raise fifty thousand dollars if the executive directors of the national organizations jointly sign a letter," she said. The line of activists and donors standing around the edge of the pool broke into applause.

After the microphone reached the far end of the pool, a waiter brought it back to Mixner. Before handing it over, he spoke into it: "I'm just a cater waiter, and I don't have much money, but I want to donate the fifty dollars I'm getting paid to work here today."

The "No on 64" letter I wrote was the first and, I think, the only time all the largest national LGBT and AIDS organizations came together on a joint fund-raising appeal. It raised over a hundred thousand dollars. The "No on 64" campaign was also the first time I asked Keith Haring, whom I had met through friends, to donate an image for an AIDS-related cause. Keith's career was hot, and scoring a design of his for a "No on 64" T-shirt was a big coup.

Despite an early polling disadvantage, we beat Proposition 64 by a wide margin. Absent our campaign to defeat it, it almost certainly would have passed.

In the late 1980s, I felt personally threatened by the efforts to quarantine us, restrict our travel, force mandatory testing, prohibit us from certain professions, kick us out of schools and swimming pools, deny us insurance, beat us up in the street, and call us names.

While we were fighting the political and cultural battle, we also had to deal with death and physical suffering on a scale that remains difficult to describe. When I ran into someone I hadn't seen in a while, I was relieved that he was still alive. Before inquiring about a mutual friend or acquaintance, I had to steel myself for a potentially sad answer: "Oh, didn't you hear? Jimmy died last week." Or "I thought you knew, Gary's ill." Or "Grant went back home to Minnesota a couple of months ago so his parents can take care of him." Or "Jack's at Lenox Hill; you better get over there fast if you want to see him before he goes." These exchanges, on the sidewalk, in the produce aisle at the grocery, or between sets at the gym, became routine, the information shared matter-of-factly.

I became intimately familiar with the floor plans at Roosevelt, St. Vincent's, NYU Medical Center, Columbia Presbyterian, and other hospitals around the city, spending countless hours visiting ill friends and accompanying other friends when they were visiting someone. Visits were scheduled during lunch hours and around our gym workouts and evening plans; on some wards, if you got to know the nurses, they were flexible about the visiting hours. Wandering hospital hallways, I always glanced at the names on the doors on the way to whomever I was visiting. Several times, I went to the AIDS ward at St. Vincent's Hospital without intending to visit anyone in particular, knowing there would be someone I knew who was there. I missed a lot of funerals and memorial services—sometimes it was too hard or there were too many—but few of my friends were sick or hospitalized without me spending time with them.

Tim Dlugos and I kept our list, but lots of people kept Rolodex cards of the dead in those days, little white cards pulled from the deck but not thrown away, sometimes bound together by a rubber band. "That's my Rolo-dead file," one friend said. Many had address books with lines crossed through the names of those who would never again answer a phone. I used a yellow highlighter, which created a fluorescent pattern of zebra stripes on page after page.

There were painful encounters with homophobic families after someone had died: A relative might fly in from somewhere and lock a partner out of the apartment he had shared for years with the deceased. There were fights over who could visit the patient in the hospital or who had the right to dispose of clothing and possessions. I remember a rush from the hospital to remove a porn collection from a dying friend's apartment before his family arrived.

There were also deathbed confessions, reunions, and reconciliations. Some of the memorial services we held for our dead friends were festive celebrations, parties honoring the deceased's too-short life. Most services were somber and profoundly sad, with pained and confused parents just in from Kansas City, say, or Tuscaloosa, or Cedar Rapids. Perhaps they'd never known their son was gay; some continued to deny it even after the truth was obvious.

When the minister chosen by the family eulogized a gay man, noting that he had "finally escaped his sinful lifestyle," the deceased's friends spoke up and took over the service, over the minister's protests, standing up one by one to talk about his virtues and compassion. More often in circumstances like that, friends, lovers, and even other family members would stand mute in horrified sorrow, tradition and the law squarely on the parents' side.

I was still in my twenties, and like tens of thousands of others, death and dying were as much a part of my days as they are for any soldier on a battlefield. We developed coping mechanisms and compartmentalized our grief so that we could use it sparingly. One way to avoid becoming immobilized by sorrow and fear was to go to work emptying bedpans, making meals, washing dishes, wiping sweaty brows with a cool cloth—or engaging in activism.

■   ■   ■

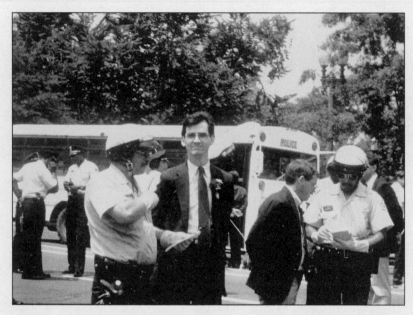

Sixty-four of us were arrested during the third International AIDS Conference, June 1, 1987, in front of the White House. It was my first arrest for civil disobedience and the last one for which I wore a suit and tie. When the police put on long yellow gloves, we chanted, "Your gloves don't match your shoes! You'll see it on the news!"

CHAPTER 14

Silence=Death

Early in 1987, I was struck by the ominous gravity of posters with a hot pink triangle against a black background and the slogan "Silence=Death" emblazoned in white type. They were wheat-pasted on abandoned buildings, the sides of phone booths, and over subway advertisements. First they showed up in Chelsea and the Village, then citywide. The word *AIDS* was conspicuously absent, but few gay men needed to be told what it meant.

The pink triangle was a familiar symbol of the gay-liberation movement. It had been appropriated in the 1970s from the pink inverted-triangle patches with which the Nazis branded homosexuals in concentration camps. By pairing it with a provocative slogan, the posters took the pink triangle one step further. At the bottom, in small white type, was the phrase "Turn your anger, fear, grief into action." It was political messaging rendered with sophistication and style. Many of my gay-activist friends speculated about who had put them up. Was it someone we knew, or a new, bolder group?

When ACT UP—the AIDS Coalition to Unleash Power—held its first demonstration in March 1987, it earned a photograph in *The New*

York Times, with a caption about the arrests of "homosexual activists" blocking traffic on Wall Street. I was sure the mostly young, good-looking gay guys in that photograph had something to do with the "Silence=Death" message.

It turned out that the poster image, which slightly predated ACT UP but quickly became its flag of defiance and protest, came from a collective of six gay artists, including Avram Finkelstein, Chris Lione, and others. They felt compelled to fight back but were uncertain whether anyone else would listen. The timing was right, and when Larry Kramer became a last-minute replacement for a talk at the Gay and Lesbian Community Services Center, his call to action launched the most aggressive and visible stage of AIDS activism we had seen.

By that point, six years into the epidemic, we had absorbed inconceivable losses. I saw a whole wave of friends in summer-share houses on Fire Island, at the Jersey Shore, and in the Hudson River Valley erased; in some cases, entire houses of four or five or six men all died. An annual summer campout I hosted at my house in Bucks County starting in 1983 had a core group of about thirty-five; by 1989, a third had died. Fewer than half survive today.

The devastation was no longer felt only in urban gay ghettos or nearby gay resort and weekend communities. The epidemic had begun to hit small towns and rural areas, where the bigotry and intolerance were worse and there was almost no contact with other people who had AIDS.

The epidemic's toll mounted in tandem with a political and cultural backlash against gay people. "Gay=AIDS" was sometimes scrawled over the pink triangle in the "Silence=Death" posters.

In the months following the *Hardwick* decision, a simmering discontent nationwide began to focus on the nation's capital. AIDS service organizations started to coordinate lobbying efforts for federal funding; the National Association of People with AIDS had an office in D.C.; and activists across the country were organizing for the third International AIDS Conference, scheduled for June 1987 in Washington. The president had not deigned to say the word "AIDS" in public. Tim Dlugos and I talked, only half in jest, about a potential deadly stunt: chaining ourselves to the White House fence and threatening suicide by taking pills every half hour until President Reagan agreed to meet with us. We were desperate.

Jean O'Leary was part of the Book Study Group, an informal network of prominent gay men and lesbians in Los Angeles, many of whom I had gotten to know on my frequent trips to L.A. They became interested in organizing a civil disobedience action during the upcoming AIDS conference in Washington. They joined forces with San Franciscans, including Marty Delaney at Project Inform and Paul Boneberg at Mobilization Against AIDS and eventually other groups across the country to plan the first national AIDS civil disobedience action.

I was working with Jean to obtain commitments from the community leadership—the "suits"—to agree to participate in civil disobedience; the arrest of the leadership was sure to attract the attention of the media and government officials.

When the conference opened on the last day of May 1987, a few blocks away from the White House, it had been less than ninety days since Larry Kramer's fiery speech launched ACT UP in New York, but scores of newly minted ACT UP activists were coming by bus to join the demonstration at the White House.

The conference was the first to bring scientists from around the world, celebrity advocates, and mainstream AIDS organizations, as well as grassroots activists, to the politicians and federal bureaucrats who largely defined the fate of people with AIDS during the next decade.

Commanding the attention of the international media at the conference would be our best shot at showcasing the community's anger and commitment. With our leaders risking arrest, we were confident that our message would resonate not only with gay people but also with other Americans who had turned against the Reagan administration and the hateful rhetoric of the homophobic right.

The night before the demonstration, President Reagan and Elizabeth Taylor starred at a glamorous tented benefit for the American Foundation for AIDS Research (AmFAR). Nearing the end of his second term, Reagan finally spoke the word "AIDS" in public, after twenty-one thousand Americans had died of it. Even as his words acknowledged the crisis, he was working to cut federal spending on AIDS research by 11 percent. AmFAR had provided us with some standing-room passes to the gala. It was glamorous and exciting, but when we booed Reagan from the back of the tent, some of the attendees hissed and glared at us, angry that we were heckling the president.

By noon the next day, dozens, then hundreds, of protesters covered the sidewalk in front of the north fence of the White House. I had on my corporate-style wire-framed glasses and wore a suit and tie, as did many of the other "older" activists. I had just turned twenty-nine.

"We've got the power! Fight back!" we chanted. Television cameras and microphones were everywhere. When we spilled onto Pennsylvania Avenue, police loudspeakers announced that we were risking arrest. The police warning was our cue to sit down in the middle of the street, protected from the grimy pavement by small squares of carpet scraps that someone had the foresight to bring. Jean O'Leary's staff at NGRA had prepared a flyer detailing our Miranda rights and providing information about the legal monitors and lawyers available for those who were arrested. I got arrested along with Jean, Michael Callen, Steve Endean, Leonard Matlovich (the early out gay soldier who had been on the cover of *Time*), Cleve Jones, Ginny Apuzzo, and many others. When the police put on arm-length yellow rubber gloves, ostensibly to protect themselves from HIV as they arrested us, we replied with a chant: "Your gloves don't match your shoes! You'll see it on the news!" My heart was pounding as the police picked me off the ground and held my hands behind my back to fasten them with plastic handcuffs. It was the first time I was arrested and it felt like I was taking a step I could not retract. I thought about how my parents would react to the news that I was arrested at the White House, how it might affect my career or whatever political ambition I still secretly harbored, but mostly it felt good and I was proud.

I was also inspired by a group of young people I had never seen before who joined in the civil disobedience. They were passionate and didn't seem nervous at all about getting arrested. One of them had a glorious thousand-watt smile, with thick dark locks and a beautifully muscled body. He was wearing bright red shorts and a tight white T-shirt. After we both were arrested, I learned that his name was Stephen Gendin. He would become my comrade in arms, close friend, protégé, and business partner. In subsequent years, I often heard others date friendships and romances to a specific action or demonstration where they first met, sometimes a jail cell they shared after getting arrested. Our activism became the calendar against which we measured our lives.

Later that summer, the telephone rang at my office and a brisk voice asked, "Is this Sean Strub, the gay direct-mail guy?" The caller introduced himself as Peter Staley and asked for an appointment to talk about fund-raising for ACT UP.

At that point, ACT UP was organizing demonstrations every few weeks and persuading scores of people to risk arrest. Within months of the group's launch, a hundred people were showing up every Monday night in the rundown redbrick building on West Thirteenth Street that housed the Lesbian and Gay Community Services Center, many of them young and with little history of involvement with established groups.

When Staley called me, I hadn't yet attended an ACT UP meeting, but I agreed to meet with him. I wanted to know how ACT UP was able to engage so many people with so much passion.

My firm was already working with a dozen national AIDS organizations with their direct-mail fund-raising, several on a pro bono basis. We were mailing out millions of letters a year. I was reluctant to take on another pro bono client, and a grassroots group of angry street activists that declined to incorporate as a legal entity or designate official leaders sounded less than ideal.

Staley surprised me when he showed up at our meeting carrying a briefcase. He had the look and manner of the precocious Wall Street bond trader he had been until his recent diagnosis; I saw no trace of the mediagenic activist face of ACT UP that he would soon become.

He explained to me how ACT UP worked: The weekly meetings were open to anyone and run by consensus; demonstrations were carefully planned, with civil disobedience training, the cutting-edge graphics, and the inclusion of marshals, attorneys, and video activists documenting not only the event but any police abuses.

I would learn that many of the participants were professionals with highly developed skills and connections. The public image of young "militant queers" blocking traffic, standing up to the cops, and seizing government buildings was entirely accurate. ACT UP was also a well-oiled machine with strategic, logistical, and management expertise.

Despite having been arrested in my suit in front of the White House, I had not yet embraced the idea of street activism having a central role in battling the AIDS crisis. The other AIDS organizations that had sprung up were focused on providing direct services or changing public policies; media spectacles and demonstrations seemed ancillary, not an end in themselves. Through my fund-raising work, I saw that people who weren't part of the LGBT community were starting to give money to AIDS organizations; I wondered if angry militant activism might jeopardize that support. I also felt like an old hand at the epidemic, having been involved for several years; many of the ACT UPpers were in their late teens or early twenties, their epidemic history was more limited and their perspective different from my own.

Staley persuaded me that ACT UP might be a viable client, so I wrote a proposal for a mailing, and he presented it "to the floor." To my surprise, it was accepted.

Attending my first ACT UP meeting felt like entering an alternate universe. It was thick with sexual and intellectual energy. I knew virtually no one but felt immediately at home. I arrived a fund-raising consultant and left three hours later a committed volunteer.

Staley had convinced playwright Harvey Fierstein, who wrote the hit play *Torch Song Trilogy*, to sign a fundraising letter. Fierstein wasn't a household name yet, but he was recognized in gay circles and known for speaking his mind, which gave the appeal credibility.

A great letter and an influential signer weren't enough if it was perceived as junk mail and never opened. At the time, no organization would let us use its mailing list if our mailing envelope included the word "gay," "lesbian," or "AIDS." But I could use the "Silence=Death" logo, with its distinctive pink triangle, signaling to those who recognized the image that the contents were important. It was clear enough to get the letter opened but discreet enough to pass muster with the list owners.

The letter was successful, and my company and our vendors were paid. That was the only time ACT UP was a paying client; after the initial mailing, my work for ACT UP was as a volunteer.

I had to personally guarantee the bills to the printers, mail shops, and other vendors and sometimes advance the funds for postage, which was stressful. Start-up groups without a list of previous donors were the highest risk, and sometimes we took a beating. Other clients, like National Gay Rights Advocates and National Gay and Lesbian Task Force, had more resources and could invest in acquiring new donors who would become profitable over time through resolicitations. ACT UP had to earn a net profit from the first mailing; if they didn't, the difference came out of my pocket.

It was frustrating to me that no matter how transparent the arrangement was between my firm and ACT UP, there were always members of the group who were convinced we were profiting. I finally came to accept—not without some bitterness—that no amount of transparency can dissuade those who are impervious to the facts. I chose to be both an entrepreneur and an activist, so I tried to remember that when I was criticized, it was a situation of my own making. But it was a price I was willing to pay, in part because I believed no one else could raise money through the mail for AIDS causes as successfully as I could. I tried to take the criticism as a sacrifice I made for something I believed was more important than my own feelings, but it wasn't always easy.

For two years, from the summer of 1987 to 1990, I was at ACT UP meetings most Monday nights. I sometimes found it amusing how the meetings bore similarities to the Catholic Masses of my childhood, with fixed weekly gatherings replete with peculiar rituals, chants, and costumes. Both featured a man in a dress at the front of the room. In ACT UP that was David Robinson, a Princeton grad and aspiring dancer in the first full flower of coming out. He generally donned a '60s mod dress and earrings of daunting length to go along with his two- or three-day growth of beard.

Each regular meeting moderator had his or her distinctive style. Maria Maggenti presided with a schoolteacher's authority and a wry sense of humor. Ann Northrop, a preppy former debutante and CBS news producer, trained us in the art of being interviewed, reminding us before every demonstration, "You don't speak *to* the media, you speak *through* the media."

The meetings began with a reading of our mission, led by the moderator but often accompanied by members of the group, just as parishioners join the priest in the recitation of prayers: "We are a diverse, non-partisan group of individuals united in anger and committed to direct action to end the AIDS crisis. We meet with government and health officials; we research and distribute the latest medical information. We protest and demonstrate; we are not silent." Every meeting ended with a raucous rendition of our trademark chant: "ACT UP! FIGHT BACK! FIGHT AIDS!"

The meetings were guided partially by Robert's Rules of Order, in an effort to impose a productive procedure on a group of people with a shared purpose but wildly conflicting viewpoints. Those who were clearly ill or infrequently spoke were sometimes given greater leeway.

When I arrived, I always walked past the tabletops covered with neat stacks of literature, including the best available guides to the New York AIDS community, from clinical trial updates to new age lectures and memorial services. There were also personal testimonies, often about a friend who had died. And always ACT UP's insider's newsletter—*Tell It To ACT UP*—filled with gossip and complaints. I picked up whatever looked interesting so I had reading material if the meeting got boring, but that didn't happen often. The most interesting items I faxed to friends around the country the next day.

ACT UP meetings did become known for their sexy vibe and the many hot men and women who attended. The cruisiness of the packed room was great for recruitment, but the meetings sometimes went on for three or four hours. Not everyone had the stamina for long, detailed discussions about drug approval processes and government AIDS budgets—or the tolerance to endure all the anger, passion, and differences of opinion on display. Activism can sometimes be an extreme sport.

Cute boys in their twenties became the "face of ACT UP," as Larry Kramer described them, though the meetings and demonstrations were more diverse. Longtime social-justice activists would find themselves sitting next to someone who had never given any thought to politics until he found himself dying. Buff gym bunnies painted protest signs with schlubby guys they'd never look at twice in a bar. There were lots of middle-class suburbanites who drove back to Plainfield or Parsippany after the Monday meetings. The struggle to survive is a great leveler.

There were various committees—treatment and data, media, majority action, and others—but I, naturally, joined the fund-raising committee and served with Staley as its cochair. To my great, yet concealed delight, my fellow White House arrestee, Stephen Gendin, was also a member.

The composition of the committee changed frequently, but there was a core group of four or five of us who organized tables for selling ACT UP T-shirts and posters; produced art auctions, concerts, and other events; and oversaw the direct-mail program.

At twenty-nine, I was the committee's oldest member except for a former Broadway dancer, Swen Swenson, who had assumed the role of ACT UP's kindly but righteous uncle. In the 1960s, Swen won a Tony nomination for his role in a Broadway production of *Little Me*, in which he sang and danced to "I've Got Your Number." His claim that it was the first striptease by a man on a legitimate Broadway stage earned him street cred with ACT UP's young "sex-positive"—in word and deed—crowd.

Long retired, Swen, tall and thin, moved across the floor during meetings with great agility and grace. His dog, Fever, a medium-sized Shepherd mix, sometimes joined him. Later, after Swen had moved to Los Angeles, he spent Saturday evenings in front of the gay bars on Santa Monica Boulevard, shaking a donation can for ACT UP/Los Angeles. Fever was his escort, wearing a white T-shirt that read "GAY DOG." "Fever's the one who raises the money," Swen said. "People can't resist a gay dog!"

Other members included David Gross, a taciturn workhorse who managed our merchandise inventory and sales; Steve Petoniak, the copywriter I met through GMHC; and photographer Scott Morgan, who helped organize concert fund-raisers starring Grace Jones and Jimmy Somerville.

I was surprised to discover that Stephen was almost pathologically shy. I had thought he would have self-confidence and social ease to match his good looks. It was difficult for him to look others in the eye for longer than a moment, but if you were lucky enough to catch a brief flash, you saw his eyes were dark, deep-set, and bordered with long lashes.

When he told me sheepishly that his day job was working in the fund-raising department at the Catholic Archdiocese of New York— where he was closeted—I was appalled. "We've got to get you out of there," I said, and started thinking I might hire him at my company. I like hiring promising young activists, helping them hone their skills, and watching with pride as they contribute so much to the community.

My company usually helped our clients raise money and then watched from afar while they spent it as they chose. But at ACT UP, I saw each week how priorities were decided and the funds I helped raise were spent. When we planned an action, we knew we had to raise the money to pay for it. When we reported to the floor the results from a mailing, event, or a tally of merchandise sales, we were greeted with an appreciative cheer, which was sometimes the highlight of my week. After years of participating as an outsider, or advising and fund-raising behind the scenes, I was enjoying this more public role.

With my fund-raising business, there was always an individual— usually a group's executive or development director—to whom we reported. With ACT UP, I instead felt accountable to the passionate "floor" that assembled every Monday night. I had always felt a responsibility to my community, but my close contact with grassroots activists heightened that obligation as well as nourished my resolve.

CHAPTER 15

Unexpected Expire

I lost several close friends between 1987 and 1989, but 1988 was particularly difficult, beginning with the drawn-out agonizing death of Bobby Barrios in January. Bobby and I dated briefly in the early 1980s, and he moved into the building on West Fifty-eighth Street where I lived. He was a beautiful olive-skinned, almond-eyed Princeton grad. When he wanted to join the Foreign Service, he carefully orchestrated a referral tree for his background check so they wouldn't find out that he was gay. After posts in El Salvador and Portugal, he took a copyediting job at *The New York Times*.

The last time I saw him at home was in the fall of 1987. Michael cooked for the three of us at Bobby's apartment. Bobby was lying on his couch but able to sit up to have dinner. Though he was in pain, he seemed glad to see us. However, moments after Bobby complimented Michael's cooking, his face turned an odd shade, and he vomited up the entire meal in a series of painful spasms.

The next time I saw him was right before the holidays, in the intensive care unit at Roosevelt Hospital. He had been unconscious for days and had no idea I was there. There were tubes running in and out of his nose and mouth, and another poked through a hole in his stomach. His body was yellowish-green and purple. No memory haunts me more than seeing Bobby for the last time. It reminded me of my own fragility and how quickly and painfully life can change.

Bobby died on January 7, 1988, while I was in Iowa helping to highlight AIDS issues in the presidential campaigns prior to the pre-cinct caucuses. My mother and her close friend Karlen Fellows orga-nized a fund-raiser for the Washington-based AIDS Action Council at the University of Iowa Art Museum. Karlen's brother, Burleigh Sutton, was sick with AIDS in San Francisco and would die later that year. Such a strong and public expression of support from my parents, and their friends, in my hometown, meant a lot to me.

Bobby's death gave Michael and me the urgent sense that anything we wanted to do with our lives, we needed to pursue immediately. After years of enduring an insufferable boss, Michael quit his job in early summer and turned his attention to opening a small antique shop in Piermont, New York, where I had bought a house after selling the one in Bucks County. Piermont is fifteen miles north of the George Wash-ington Bridge on the west side of the Hudson River, a quick commute to the city. It was enjoying a revival, spurred in part by Woody Allen having recently filmed *The Purple Rose of Cairo* in its quaint downtown.

It was a huge step for Michael to go into business. We leased space on Piermont's small main street and left for a buying trip throughout the Midwest with a ten-thousand-dollar budget. We scoured antique shops, flea markets, and yard sales, buying furniture and paintings and bric-a-brac for inventory, packing tight a U-Haul trailer we dragged behind my Saab.

We made a stop in Iowa, where my family and Michael finally met, three years after we had started dating. At my parents' cottage on a lake in northwest Iowa, Dad sat across from Michael on the screened-in front porch, valiantly trying to make conversation. Since we'd arrived, Michael, naturally shy, had hardly said a word. I was worn out with try-ing to facilitate, so I just kept my nose in the newspaper.

"Do you like football?" Dad asked Michael.

"Nope," Michael replied, shaking his head.

After a pause, my dad tried again. "Ever go hunting?"

"Nope," said Michael, tongue-tied, realizing my father was trying to be friendly but not knowing what to say in response. After an even longer silence, Michael finally piped up and asked Dad, "Do you enjoy the ballet?" The three of us burst into laughter.

When we got back from our summer sojourn, Michael painted his new shop a precise shade of salmon, sanded and polished the floors, and built display fixtures. It was a happy time for us, but the headaches Michael occasionally had complained about since we met seemed to have worsened. The only thing that relieved the pain was when I massaged his head and neck. I kneaded his scalp while we were watching TV, lying in bed, even while I was driving, with my right arm stretched across the top of the seat.

That Thanksgiving was to be a big celebration in Piermont; it was the first major holiday we were together in a truly shared home, and a large group of friends and relatives was joining us. Michael spent the week preparing a spectacular feast. He had a few tasks for me every day: a run to the store for a forgotten spice, polishing a silver tray, fixing the long-broken seat of a chair. He was worried that it might rain on Thanksgiving, so he made sure we had enough dry firewood inside so the fireplace could roar all day.

Our guests arrived, including Jean O'Leary from California, and it felt like a perfect holiday, one everyone would remember. The dining room was set up beautifully; I teased Michael that he was channeling Martha Stewart. During the meal, however, Michael barely said a word. After we finished eating, he excused himself and went upstairs to lie down, saying his head hurt. After the dishes were done and the guests left, I joined him. The lights were out, but Michael was awake. "I think something's wrong," he said, "my head really hurts." I massaged his scalp, and eventually, he dozed off.

He tossed and turned all night and the next morning, over his protests, I insisted on calling a doctor. I didn't think he had been to a doctor since we met, and when he suggested I call Dr. Sonnabend, I was surprised. I left a message with Sonnabend's service and he called back fifteen minutes later. After I described what was going on, Joe said to take Michael to St. Vincent's emergency room immediately, that it sounded like cryptococcal meningitis. What I didn't know was that Sonnabend knew Michael was immune-suppressed because Michael was already his patient. As I packed a small bag for Michael and got him into my car, his symptoms worsened, and he began to moan softly. At the ER, he gripped my hand and told me under no circumstances should I tell his family he was hospitalized.

Because Sonnabend did not then have privileges at St. Vincent's, Michael's official admitting physician was someone else. But it was a holiday weekend—the day after Thanksgiving—and she wasn't present. The doctor on duty got him checked in, and the hospital began running tests, but no decisions or diagnosis would be made until the admitting physician saw him. On Saturday, she still had not seen Michael yet, so I called her office and left a message on her answering machine. On Sunday I did it again. When she hadn't seen him by Monday morning and hadn't returned any of my calls, I left a pointed message.

That afternoon, I finally met her in Michael's room. After a perfunctory greeting, she told me, "I take one call per patient per day. If you do not like that, I can have you kicked out of here because you're not related to him." I was stunned at her insensitivity, but frightened for Michael and intimidated by her threat. I couldn't imagine not being able to see him while he was in pain and hospitalized. As angry as I was by her response, I nodded meekly.

Sonnabend's telephone diagnosis was confirmed on Michael's fifth day in the hospital, after a painful spinal tap. It was also confirmed that he had HIV, as Michael and I had assumed.

I routinely heard terrible news about friends getting sick or suddenly dying. This time it wasn't just a friend. It was Michael, the man I loved. Though I had many good friends, few of them knew Michael well, and some were dealing with their own failing health or ill friends. My sister Megan was my unfailing support. She had moved from my house in Bucks County into an apartment in Chelsea, a few blocks from the hospital. If she wasn't accompanying me to see Michael at the hospital, I usually stopped to see her before or after.

The typical treatment for meningitis at the time was amphotericin B, with its awful side effects of shaking chills and high fevers; among people with AIDS, it was known as "amphi-terrible." Michael's case was severe and his system weak; we weren't sure he could survive the treatment.

A less toxic and equally effective treatment, Diflucan, was available in Europe but not yet approved in the United States, pending completion of a clinical trial. St. Vincent's was one of the trial sites. I wanted to rummage through every cabinet and closet in the hospital until I found it; but I knew that would get me kicked out. The only way to get it, I was told, was to enroll Michael in the trial; there was a 50 percent chance he would get the drug.

In desperation, I called Dr. Mathilde Krim, the head of AmFAR, to see if she could get Diflucan for Michael. She was aware of the clinical trial at St. Vincent's and said she'd see what she could do. Meanwhile, Sonnabend offered to write a prescription we could have filled in London, where he was licensed and the drug was available. We needed to take a hard copy of the prescription to a pharmacy there and have someone carry the medication back to New York, so Megan applied for an emergency passport on a rush basis.

About a week after Michael was admitted, while Megan was waiting for her passport, he lost consciousness. I was concerned that he was being overmedicated. When a nurse gave him methadone, an opiate typically used to treat narcotic withdrawal, I knew it was an error. The hospital got his admitting physician on the phone, but she denied prescribing methadone and blamed the nursing staff. The nurse showed me the doctor's handwritten instruction on Michael's chart.

I had respected Michael's wish that I not notify his family of his hospitalization, but when he lost consciousness, I phoned them and said he had cryptococcal meningitis, without mentioning AIDS, and that I thought he would be released in a couple of days. Though his mother wanted to visit, I told her that he had pleaded not to have anyone visit him. "That's Michael," she said, with resignation in her voice, "but will you call me every day to let know how he is doing?" I promised I would.

When Michael had been hospitalized for about ten days, Krim called and told me to enroll Michael in the Diflucan trial at the hospital. "But what if he's put in the placebo arm?" I asked. She spoke slowly and deliberately, instructing me with authority in her fricative Swiss accent: "Sean, listen to me. Enroll him in the trial. I will make sure he gets what he needs. Do you understand?"

It took a moment to sink in. She was clearly implying she was able to break the double-blind trial protocol to make sure Michael got the actual drug. That would have been a serious ethical violation on her part, but I didn't care. I wanted Michael to get better. I later wondered if she really would have done that, or if she was just trying to give me some hope.

I didn't get to Michael's room until late that evening. I turned down the bright lights, straightened his bed linens, pulled a chair close to his bed, and pressed a damp cloth to his lips. I told him he would soon have the medicine he needed. He hadn't been conscious in several days, and I didn't know if he could hear me.

I always stayed with Michael past visiting hours, usually climbing into the bed to hold him or doze off next to him. That night around ten-thirty, I straightened his bedcovers, kissed him, and drove back to Piermont.

At one A.M., I was jolted awake by the ringing telephone. Five years earlier, a call at that hour might have been from a friend trying to cajole me into meeting him for a late drink at a club, but by 1988 it meant something entirely different. My throat tightened before I picked up the receiver. As soon as I heard Sonnabend's gentle voice, I knew. The hospital had just called to inform him that Michael had died. I couldn't speak. My chest heaved as if to release sobs or an anguished wail, but nothing came out.

After I hung up the phone, I closed my eyes and tried to regulate my breathing for a few minutes before calling Megan. She said she would meet me at the hospital. I tore down the Palisades Parkway, venting my grief through the gas pedal. Tears streamed down my face. I pounded the steering wheel of the car; it took a few days before I noticed the bruise on my palm.

At the hospital entrance, Megan looked as frightened as I felt angry. The guards at the front desk allowed us in because Michael's death was classified as an "unexpected expire." I knew Megan never had touched a dead body, so while we were going up in the elevator, I told her that I wanted her to touch Michael's. I couldn't help but think that soon she might have to claim mine. I didn't want to be her first.

When we arrived, the lights in his room were off, but Michael's body was in the bed, still faintly warm. His personal effects had already been placed in a black plastic garbage bag on the chair next to the bed. I kissed his lips and put my arms around him, squeezing him tight, stifling my sobs. Megan wept silently. Michael was the first person I'd dated whom she had known well; she was losing a friend, too. Because of me, Megan's world had become filled with death. I had just turned thirty; she was only twenty-two.

I put her hand gently against Michael's face. I told her that someone from Redden's Funeral Home would come to get his body. Unlike so many other funeral homes, Redden's didn't assess a "biohazard" surcharge on bodies with AIDS, gouge the grieving, or impose other exploitive fees.

Every day I called Michael's mother and felt her anguish. When I called the morning after he died, I was relieved that his brother, Paul, answered. Paul had polio as a child and now was battling lung cancer, divorced and living with his parents. Michael's sister had already died from cancer. When I told Paul, he was quiet for a moment and then said his mother was at Mass, praying for Michael. He would tell her when she got home.

Later that morning, at Redden's, I couldn't help but notice the beautifully sunny day. I had been to services there more times than I could count, but this visit was different. I was sensitive to every detail, from the frayed trim of a carpet and the paint-worn counter by the pay phone to the peculiar smell. Michael hadn't written a will or left any written instructions for disposing of his remains. I told Redden's that I wanted his body cremated. I put the $575 charge on my Visa card. Then it felt strange to use that Visa card again, so I threw it away and closed the account.

When I saw Michael in the viewing room, I realized I had never seen him with even three days' growth of beard. I felt a pang of regret that I hadn't asked Redden's to shave him. This time he was stone-cold when I touched him, but he still smelled like Michael, and I breathed deeply. His brother called and said he and his parents were driving to the city from their home upstate and would arrive midafternoon. I met them at Redden's, and they invited me to join them in saying a rosary over his body. I declined but arranged to meet them later at a nearby diner.

The meal was awkward, and we were mostly silent. I answered their questions and tried to reassure them that Michael hadn't suffered. I said he had meningitis and HIV, and they didn't probe further. Michael had never come out to his parents, let alone told them he had HIV, but they knew we lived together and that he did not date women.

Michael's father had barely uttered a word until he said he didn't want the body cremated; he intended to take it upstate for a funeral Mass. I had expected this and had rehearsed in my head how to respond, but I didn't get the chance. Michael's mother spoke up and said that if I felt Michael would have preferred cremation, then that's what would be done.

For the next few weeks, I was on autopilot, coping with his death and cleaning out his apartment while also moving my company from midtown Manhattan to Westchester County. Numb, I masked my grief with immediate tasks and by deflecting interaction with other people. Though friends called, no matter how well intentioned, too many seemed to say exactly the wrong thing. Michael's death made me much more sensitive to what is and is not useful to say to someone who has lost a loved one.

I didn't break down until two weeks later—just before Christmas—when I received a beautiful letter from Michael's mother, thanking me for taking care of him and for being his "special friend." It was written in careful Catholic-school penmanship with a shaky hand. No response to Michael's death consoled me as much as his mother's gentle recognition of our relationship.

I spent Christmas that year alone, by choice. When I sorted through Michael's wardrobe and furnishings, I discovered bottles of Excedrin everywhere. They were in the bathroom, bedroom, in his coat pockets, gym bag, even in the spice cabinet in the kitchen. I wondered how long he'd had the crypto.

Michael wasn't sentimental and didn't keep a lot of mementos or photographs. What he did save shed light on his life, starting with his discharge papers from the navy that showed he'd been kicked out for being gay. He confided to a navy doctor that he thought he might be attracted to men. The doctor diagnosed him as having a "polymorphous sexual disorder" and reported him to superior officers. He was sent to a psychiatric hospital in Philadelphia and booted from the navy. I knew Michael's departure from the navy was on bad terms, but I never knew specifically why until I found those papers.

During the holidays my friend Nic Latimer—whose own partner, a native Iowan, had died of AIDS a few years before—gave me an envelope of pictures he had taken of Michael and me right before Thanksgiving. One is on the cover of this book. For a few months, between when he quit his job and his death in December, we had been happier than I ever thought possible.

Looking at the pictures, though, I realized Michael had lost weight in the months prior to his death. I wondered if his decision to quit his job, move in with me, and open a shop was driven by an awareness that his time was running short. The shop never opened, as Michael died three days before the planned grand opening. Later, a friend took over the lease and bought our inventory. That friend died of AIDS fourteen months later.

When Michael and I had walked to work together from his apartment, we sometimes passed the Soldiers', Sailors', Marines', Coast Guard, and Airmen's Club on Lexington Avenue at Thirty-seventh Street. Founded in 1919 in two adjoining mansions by General George Pershing and Mrs. Theodore Roosevelt, the club served as a home away from home for those in military service. It was where Michael lived when he first moved to New York, and he once told me how happy he had been there. He especially liked the first-floor parlor, which he said was painted a beautiful shade of yellow. After he died, I called the club to see if they might make a room available for a memorial service: The yellow parlor was precisely as Michael had described it.

We had the service around his birthday in April. A nun drove Michael's parents to the city. As they got out of the car, they looked as though they had aged several years since Michael's death. His mother, leaning on a cane, hugged me tightly and walked slowly to the entrance. We had saved a place for her on a small settee near the fireplace. One by one, our friends introduced themselves, expressing their sorrow or sharing a memory of Michael. I simply thanked everyone for coming and introduced Michael's family. His brother spoke briefly, saying how gratifying it was to Michael's family to know that he had so many loving friends in New York.

At one point, Michael's mother waved to me and patted the empty space next to her on the settee. "Please, Sean, sit here," she said. I did so, and she grasped my hand and held it tightly, looking at me through blue eyes the exact color as Michael's, now misty with tears. Then she said one of the most affirming things anyone has ever told me: "When you are sitting close to me, I feel like I am so much closer to my Michael."

Michael had always sent his mother a dozen yellow roses on January 7, her birthday. Yellow was her favorite color, and Michael had said he was sure it was the only time all year that anyone gave her flowers. So on January 7, a month after his death, I called a florist in Kingston and had a dozen yellow roses sent to her with no card.

I did that every year, until one January a decade later, when the florist said, "Oh, Mr. Strub, I've been waiting for your call. I'm so sorry, but Rose Misove died last fall." The florist told me that Michael's mother once asked her who sent the roses. Before the florist could answer, she said, "Never mind, I don't really want to know. I want to just believe Michael's sending them from heaven."

■   ■   ■

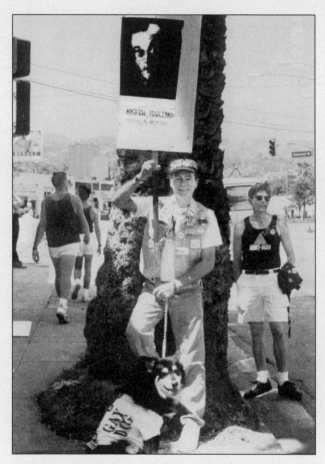

Swen Swenson shaking a can on Santa Monica Boulevard in West Hollywood raising money for ACT UP/LA. He's holding a sign memorializing his close friend, artist Keith Haring, who had died earlier that year. Swen's dog, Fever, is wearing a T-shirt that says "Gay Dog."

CHAPTER 16

Keith and Swen

After Michael's death, my life became unmoored. My apartment was sublet and I couldn't move into Michael's because I wasn't on the lease. So I lived full-time in Piermont, but without Michael I was lonely there.

As is my way, I buried my painful feelings in constant activity, including expanding the scope of ACT UP's fund-raising. I felt a deep-seated need to be in that room at the LGBT Community Center every Monday throughout 1989 with hundreds of others who understood the loss and grief I now felt more acutely than ever. Swen Swenson became one of my closest friends and we had dinner at least once a week. He never met Michael, but he encouraged me to talk about him. Swen also gave me a piece of advice that sounded strange at the time but that I came to appreciate. He suggested I freeze or put in plastic baggies a few things that carried Michael's scent—such as T-shirts, a scarf, his gym gloves—so I could later have what Swen called "fresh Michael smell" to remember him. The last scent of Michael was on his favorite silk scarf; I slept with it for weeks.

One of Swen's most important contributions to ACT UP was helping to obtain Keith Haring's support. Swen and Keith had an improbable friendship that began after Swen put his Minetta Lane town house on the market. Keith fell in love with the cozy town house, tucked away on a leafy, almost secret side street not far from the SoHo loft where he painted. An agreement was reached, and contracts were signed.

When Keith found out that he had HIV and his CD4 count was dangerously low, all bets—and deals—were off. He didn't want to take on renovating a town house. When he told Swen about his diagnosis, Swen confided that he, too, had AIDS. The retired sixtysomething Broadway "gypsy" and the global art scene's current "it boy"—just thirty years old—bonded over their diagnoses.

Swen became a mentor to Keith, helping him manage the combination of a life-threatening condition and meteoric fame. Keith kept his diagnosis a secret, in part because he didn't want to drive speculation in his work. His self-imposed isolation limited his access to the support, information, and resources of the AIDS community; Swen became an important link for him.

Every Monday, Swen took literature distributed at the ACT UP meeting to Keith's studio, where Swen often stayed through the night while Keith painted. I asked Swen when Keith would come to an ACT UP meeting. "I'm working on it," Swen said.

Some celebrities dropped by ACT UP meetings in 1989, including Susan Sarandon and Martin Sheen, who both wore "Silence=Death" pins on late-night TV talk shows and at awards ceremonies. That visibility conferred legitimacy as well as glamour to our efforts.

What finally brought Keith to our meetings was a poster designed by ACT UPpers Richard Deagle and Victor Mendolia for an upcoming demonstration against New York's John Cardinal O'Connor, who led the Catholic Church's campaign against gay people and people with AIDS.

The poster featured two large black-and-white images. On the left side was a photograph of the head of Cardinal O'Connor, wearing his pointed miter; on the right, comparable size and shape, was an image of a used condom. At the top, a headline screamed in red: "KNOW

YOUR SCUMBAGS!" Underneath the condom, small type read: "This one prevents AIDS."

Even I, far removed from the Catholic faith of my childhood, felt a momentary wave of shock. Among ACT UP posters, it was tough to top one by Gran Fury, an artists' collective, that featured a large, erect and erotic penis with the tagline: "Use a condom or beat it." This poster was close and when it was unveiled at a Monday meeting, the room hooted and hollered. When Swen took one to Keith's studio that night, Keith was sold. "Okay, that's it, I have to check out a meeting," he told Swen. "Do you think I can get some extra copies?"

When Keith showed up, there was a buzz in the room.

I didn't know for sure that Keith had AIDS until Swen told me. When Keith agreed to sign a fund-raising letter for ACT UP, I hoped he would agree to disclose his HIV status. I wasn't sure how to suggest it without betraying Swen's confidence. I needed to talk to him face-to-face, but scheduling time with Keith was difficult. He was constantly traveling or painting, with a nonstop flow of requests for meetings and interviews. When Julia Gruen, his assistant, said he would be in Europe for several weeks, it coincided with a trip I was taking. She scheduled a time for us to meet in Paris in August 1989.

I met Keith at the Hotel Ritz at Place Vendôme, where Proust had studied Parisian society, Coco Chanel had lived, and royals had stayed for over a century. Keith's suite was opulent, in white and gold Louis XV style, contrasting with Keith's humility and down-to-earth manner. It was early afternoon, but he was in a long white terry-cloth robe draped over cotton pajamas. "We had a late night," he said softly, Gil's not even up yet," referring to his friend and traveling companion, Gil Vasquez.

I sat on a settee and Keith was in an armchair to my left. I had worked with celebrities on fund-raising letters and was accustomed to feeling like a supplicant. But Keith was another gay man of my own generation; a peer who also had HIV and was a member of ACT UP. He was a comrade.

"What did you think of the meeting?" I asked, referring to his recent first ACT UP meeting. He casually disclosed his HIV status in his response: "[It was] one of the first times that made me feel good about, or feel comfortable with, the fact that I was sick, because, I don't know, there's more strength in numbers."

I steered the conversation to the fund-raising mailing. "We want to send your letter to two hundred thousand subscribers to art magazines, donors to gay and lesbian groups, and others. If they were all in a room, what would you say to them?"

He closed his eyes for a moment. "I would tell them that to dwell on the negativity and cynicism and pessimism of the situation is very easy, because it is so evil and morbid, but that is not going to do anything productive. The only way to deal with something negative is to change it, turn it into positive action," he said.

We talked about the AIDS empowerment movement, the People With AIDS Coalition, and other "positive action" efforts, including Michael Callen's work. Keith knew of Michael, and when I told him that Michael was battling KS, Keith said, "Me, too," and lifted a pajama leg, exposing dark purple KS lesions on his shin and calf, one the size of his hand. I knew in an instant that Keith was extremely ill. Lesions that advanced were typically associated with end-stage AIDS.

I asked if he was comfortable with referencing his KS in the letter. He consented, reluctantly. "I don't want to be pitied," he said. "It's not because I am sick that I think people should feel terrible about AIDS. It will come off sounding obnoxious if I'm just sort of crying, 'Oh, now I won't be able to work.' "

He told me about his trip and the effect that rumors about his health were having on the market for his work. "It's really disgusting how people are like vultures," he said. "After Jean-Michel [Basquiat] died, his prices went so high, and Andy [Warhol], too. Right now I could sell anything, and I'm not doing it."

Back in New York a few weeks later, I met Keith at his studio with graph paper so he could write out the alphabet in his distinctive handwriting. I then scanned and used it to laser-image recipients' names and addresses for the mailing. On the outside of the oversize envelope, we printed Keith's red "hear no evil, see no evil, speak no evil" imagery in his signature line drawings.

The mailing went out in October 1989. It raised a fortune by ACT UP's standards, enough to fund several major demonstrations. The news of Keith's HIV status—which broke in *Rolling Stone* right before our mailing dropped—helped boost the response.

In addition to the mailing program, I was coproducing the Auction for Action to raise funds for ACT UP's Stop the Church! action, scheduled for a week after the auction, on December 10. I was finally coming out of my grief about Michael's death a year before, aided by Zoloft, an antidepressant.

The auction benefit was cochaired by photographer Annie Leibovitz and painter David Hockney, and more than a hundred pieces of art were solicited from ACT UP's extended network of artists, galleryists, critics, and collectors. We had work from the Robert Mapplethorpe Foundation, artists Robert Rauschenberg, Robert Gober, Barton Benes, Christopher Makos, Jenny Holzer, Barbara Kruger, and many others.

Keith offered a wooden piece from his *Totem 89* series. When we picked it up at his studio, Julia told us to put an estimate of twelve thousand dollars on the piece. A few days later, she called and said we should increase the estimate to twenty to twenty-five thousand. As Keith had predicted, when news broke that he was sick, there was a frenzy of speculation in his work, driving prices higher.

The December 2 auction was held at American Ballet Theatre's rehearsal space on lower Broadway, in a building that ACT UP treasurer Marvin Shulman once owned with Michael Bennett, the creator of *A Chorus Line* and an early AIDS casualty. Several hundred people showed up, mostly ACT UPpers and familiar faces but also a number of expensively dressed strangers who we assumed were art dealers or collectors.

Among the ACT UP membership, one could find virtually any talent imaginable. When we needed an auctioneer, we discovered that member Aldyn McKean had been trained as a cattle auctioneer in his native Idaho. Aldyn presided that evening with my friend Ernest Quick, an elegant silver-haired antiques dealer more accustomed to auctioning rare silver and eighteenth-century furniture with his clipped, crisp, and understated style. Aldyn had the booming singsong chant typical of livestock sales. They were a perfect "high-low" pairing.

I served as the "ring man," soliciting bids from the crowd, then pointing or hollering when I spotted a bidder. I waved my arms to encourage a higher bid and, when I got it, yelled out "YEEEEEEEEESSSSSSS!!!" or "TWENTY-FIVE HUNDRED, NOW!"

About halfway through the evening, it became apparent that a portly, balding man with a fringe of red hair, a tweed jacket, and horn-rimmed glasses was bidding more frequently than anyone else, especially on sexually explicit pieces. If a painting, photograph, or sculpture depicted any sexual act or a penis, vagina, breast, or anus—and there were plenty such pieces—he was a sure bidder.

On one hand, this was great, as the serious money in the room was waiting to bid on Keith's *Totem 89* and other important pieces by famous artists. Having someone buy the erotic and more difficult to sell pieces was a relief. But after a while, Marvin Shulman, who watched our finances like a hawk, grew nervous. At one point he whispered in my ear, "We don't have that guy's credit card information or even a driver's license, just the name he gave, Walter Hardgraves."

"Check directory assistance," I said. "See if we can at least find out where he lives."

In a few minutes, Marvin was back. "He's not listed! Stop taking bids from him. I'm afraid he'll run out and not pay. Maybe he's a plant from someone who wants to sabotage our fund-raiser!" From that point, I did everything I could to work around the mysterious Hardgraves. Whenever he bid, I went back to the crowd, pleading and cajoling others to raise their paddles. The prices went higher and higher. More often than not, Hardgraves stuck it out and topped the other bids. Marvin and the volunteer team kept careful watch, lest he try to sneak out without paying.

Totem 89 arrived on the block near the end of the sale. The bidding started out furiously, rapidly advancing in $5,000 increments, exceeding Julia's high estimate of $25,000 in the first few minutes. When it hit $50,000, the crowd applauded and then fell hushed. By the time bidding hit $70,000, the crowd had started to chant softly, "Do it! Do it! Do it!" to urge on the two remaining bidders, neither of whom any of us knew. When the gavel came down at $74,000, the room spontaneously exploded, with everyone leaping up, fists in the air, chanting, "ACT UP! FIGHT BACK! FIGHT AIDS!" like it was an anthem. The frenzy went on for several minutes, and many of us were in tears; it was one of the most exciting moments in my life.

The entire evening netted over $300,000, after expenses of about $25,000—the most successful ACT UP fund-raising event ever. As buyers packed up their purchases and lined up to pay their tabs, Marvin and I kept our eyes on Hardgraves. His tab came to $22,000, making him one of the evening's biggest spenders, aside from the buyer of the Haring piece. When he was handed his bill, Hardgraves put on reading glasses and reviewed it. Then he pulled a fat envelope out of his jacket's breast pocket and counted out, to our great relief, 220 brand-new $100 bills. Later we learned that Malcolm Forbes, the closeted gay publishing magnate, had given Hardgraves, his art consultant, $25,000 and instructed him to spend it at our auction.

Forbes had hit ACT UP's radar earlier that year, when he published an article about heterosexual transmission of HIV that addressed important points but did so in a homophobic manner. ACT UP protested on the sidewalk outside his Manhattan office, until Malcolm himself invited the ACT UPpers inside to chat, which led to a follow-up in their next issue. After Forbes died in 1990, ACT UP member Michelangelo Signorile wrote an exposé of his secret gay life for *Outweek* magazine. I've sometimes wondered what happened to all of the homoerotic and sexually explicit art Forbes collected.

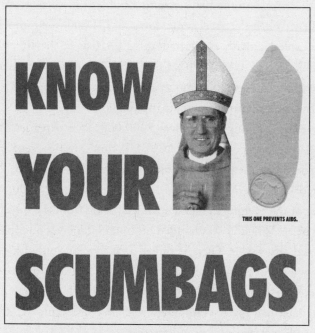

THIS ONE PREVENTS AIDS.

This is the poster designed by Richard Deagle and Victor Mendolia for the December 1989 "Stop the Church!" demonstration at St. Patrick's Cathedral. It was this poster that finally inspired Keith Haring to start attending ACT UP meetings.

CHAPTER 17

Cardinal Sin

In addition to the Keith Haring mailing and the auction, I was also participating in what turned out to be the most controversial demonstration in ACT UP's history. From a perch of exceptional power, the New York Catholic Archdiocese's Cardinal O'Connor condemned LGBT activism, opposed anti-discrimination statutes, and called homosexuality an "intrinsic evil." He prevented groups of gay Irish-Americans from participating in the annual St. Patrick's Day parade and kicked Dignity, the gay Catholic group, out of all facilities controlled by the archdiocese, where they had celebrated Mass for many years.

O'Connor's most damaging action was campaigning against condom usage. He stopped church-run hospitals from distributing condoms or discussing safe sex with patients—an edict widely ignored by doctors, nurses, and nuns on staff—and he funded a disinformation campaign on billboards, buses, and subways that claimed "condoms don't work," citing statistics from discredited studies that suggested condom failure rates of 50 percent or greater. He even opposed condom use between two partners when one was known to be HIV positive.

At the same time, O'Connor took every opportunity to boast of the Church's compassion toward people with AIDS who were dying in church-run hospices. His hypocrisy was galling; he acted like he hated gay people when we were healthy and sexually active but was eager to love us as dying "AIDS victims." When O'Connor prevented New York City schools from educating students about protection from HIV through the use of condoms, we knew we had to do something.

From the moment it was proposed in the summer of 1989, the Stop the Church! action was even controversial within ACT UP. Protesting *outside* Manhattan's St. Patrick's Cathedral was one thing—activists had done that for years—but interrupting a religious service *inside* the church was, for some members, beyond the pale. An internal debate raged throughout a sweltering summer heat wave. The unair-conditioned ACT UP meeting space at the Center provided no relief.

Some ACT UP members thought interrupting a Catholic Mass was deeply disrespectful. They feared it would jeopardize our credibility and fund-raising; I predicted it would do the reverse by raising our profile dramatically and tapping into anger at the Church. Catholics in ACT UP—both the faithful and those who had fallen away from the Church—were split, some from each camp vehemently opposed and others as strongly in favor.

By the time the Women's Health Action and Mobilization (WHAM) came on board as a cosponsor, the debate was over, a vote was taken, and the action was on. Flyers and posters were designed, and momentum and anticipation mounted all fall.

Clusters of ACT UP members formed affinity groups, cells of five to fifteen, each planning a mini-action within the overall demonstration. Some would infiltrate the cathedral, posing as regular Sunday Mass-goers, so they could stage actions during the Mass. They kept their plans secret, so there wasn't any one person in ACT UP who knew everything. Some actions were risky, in terms of legal consequences, so plausible deniability was important.

On a bitter cold December 10, the day of the action, forty-five hundred protesters packed Fifth Avenue, chanting and waving placards. Fists pumped the air, bullhorns blared, and our voices echoed into the cathedral every time the door opened to let someone in or out. Guerrilla theater on the sidewalk featured protesters dressed as clowns, nuns, priests, and as Christ himself.

As parishioners wove their way through the demonstrators, they were handed flyers detailing the harms perpetuated by Cardinal O'Connor and the Catholic Church. Few were surprised by our presence, as there had been media alerts all week, and we had distributed similar flyers the Sunday before, explaining why we were coming to St. Patrick's. Some were overtly hostile, but others expressed support for our cause, if not our crude criticisms of O'Connor.

Police officers expected disruption inside the cathedral, so they formed a line from just inside the Fifth Avenue entrance all the way to the elevated apse at the easternmost end. Another line of men in uniform, wearing white-and-gold-robed vestments, stood in front of the altar.

We were there to witness and protest, not worship or confess. Parishioner, protester, or observer, it was difficult not to be moved by the drama of the scene. Cardinal O'Connor tried to proceed with the Mass and ignore the persistent interruptions of the protesters, but he eventually gave up and retreated to his thronelike chair. Ushers handed parishioners printed copies of O'Connor's homily—prepared in advance, anticipating the disruption—and the Mass continued.

My friend Tom Keane was part of the Hail Marys affinity group, and he invited me to join them. We had dressed conservatively, dispersing throughout the pews and participating quietly in the Mass, readying ourselves for the communion ritual. Our plan was to make political statements as we accepted the wine and wafer—"the blood and body of Christ."

I was nervous. It had been a long time since I had taken communion—the holiest of sacraments—and now I was doing so only as an act of protest. As the minutes passed and the first wave of protesters was arrested, my apprehension grew. I knew my participation would deeply offend my parents, particularly if my name appeared in the press. Duty to the church had shaped my family for generations; we had the devotion of feudal serfs, obeying an authority beyond question. But when the time came for me to stand and join the line for communion, I did. As I neared the head of the line, I unbuttoned my coat, exposing the ACT UP logo and pink triangle on my shirt, daring the priest to deny me communion. He looked at my shirt and hesitated, then held up the host and declared, "The body of Christ." I wasn't sure what I would say in response until I heard myself summon Michael: "May the Lord bless the man I love, who died a year ago this week."

As I walked back to my pew, someone opened the main door to the cathedral at the far end of the church, letting in the bright sunlight. I thought about walking all the way down the aisle to join the protesters outside. But I didn't want to look like I was either ashamed of what I had done or fearful of what came next, so I returned to where I had been sitting. Once seated in my pew, I felt a surge of relief, like I had just shed a heavy burden. I felt Michael's pride in me, too.

In the demonstration's most notable moment, Tom Keane took communion, said, "Opposing safe-sex education is murder," and crumbled the consecrated host in his hand, which he later referred to as "snapping the cracker." The priest serving him frantically dropped to his knees to pick up the pieces, while a blue blur of cops rushed Tom. A former seminarian, John Wessel, also snapped his cracker, but not until he was returning to his pew, when he tossed the pieces toward the altar, over the heads of the seated parishioners.

My verbal protest at communion didn't qualify for an arrest, but 111 other protesters were arrested, 58 outside and 53 inside the cathedral. When I scanned the names, I noticed those arrested inside the church had a preponderance of Irish, Italian, and Polish names, much more likely to have been raised culturally Catholic than were those arrested outside the church.

By the next morning, ACT UP was being criticized from all corners, including elected officials, *The New York Times*, and most major media. Even other ACT UP chapters and AIDS organizations were quick to disassociate themselves from the demonstration. GMHC issued a statement calling the action "a mistake" but did note: "If the cardinal cannot accept scientific facts about AIDS, he should stay out of the debate. And if he makes political statements, he must expect a political response."

Some members of ACT UP characterized Stop the Church! as a strategic failure. They claimed that the cost to our public image, which had been increasingly favorable, was not worth whatever benefits we'd gained by publicizing the church's propaganda against reproductive rights and HIV prevention.

I think the demonstration inspired and reflected a major change in the LGBT community's relationship to the Catholic Church and the Church's role in American politics. If the 1969 Stonewall rebellion was a milestone in protesting the civil authority that oppressed us, the St. Patrick's action was a milestone in protesting the religious authority that oppressed us. The Church's influence in AIDS policy remains substantial, but nowhere near what it was prior to the Stop the Church! action. But I may be overstating the significance of this one action, because my own participation had such a deep significance for me.

Two years later, my brother and his wife had their first child, Joseph, and asked me to be his godfather. I was surprised and pleased but wasn't sure I was the right choice. My brother and sister-in-law weren't especially devout Catholics, but they knew my views about the Church.

When my dad picked me up at the airport in Cedar Rapids, he said I was supposed to be at St. Mary's rectory an hour before the baptism to meet with the priest. I assumed this was routine for godparents-to-be. St. Mary's rectory is next door to the church, in a Victorian frame house with a wide front porch. I was led to the parlor, where the priest was waiting for me.

He wanted to know about the action at St. Patrick's Cathedral. I could tell he was both fascinated and horrified; he grilled me about the crumbled host and wanted to hear about ACT UP's internal debate over whether the demonstration should have happened.

When he learned that was the last time I had been to Mass, he said, "to be safe," he wanted to "rebaptize" me (there is no such Catholic sacrament). I had a fleeting urge to refuse but didn't want to distract from the day's celebration. After he prayed and sprinkled holy water on me, I said, "See, I didn't burst into flames!" and the priest laughed.

I wasn't so well behaved a few years later, as far as my parents were concerned, when I agreed to speak at the Iowa City Lesbian, Gay, and Bisexual Pride Rally. The rally was on the east-facing steps of the Old Capitol; a restored 1842 Greek revival limestone building that had served as Iowa's territorial capital. My German émigré great-great-grandfather was a stonecutter who moved into the Iowa Territory to cut stone for the capitol building. The Iowa Constitution, one of the most progressive state constitutions, was written inside the building he helped build.

The steeple of St. Mary's, where seven generations of my family have worshipped, was visible a few blocks to the east, heightening my emotions. I spoke off the cuff, telling stories about growing up as a queer boy in Iowa City. Marlene Perrin, a local journalist who has known me most of my life, covered the event for the *Iowa City Press Citizen*:

"I'm a Hawkeye and a homo with AIDS," he told the crowd. "And I'm very proud to be here. For many of us, a return to our hometown is often a return to the emotional and psychological battleground of their youth—the scene of the crime, if you will."

For Strub, too, a visit home brings back some painful memories of the speech therapist at Penn School, who treated him for a lisp. The therapist told him he sounded like a girl. He remembers the physical education teachers who told him he threw a ball like a girl. He remembers the vice principal at Central Junior High School who told Strub he should quit talking about antiques because "the other boys will think I'm funny."

And he remembers a session led by a priest and a nun when he was an altar boy at St. Mary's Church. "The nun said the souls of sex perverts and homosexuals were the very most difficult to save."

It had taken years, but I had come to terms with my identity, gotten past the shame, and was no longer afraid to come home and reveal myself. In fact, I was anxious to speak out, especially since I didn't know whether I would ever have another such chance in my hometown.

CHAPTER 18

Hope Is Hope

Every meeting of ACT UP began with a reading of the names of members and friends who had died in the previous seven days. If it was someone I knew, it seldom was a surprise as I usually was already aware they were ill. But sometimes it was a shock, particularly when people hastened their own deaths. The prognosis Dr. Pier gave me when I was diagnosed, "These days, Sean, you can have two good years left," was similar to what many others heard; when ACT UP started, two years later, it wasn't much different. Few thought survival was possible.

Michael Callen, through his work with PWAC, was aware of many people who had survived longer and were leading vibrant lives, despite the burden of illness. His doctor, Sonnabend, had said he didn't think AIDS would ultimately turn out to be 100 percent fatal; some unknown number would survive.

Mark Harrington, an ACT UP treatment activist, was also a patient of Sonnabend's and wanted to get the federal government to study long-term survival. Harrington wrote Fauci, requesting a meeting to discuss the phenomenon. But in 1991, when Sonnabend, Harrington, and Gregg Gonsalves, another ACT UP treatment activist, went to

Bethesda to see Fauci and about a dozen of his NIH colleagues, they were met with polite but dismissive disbelief, only getting a vague promise that they "would look into it."

A decade after AIDS was identified, the people leading the federal response didn't even know there were patients living five, six, seven years or more, let alone initiated any research to understand why.

Sonnabend says he was treated with "derision and scorn" at the meeting, as though he wasn't a scientist. When he began to share data about long-term survivors from his practice, one member of the group asked, "Who's he?"

When Callen's book, *Surviving AIDS*, was published in 1990, it had a tremendous influence on my attitude and thinking about my own prognosis, especially after I had outlived Dr. Pier, who died in January of that year.

In *Surviving AIDS*, Callen interviewed people with AIDS about why they thought they were alive. He found that those who had survived the longest shared three important traits: They *believed* survival was possible; they could identify a reason to get up in the morning; and when asked how they treated their illness, they could rattle off a list of different strategies. What was on the list wasn't important. Survivors sought survival; seeking and experimenting with various treatments and strategies was the key.

Callen told me he was accused of offering people with AIDS "cruel hope" by suggesting that survival was possible. "I tell them there's no such thing as 'cruel hope,' " he said. "Hope is hope—either you have it or you don't."

I hadn't considered it in those terms, but in reading Callen's book, I recognized myself. I always believed Sonnabend's conjecture that someone would survive, even at those times when I thought I might not be among that group. I read an article once that described "the most fatal forms of cancer" as 96 percent fatal. That meant 4 percent, one out of twenty-five, survived. Not great odds but a far cry from impossible, and I hadn't heard anyone suggest that AIDS was more fatal than the most deadly cancers.

I never had any trouble finding a reason to get up each morning. My life was full of friends, activism, entrepreneurial activities, and projects.

Callen's third point—that survivors were never passive patients who simply followed a doctor's instructions—resonated most strongly with me. Survivors, Callen wrote, were people who were engaged, curious, and willing to experiment. They pursued treatment strategies independent of, and sometimes against the advice of, doctors. There were several anti-retroviral treatments available in 1990, but the long-term survivors Callen interviewed didn't list just medications; they cited alternative and complementary therapies, such as acupuncture, massage, visualization, herbs, prayer, exercise, positive thinking, and more. I realized that those surviving had become well enough informed to take their lives into their own hands.

Though the public still thought of AIDS as a death sentence, by the time *Surviving AIDS* was published, the gay community and many frontline doctors had seen people who had become outspoken activists, looking healthy and vibrant as they protested or got arrested at AIDS demonstrations. Many of the newly formed AIDS service organizations emphasized survival and empowerment rather than a retreat from life and preparation for an impending death. Even so, I knew that many of the people in my life expected me to die, and on bleak days I expected the same.

I was raised to trust doctors and to believe that "alternative" practitioners were, almost by definition, quacks. But with support from other people with AIDS, I pursued my own treatment trajectory, one that wasn't about waiting for scientists and drug companies to come up with the right combination of pills. I knew I didn't have the time to wait so I learned how to listen to my body and actively seek survival.

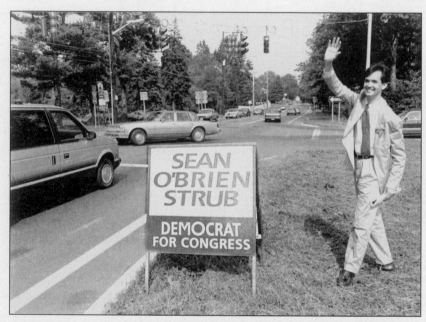

During my campaign for Congress in 1990, I stood on busy street corners during rush hour waving at passing traffic. It was beastly hot that summer. I noticed that passengers in expensive cars, with their windows rolled up and the air-conditioning on, looked at me with suspicion, like I was dangerous or mentally ill. But trucks with construction workers who sweat for a living always waved at me or cheered me on. I think they liked seeing a candidate standing in the hot sun, asking for their support.

CHAPTER 19

Running Man

Even as I sought survival, and believed it was possible for some, I never was sure I would be among them. No one could be sure, because while some deaths were expected, others felt random. Someone would look fine on Tuesday and be dead a few days later. In 1988, when Michael made that magnificent Thanksgiving dinner for a dozen people, he had no thought that he was so sick and would be dead ten days later.

Over the next two years, I embarked on a frenzied rush of activity. I wanted to do everything at once, cramming decades of life and accomplishment into just a few years. But instead of being a finale, the '90s opened up a new chapter in my life during which my politics and activism became much more important than building a business.

Early in 1990, my friend David Hochberg considered running for the U.S. Congress from New York's 22nd district, and I offered to help. The district started at the Yonkers city line in Westchester County and ran all the way up to the Catskills' Pennsylvania border, encompassing parts of Orange and Sullivan counties and all of Rockland County, including my house in Piermont. For eighteen years the district was represented by Ben Gilman, a Republican hawk, typically reelected with big margins.

David had tremendous financial resources—his mother is Lillian Vernon, the direct-mail catalog magnate—and while considering the race, he commissioned survey research that outlined a difficult but potentially achievable path to victory. I was excited by the idea of having a close friend in Congress and began planning legislative initiatives to address the epidemic even before David made a decision about whether to run.

He ultimately chose not to, unwilling to sacrifice his privacy and time. When no other Democratic candidate appeared on the horizon, I started toying with the idea of entering the race. I thought about what it would mean to have someone in Congress who would make battling AIDS a priority. Years before, I had given up any hope for electoral office and had largely soured on partisan politics. But while I had given up the dream, I hadn't lost the desire. The prospect of winning a seat in Congress was tantalizing, and the reelection of Gerry Studds and Barney Frank after they came out in the late '80s demonstrated that sexual orientation was no longer an impassable barrier to elective federal office.

I discussed my options with Jean O'Leary one night in Los Angeles. She still ran NGRA and chaired the Democratic National Committee's LGBT caucus. "You've got to do it," she said. "Even if you lose, as an openly gay candidate, you'll be blazing a trail for others." She offered to put together a fund-raiser for me in Los Angeles, vowing, "We'll make this a national race!" We talked a lot about how to handle the media when my sexual orientation was addressed—it was never a consideration not to be upfront about it—but we didn't dwell on my HIV status. At the time, much of the public didn't distinguish between an out gay man and a gay man with AIDS; they considered them essentially the same. The major news would be that I was gay, not that I had HIV.

Jean's close friend Midge Costanza was equally enthusiastic. Midge was well known from her time working as a special assistant to President Jimmy Carter, and she was a charismatic and fiery speaker, in demand at Democratic rallies and events. I asked if she would fly out and help me on the campaign. "Honey," she said, "I'll come speak for you anywhere, anytime. There are a lot of Italians in that district. They'll love me—and everyone else, well, they won't know what hit them after I've been there!"

That evening, Jean and Midge made me feel like a candidate. I knew the political odds were against me, but the chance of victory, no matter how slim, and what that could mean for people with AIDS was a powerful draw.

I made my decision at a memorial service for my friend Jay Johnson. When Michael died, Jay and his partner, Rubens Teles, had taken over the antique shop Michael was preparing to open. After the service for Jay, Rubens and I and a few other friends were sitting in Rubens's folk art–filled house, reminiscing about Jay and discussing the epidemic. When someone asked if I had made a decision about the campaign, Rubens brightened, turned to me, and said, "You have to! You have to tell them what we're going through!"

In that moment, I knew that if I didn't run, I would feel like a coward. I went from considering it an opportunity to thinking of it as an obligation. Washington, D.C., was where I came out of the closet and gave up on my dream of serving in Congress; it was tantalizing to think about going back as openly gay.

When I mentioned the potential campaign at an ACT UP fundraising committee meeting, we joked about ACT UP friends working in congressional offices, wearing "Silence=Death" T-shirts under their suits, maybe staging an action in the members' dining room.

Not long after I met him, I hired Stephen away from the archdiocese to run a division of my direct-mail company that published cardpacks, decks of advertising cards that we sent to gay and lesbian households across the country. When I discussed the prospect of the campaign with him, he was enthusiastic and agreed to head up fund-raising. Another member of the ACT UP fund-raising committee, Dan Baker, known for his organizational skills, became my campaign manager.

In those first few weeks, I ricocheted between my two lives. Part of the time I was in the district, driving around the lower Hudson River Valley to kaffeeklatsches, firehouses, and senior-citizen centers; the rest of the time I was in Manhattan, attending ACT UP meetings, demonstrations, and fund-raising events for my campaign.

I knew Robert F. Kennedy, Jr., through the Natural Resources Defense Council, a client of my firm. I went to see him to try and get his endorsement of my campaign. We shared an interest in protecting Sterling Forest, a twenty-thousand-acre pristine wilderness in the district that straddled the New York/New Jersey border. A developer had proposed turning it into the largest planned community in New York, with a projected population of fifty thousand.

We met at Kennedy's home in Westchester County and sat in comfortable chairs in his den. I was in a suit, trying to look like a candidate; Kennedy was dressed casually. He was skeptical about my chance of winning but encouraged my effort. "Gilman's been there forever; he'll be tough to beat," he said. "But it'll focus attention on Sterling Forest, and that would be great."

He knew I was gay and an AIDS activist. I wondered if he would bring it up, particularly since he was a devout Catholic. He eventually did. "They're not going to like your ACT UP stuff. Were you at that protest at St. Patty's?"

I'd known he wouldn't approve of the St. Patrick's action. "Yeah, but I didn't get arrested," I answered. I tried to make a joke: "That's the most spiritual time I've spent in a Catholic church in years."

He didn't laugh. "Interrupting a Mass is a big mistake. That's not going to help your campaign. A lot of people won't forgive it." After a pause, he added, "I'd be really furious if someone did that while I was at Mass."

Scrambling to salvage the possibility of his endorsement, I explained why we had focused the protest on Cardinal O'Connor and the institution of the Church and how we had gone out of our way to be respectful of the parishioners. He smiled slightly but said, "I still don't think it was a good idea."

We went out to a small ramshackle barn behind his house, and he showed me the falcons that he trained and the injured raptors that he was helping to heal. It wasn't until I was leaving that I asked explicitly if he would endorse me. He was hesitant, then asked, "You don't think you're going to have opposition?" I told him no other Democrat had announced for the seat, and the county chairs had already said they would support me.

"Okay, then you can go ahead and say I'm supporting you, too," he said. "But I can't do any events until closer to the election."

I was elated. RFK Jr. didn't get involved in many races, especially not before the primary. His support would underscore my commitment to save Sterling Forest, which I intended to make a major issue in the campaign. From the beginning, the largest circulation daily paper in the district, the Rockland County *Journal News*, reported on my campaign as a serious effort. They not only noted RFK Jr.'s support but called my announcement speech "Kennedy-esque" and cited my advocacy on behalf of Sterling Forest. With strong press coverage of the campaign launch, Kennedy's endorsement, and Midge Costanza nominating me at the county conventions, we were off to a great start.

But there were obstacles, starting with the facts that I had lived in the district only a couple of years and, of course, that I was gay and had HIV. I knew if I brought up these issues first, I would be labeled the "gay candidate" or "AIDS candidate" and not taken as seriously.

My campaign biography and literature listed LGBT and AIDS groups with which I had worked. So many of my volunteers wore the de facto ACT UP uniform—T-shirts with activist messages, jeans, and black boots—that our campaign events sometimes looked like ACT UP rallies. We didn't mention my sexual orientation or health status in press releases, and when speaking to groups, I brought up these facts only when it felt appropriate. I was more curious than worried to see how it would play out.

The first time I was asked about my short residency, it was in front of a friendly crowd, at a small fund-raiser where most people also knew I had HIV. I responded simply, noting that while I was new to the district, I wasn't new to the issues I held dear or the values I espoused. Then I made an oblique reference to my health, saying that I didn't feel like I was in a position to wait a few years to run for office.

The five-month campaign was funded by several thousand donors who each gave on average forty-five dollars in response to appeals sent to LGBT and AIDS donors nationwide. I also solicited my personal friends and family and received some memorable responses. A month into the campaign, I got a note in the mail from one conservative Republican friend that said, "Dear Sean, I disagree with almost everything you stand for. Love, Joe." Enclosed was a check for a thousand dollars.

Other contributions were memorable because they came from people who once felt like adversaries. About a year before the campaign, my assistant came into my office and said there was someone on the line who "sounded important." When I picked up the phone, the caller identified himself as Robert Woolley. He said, "I understand that ACT UP is going to throw blood on my dear friend Pat Buckley at the Skating for Life benefit. Ashton Hawkins says you can get them to stop it. I command you to do so. Now!"

I knew the cast of society characters in this bizarre tirade: Woolley was a socially prominent openly gay auctioneer at Sotheby's; Pat Buckley was the high-society wife of ultra-right conservative William F. Buckley, editor of the *National Review*; and Ashton Hawkins was an executive at the Metropolitan Museum who was Jacqueline Kennedy Onassis's occasional escort at public functions.

But Woolley's "command" was pointless. I told him that he didn't understand how ACT UP worked and was misinformed about my influence in the organization; that ACT UP had never thrown blood on anyone; and in any case, non-violence was fundamental to our activism. I also said Pat Buckley had a lot of nerve hosting an AIDS benefit when she refused to repudiate her reactionary husband's call to tattoo the buttocks of people with AIDS. Woolley slammed the phone down.

Later, during the campaign, Bob MacLeod and Steve Byckiewicz, who owned the Kiss My Face cosmetics company, hosted a cocktail-party fund-raiser for my campaign at their Manhattan apartment. Though I was appreciative, my expectations were low: I knew that many of the straight-acting, straight-appearing white "A-gays" in attendance weren't eager to support me. I did my best, though, giving my impassioned "apathy of the affluent" speech.

"Good speech," muttered a bearded, portly man wearing a silk ascot. He stuffed a check into my front shirt pocket and introduced himself as Robert Woolley. I recognized his name from the call a year earlier, but I wasn't sure if he realized we had previously spoken. After a few minutes, my curiosity got the best of me. Did he remember, I asked, our earlier conversation?

"Yes, I thought you were a real asshole," he said without smiling. Then he added, "I've changed my mind." I didn't realize Woolley was ill with AIDS at the time. By the time he died in 1996, we had become good friends.

Two fund-raising events held in Los Angeles illustrate the economic divide that ultimately was defining for LGBT politics in the '90s. One was a barbecue hosted by Torie Osborn, then the head of the L.A. Gay and Lesbian Center. It was a grass-roots event, diverse, and a lot of fun. Many of the checks were for small amounts, but donated with great sincerity and we raised more than $1,000.

The other was the event Jean O'Leary promised, a fancy cocktail party hosted by Scott Hitt and his partner, Alex Koleszar, at their lavish home in Beverly Hills. Hitt was a warm and talented physician who later was appointed by President Clinton to chair the Presidential Advisory Council on HIV/AIDS.

The cocktail party guests were mostly affluent gay men from Beverly Hills and West Hollywood, many of whom were getting involved in politics for the first time. They were interested in meeting these street radicals from ACT UP and, just in case I won, didn't want to miss being on my list of early supporters. Stephen joined me on that trip, and we felt like celebrity activists. We raised about $7,000.

The gay and lesbian magazine *The Advocate* interviewed and photographed me for a profile while I was in L.A. The daily newspapers in my New York district had been wrestling with how to report I was gay. They hadn't found the right angle to break the story without looking like they were unduly focused on my sexuality. When the *Advocate* profile came out, it provided the necessary opening. The *Journal News* ran a headline reading: "Strub: Homosexuality 'Not an Issue.'" This "nonissue," however, covered the top half of the newspaper's front page.

The article came out at a time when my campaign had serious momentum; I had strong endorsements, was raising money, and was getting under my opponent's skin. The state's old-line conservative Democratic establishment hadn't cared if a gay guy got the Democratic nomination for the 22nd Congressional District when nobody wanted it and they thought it was a futile race. Once my energetic campaign made the race look viable, the politicos started having second thoughts.

The growing awareness that I was gay emboldened the opposition to my candidacy within the Democratic Party. A retired member of Congress, John Dow, was talked into entering the race a few days before the filing deadline. He was in his eighties and hadn't served in Congress in two decades, but he was spry and passionately single-minded about the need to raise taxes. He was delighted to have the opportunity to talk to Democrats in the region.

I had admired Dow as a principled civil libertarian who was one of the earliest members of Congress to oppose the Vietnam War. When we met face-to-face at a campaign event, I felt like I had made a new friend, even though he was my electoral opponent in the primary. We couldn't really have a debate, because we agreed on almost everything. He didn't like to drive at night, so on several occasions I picked him up at his home in Nyack and took him to events where we were both scheduled to speak. People were surprised when opposing candidates showed up in the same car.

In my stump speech, I quoted from *The Politics of the Rich and Poor*, a recently published book by conservative theorist Kevin Phillips, who warned of the growing income disparity in the United States that had emerged during the Reagan administration, resulting in a rapidly shrinking middle class. I bought twenty-five copies and gave them to donors and members of the media. I also gave a copy to Dow, and the next time I saw him, we sat in my car talking for almost two hours about the relationship between social and economic justice.

The most damaging media disclosure was not the revelation that I am gay but the allegation that I had sent out literature promoting "safe hot sex" between men.

My company's Community Cardpack was sent to one hundred and fifty thousand LGBT-involved households across the country. One card advertised an HIV-prevention program at GMHC that referenced "safe hot sex." An Associated Press reporter was one of the recipients, and she called, angrily demanding to know how she got on our list. The snarky story she wrote called my judgment into question by suggesting that my campaign had sent sexually explicit material to voters in my district. That story probably cost me the election. Ironically, my participation in the highly controversial St. Patrick's demonstration never came up during the campaign.

At the same time, the incumbent Republican's campaign mobilized conservative religious voters—mostly Catholics and Orthodox Jews—to support Dow in the primary. They called newspaper editorial-board members to urge them to report I was gay, had AIDS, and was pursuing a secret "radical gay agenda." They also distributed flyers at Catholic churches the Sunday before the election prompting parish priests to oppose me from the pulpit.

Dow won with 54 percent of the vote to my 46 percent. I had the newspaper endorsements, more volunteers, a better organized voter-turnout effort, and I spent more on television and media. Dow had religious conservatives determined to defeat an openly gay candidate as well as a base of older voters who knew him from past campaigns. In my concession speech, I pledged my support to Dow in the general election (where he got creamed) but made it clear that I'd been defeated by homophobia, not John Dow.

As O'Leary, Costanza, and Kennedy had predicted, good things can come out of a loss. One of them was our success in protecting Sterling Forest. We alerted the public to the risks, helped coalesce and organize opposition, and uncovered campaign contributions from the developer that the incumbent had denied receiving. The revelations encouraged

U.S. Representative Peter Kostmayer, a prominent environmentalist and gay man who represented Bucks County, to get involved, and the dynamic changed dramatically. Kostmayer held district hearings on Sterling Forest, bringing attention to the issue and, by extension, to my campaign. Then Kostmayer and others persuaded House Speaker Newt Gingrich to support protection of the property. Today it remains a pristine wilderness.

My race also broke ground in terms of how the district and the incumbent viewed issues concerning sexual orientation. Until my campaign, Gilman's voting record had never received greater than a 35 percent LGBT-friendliness rating from the Human Rights Campaign, but in the years after the race, his rating nearly doubled. I don't know if he saw the light or just wanted to be ready to compete with a future opponent who might be strong on those issues.

An editorial in the *Journal-News* on the Sunday following the primary revealed how the campaign helped change community attitudes. Titled "A Race of Courage: Strub's Honesty Blazed Ground," it began:

> Sean O'Brien Strub has much to be proud of despite his loss . . . He admitted his homosexuality up front; he spoke strongly about the serious issues of the economy and human need . . . We hope Strub seeks another elective office . . . After all, once an African-American or a woman couldn't seek office in this nation. Now many hold key positions as more voters realize how silly it is to reject people because of their race or sex. Now let's add sexual preference to the list.

In the years following the race, several openly LGBT candidates in the district ran for local offices. The most conservative part of the district, where the news about my sexual orientation was most damaging to my campaign, is now represented by an openly gay man who is also named Sean: Representative Sean Patrick Maloney.

■   ■   ■

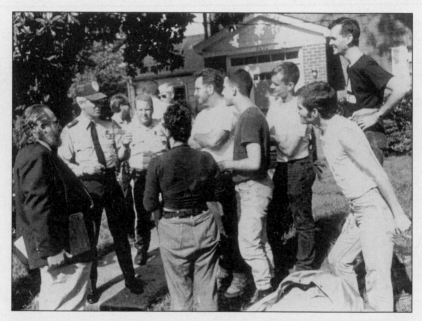

We called ourselves the "Helms 7," because seven of us had just put a gigantic condom over U.S. Senator Jesse Helms's house in suburban Washington. It was fully tumescent when the police arrived, but they made us turn off the generator and blowers. That's me on the upper right. (Photo courtesy of the *Washington Blade*.)

CHAPTER 20

Taking the Helms

In early 1991, I was living with the financial and emotional aftermath of my losing campaign for Congress. I had gone into the race knowing it was a long shot, but somewhere along the way, I drank the Kool-Aid and became convinced I could win, making the loss more painful. Though I consoled my supporters, I didn't have time to console myself; I needed to get my business life back in order, starting with paying off a ninety-thousand-dollar campaign debt.

I no longer had any business partners, and during the campaign, the company suffered. So I focused on working with Stephen to rebuild the business. Our personal and professional relationship had grown. Stephen was methodically learning everything I could teach him about direct marketing, politics, the epidemic, and LGBT history. I loved the role of mentor, especially when mentoring someone so smart, motivated, and from whom I could learn as well. The belief that I could die relatively soon gave mentorship more meaning, enabling something of what I had learned to live on.

Stephen was managing the cardpack division when an opportunity arose to start a new company that would become Stephen's focus for the next decade. One of our cardpack advertisers was a Cleveland-based mail-order pharmacy. We were friendly with their straight Republican CEO, Mike Erlenbach, and he proposed that Stephen and I start a new company to market his firm. "You know this community," Erlenbach told us. "You know what people with AIDS need from a pharmacy." His pharmacy would fulfill all the prescriptions and handle the insurance paperwork, while we would handle customer service and marketing. Erlenbach said he would split the profits with us.

As Stephen and I talked about the idea, we realized it was not only a good business model but also an opportunity to get timely treatment information to people with HIV. I had been providing it through fund-raising appeals and cardpack messages for years. Stephen had edited the first issue of ACT UP's *Treatment and Data Digest,* a newsletter geared to treatment wonks, including people with HIV, as well as doctors, scientists, and government officials.

Erlenbach offered an advance of seventy-five thousand dollars to fund initial marketing expenses. We used it to start a treatment newsletter geared to the average person with HIV, not just the science club, as we called the wonkier activists. We named the company Community Prescription Service and Stephen was a co-owner and its chief operating officer. A picture of Stephen was featured prominently in our advertising, with the caption "I don't just run the company, I'm a client, too," playing on the Hair Club for Men ads.

We established an advisory board of well-known people with HIV, including Michael Callen; ACT UP's Peter Staley; Phill Wilson, the Los Angeles AIDS coordinator who later founded the Black AIDS Institute; and Connie Norman, a transgender AIDS activist in Los Angeles. The independent, slightly rebellious approach to the editorial content in our newsletter, the CPS InfoPak, was a precursor to *POZ,* the magazine I would start in 1994.

CPS routinely waived customers' copays and argued with insurance companies to get them to cover off-label treatments. We saved our customers money, offered greater privacy than a local pharmacy, and provided more personal and knowledgeable customer service. Most of the dozen or so staffers were people with HIV, so customers calling in could always speak to someone who related to them.

Stephen and I were a good team in business as well as in our approach to treatment and activism. We both read everything we could find about HIV treatment and were interested in every idea, no matter how strange or unusual it might sound. While I viewed anti-retrovirals like AZT as a treatment of last resort, after I had exhausted less toxic options, Stephen, who possessed a scientific understanding of pharmacology, was eager to put his body on the line with every anti-HIV drug he could get.

It turned out that Callen and Sonnabend's concerns about AZT were well founded. While it did help many of those who were in the last stages of the disease, it only did so for a few weeks or months. Then the virus developed resistance, mutating to get past the AZT barrier and overwhelming the immune-defenseless body. People who did not have advanced disease were made sicker faster by AZT's toxicity.

Stephen missed much of this debate, which started before he tested HIV-positive in 1988, when he was twenty-one. He knew few people personally who had died from AZT poisoning. My treatment decisions were driven by painful experience and hardened skepticism. Stephen had greater faith in the scientific and medical establishment.

For the most part, we handled our philosophical differences well, but not always. During my campaign for Congress, when I wasn't paying close attention to the business, Stephen accepted an ad promoting HIV testing from Burroughs Wellcome, the company that marketed AZT. Burroughs Wellcome had launched a massive ad campaign that never mentioned AZT or any treatment but urged gay men to contact certain AIDS service organizations to get tested for HIV.

In the mid-'80s, when the HIV test was introduced and especially controversial, I created a mailing for San Francisco's Project Inform that said on the envelope: "There are two ways to find out. 1) Get tested; or 2) Get sick." I opposed the Burroughs Wellcome campaign because it was deceptive. The AIDS service groups recommended in the ad all received funding from Burroughs Wellcome and were friendlier to BW's pro-AZT message than they should have been.

So when I saw the ad, I felt compelled to explain to our readers in the next issue why I opposed the campaign. I didn't blame Stephen; his job was to sell advertising. It was my fault for not reviewing the ads before we went to print. I knew my note would infuriate the advertiser and potentially embarrass Stephen. The advertising agency went ballistic, threatening legal action and saying they would never do business with us again. I knew it might jeopardize our viability—attacking any advertiser isn't a good way to inspire confidence from others—but I felt accountable for what I believed.

The New York Native wrote a news article about my repudiation of the Burroughs Wellcome campaign. People working at AIDS service organizations told me privately that they supported what I said, but they couldn't speak out publicly because their employer was funded by Burroughs Wellcome or was otherwise on board the AZT train.

The episode underscored in stark terms the specter of what we had started to call "AIDS, Inc.," the emerging AIDS establishment defined by the government and the pharmaceutical industry and the agencies they directly or indirectly funded. I didn't expect morality to play a significant role in drug pricing, but I found it shocking that Burroughs Wellcome would promote a powerful chemotherapeutic treatment to people when there was little proof they would benefit from it and considerable evidence that it could harm them.

I never thought "Pharma" hated people with AIDS or was out to kill us; we were seen primarily in terms of opportunity and profit, filtered through the religious biases found in broader society. The real religious and moralistic venom against LGBT people and people with HIV was found in extreme homophobes, such as U.S. Senator Jesse Helms.

*   *   *

By the summer of 1991, ACT UP had an ugly and fierce split between a small group—mostly the members of the treatment and data committee—and everyone else. The drama was played out between the women's committee and the treatment and data committee over issues about whether to cooperate, and in what way, with the federal research agenda.

Many members of ACT UP, including most of those on the women's committee, had a background in other social change movements. They saw the epidemic as inextricably linked with sexism, poverty, addiction, racism, homophobia, and other social ills. They believed ACT UP needed to address the epidemic in that context.

The treatment and data group that split off, mostly Ivy League–educated white men, was more focused on working with the pharmaceutical industry and government regulators to expedite the drug development and approval processes.

I wasn't engaged in the conflict—my ACT UP participation was confined to fund-raising, attending demonstrations, and the weekly meetings—but that summer I was in a house on Fire Island with Peter Staley, who introduced me to ACT UP.

Peter was helping launch the splinter group, Treatment Action Guerrillas (later changed to Treatment Action Group), or TAG, to focus solely on the narrower agenda. His plan was to mark TAG's birth with a spectacular event to capture media attention and give the new group the in-your-face cachet that only civil disobedience, with a dose of humor, can deliver.

U.S. Senator Jesse Helms, the notorious right-wing extremist from North Carolina who had built his career on racism, sexism, and homophobia, was the chosen target. He was responsible for making the United States the only industrialized nation prohibiting travel based on HIV status, bitterly opposing federal financing of AIDS research and treatment, and passing an amendment prohibiting HIV prevention funding for any program construed to "promote" homosexuality. When the mother of Ryan White, the eleven-year-old Indiana boy who died of AIDS, lobbied Congress for AIDS funding, Helms was the only member she approached who refused to see her. He wouldn't even speak to her when she was alone with him on an elevator. There has been no one in public life in the United States who was a greater enemy of people with AIDS than Senator Jesse Helms.

Peter had cooked up a scheme to construct a gigantic "condom" and inflate it over Helms's two-story brick colonial in suburban Arlington, Virginia, just outside of Washington. One of our other housemates was Kevin Sessums, *Vanity Fair*'s top celebrity journalist, who was then Peter's boyfriend. Kevin's friend, music mogul David Geffen, had a house just down the beach. A few days after Kevin told Geffen about the action, Peter was walking on the beach when Geffen walked up and pressed a wad of thirty hundred-dollar bills into his hand. "Be careful," Geffen said.

We had a technical adviser who had worked on civil disobedience campaigns with Greenpeace as well as a mole on Capitol Hill who provided Helms's address. We felt like spies—photographing the house surreptitiously, plotting the action with stopwatches and code words, and enticing the media with an invitation to an event we couldn't reveal in advance. The giant condom—complete with a reservoir tip—was made of parachute material. When it arrived, we took it upstate to a house owned by ACT UP's treasurer Marvin Shulman, in New Paltz. We unfolded it and timed how long it took to inflate using a portable generator and two blowers. On the side of it, we painted: "A condom to stop unsafe politics. Helms is deadlier than a virus."

On September 4, I drove with Peter and a half-dozen TAG members from New York to Virginia. We cruised by Helms's house to make sure the lights were out and no one was home. We spent the night in a budget motel and rose early, pumped with adrenaline. Five of us piled into the enclosed cargo box of a U-Haul truck and rolled the metal door down tight; two others were in the cab of the truck. We each had specific assignments that we had to perform with quasi-military precision. We figured we had only six or seven minutes before the police would arrive.

Reporters and photographers met us at a prearranged spot and followed us to the Helms house on a leafy suburban side street. We jumped out of the back of the truck like jackrabbits, racing to unload an array of equipment and the gigantic bale-shaped compressed condom. We positioned a ladder against the edge of the roof, and Peter and I—the fastest climbers during practice runs—carried the condom up the ladder. It was heavy and unwieldy, and we inched up slowly. As we crawled on the roof unrolling the condom, Dan Baker, my former campaign manager, was in his suit and tie on the front lawn, talking to the media.

A risk with a real condom is that it might fall off the person using it; Peter and I were concerned that *we* might fall off the condom. Some of our crew staked guy wires into the ground and pulled the balloon's fabric corners to fit over the house. Then the blowers kicked into action, powered by a noisy portable generator. The yellow-beige condom sagged lopsidedly as it became tumescent. In under seven minutes, it was fully erect, and we all cheered. It was thirty-five feet tall and covered the entire top and front of Helms's house.

The first police officer on the scene was laughing as she got out of her squad car. "I haven't even had my coffee yet!" she said. When a neighbor alerted her to the fact that it was Helms's home we were covering, she radioed her superiors, and soon the place was covered with more police, media, and neighbors. The generator was noisy, and when a lieutenant arrived, he ordered us to turn it off. As the quiet returned, the condom wilted. The police phoned Helms at his office. He didn't want us arrested, apparently fearing that it would add to the publicity. Instead, the police took down our names, addresses, and driver's license numbers and made us promise to never again set foot in Arlington, Virginia.

The only official citation that day was a ticket for parking the U-Haul truck facing the wrong direction. TAG was off to an auspicious start, although it quickly abandoned guerrilla tactics for more mainstream advocacy. A week later, Helms complained about the stunt on the Senate floor, referring to us as "radical homosexuals," but as Staley later noted, he, "never again proposed or passed a life-threatening AIDS amendment."

CHAPTER 21

Today Is a Good Day

In late winter 1992, I visited my friend Ken Dawson at his Brooklyn home. Ken was one of my first fund-raising clients when he ran SAGE, a group working with LGBT seniors, and later he became a partner in my fund-raising firm. Now he was very sick, just weeks from death. Though he was the ill one, I always left a visit with him feeling like it was I who had been comforted. He had a quiet but authoritative demeanor that reminded me he'd been a high school principal before he became a gay activist.

Ken was gaunt with AIDS-related wasting, his skin the ocher of impending death, his limp hair damp with perspiration. Confined to his bed, he needed assistance to eat, bathe, and go to the bathroom. He was forty-five years old; I was thirty-three.

As I walked into his room, he moved his eyes very slowly toward me. His head trailed his eyes, as though moving faster would cause pain. When I lightly kissed his broad forehead, I felt his fever against my lips. The medicinal smells of antiseptic and skin moisturizer mixed with the stale odor of sweat and the unmistakable stench of bodily decay.

I took a seat on a chair next to his bed and struggled for conversation. Visiting sick friends doesn't get easier with experience. The futility of hope makes typical conversation seem like trifling chatter. Mostly, Ken and I sat in silence. After one long pause, he asked, "Do you remember a few years ago, when we pitched that right-to-die group?"

I remembered it clearly. The AIDS epidemic gave momentum to the so-called right-to-die movement, which advocates for the right of terminally ill patients to have a doctor help hasten their death. We both knew doctors who had broken the law to help patients, friends, or their partners die peacefully. Ken once pleaded with a doctor to increase a dying friend's morphine drip. In fact, the morphine drip as a compassionate and painless way to ease a suffering patient's passage from life to death was an innovation of the AIDS crisis, popularized by nurses on AIDS wards. We had reached out to one of the organizations active in the campaign because we thought our AIDS-related donor database could help them raise money.

Ken's next words came slowly and deliberately. "Do you remember how we said we would want someone to pull the plug if we got terribly ill?"

"Yes," I said softly as my heart leaped into my throat. I thought Ken was about to ask me to do something I wasn't sure I could do. I knew Ken had collected a stash of barbiturates in sufficient quantity to kill himself.

"Well, I am way past the point where I would have thought I wanted to die . . . Wa-a-a-y past it," he said. Then he was quiet, pausing to let his words sink in while he summoned the energy to speak further. "But today is a good day," he went on. "I am glad to see you." He lightly squeezed my hand. "Do you see how beautifully the sun shining through the window reflects on that wall?" He nodded toward the far wall of his bedroom. "I can tell it is a nice day outside. And it is a nice day inside, too." He gave a wan smile. "I never thought I could be so sick and yet still have such a nice day."

Ken had adjusted to his shrinking realm and found that his life was still worth living even as he endured the indignities of helplessness, the agonies of his deteriorating body, and a fear of what lay ahead. It was a revelation to me what constituted quality of life for Ken in those last days.

In retrospect, I think that as younger men we were too casual—even flippant—about the issues confronting those on the verge of death. As a defense against our own anxieties, we had gone so far as to mechanize death linguistically: one "flipped the switch" or "pulled the plug." While gallows humor was our campy culture's inspired response to the otherwise-inassimilable fact of massive death, when we personally witnessed the courage and grace of loved ones in their effort to be alive for their deaths, humor seemed almost a dishonor.

Three years after my visit with Ken, when I became severely ill and was expected to die, I remembered this conversation. I knew I did not want to die in a hospital, and I was sure I would end my own life if the emotional or physical pain became too great. Recalling what Ken had said that day reassured me.

Ken died peacefully in April 1992, the same month that an FDA panel approved the third HIV drug, ddC, about six months after the approval of ddI. Many of us had the same concerns about ddI and ddC that we did about AZT: that the drugs might make people sick who weren't otherwise ill.

Over the next two years, three new HIV drugs came on the market. As I learned more about them, I began to grasp how easy it was for pharmaceutical companies to manipulate the information received by doctors and patients. That prompted me to establish new editorial ground rules for what we published in the CPS *InfoPak* newsletter, such as never making assumptions about any individual's course of either HIV treatment or HIV infection. Conventional wisdoms about treating HIV changed or were proved wrong with regularity, and the disease manifested with great variability. Over time I learned to trust official sources less and people with HIV more.

I also recognized the limitations of the *InfoPak* newsletter: It was dense with text, and the design was dry. I began thinking seriously about producing a different kind of publication, to extend the message of health empowerment, individualized treatment, and all sorts of life issues beyond which HIV drugs to take. Even though I had briefly taken AZT, ddI, and ddC, I considered activism and engagement with other people with HIV my primary treatment strategies. When friends were diagnosed, I told them—with a smile—that "Activists live longer."

By 1992, I was brainstorming with my friend Jeffrey Schaire, editor of *Art and Antiques* magazine, about creating what I was calling "a *People* magazine about AIDS." We were only half serious at first, but the topic came up every time we saw each other. Sometimes other friends were present—writers, photographers, illustrators, or others with publishing experience—and a community sprang up around the idea of the magazine long before I decided to launch it.

Since the start of the epidemic, media coverage of people with AIDS mainly portrayed us as suffering and dying as victims with no possibility of survival. We needed to hear AIDS wasn't necessarily "inevitably fatal," "an incurable terminal illness," "a dreaded disease" with "no survivors."

What I saw in my world was different. Amid inconceivable loss, I was surrounded by people who led productive lives full of courage and hope. We fell in love, pursued careers, opened businesses, raised children, traveled, and went to school. Sometimes the vibrancy of one's life was heightened by the experience of having HIV.

It was that apparent paradox that was so difficult for those "on the outside" to understand.

■   ■   ■

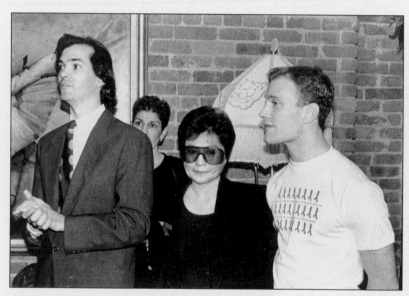

Yoko Ono hosted a benefit performance of *The Night Larry Kramer Kissed Me* on December 4, 1991, to raise money for the Treatment Action Group. That same evening, ABC's *20/20* was airing Barbara Walters's exclusive interview with John Lennon's killer, Mark David Chapman.

CHAPTER 22

The Night Larry Kramer Kissed Me

Before Dan Baker agreed to manage my congressional campaign in 1990, he recruited me to help with an ACT UP talent contest he was producing at the Pyramid Club in the East Village. The show's MC, Ryan Landry, planned on eighteen costume changes between featured talents. Dan assigned me to assist another volunteer dresser backstage to help. "Hi, I'm David Drake," the other volunteer said, smiling and extending his hand. Though I'd never had any role in a theatrical production, backstage or onstage, David patiently showed me what to do.

He was funny and a little bit campy, cracking jokes about the talents and teasing me as I got flustered rushing to be helpful as Ryan changed costumes. Then David said, "I'm next!" and closed his eyes in meditation. He stepped onstage and transformed himself into "Tommy Bobby Sherman," once a "perfect Upper West Side boy," sharing with the audience his evolution into a black leather–jacketed, Doc Martens–wearing, fist-clenched-in-the-air downtown AIDS activist.

I was in awe, watching how perfectly David channeled the activist zeitgeist with the colorful and tender story of his character's politicization. And I related to his character, as I had undergone a similar transformation. When David told me the show was one of a series of performance sketches he had written, I sensed there was an audience for his work beyond the Pyramid.

From late 1990 through 1991, I serialized David's work in my Community Cardpack. Each installment was printed on a postcard-sized insert called "The Tommy Chronicles," with the subtitle "A Short Story in Tiny Type."

David and I became good friends. While he was volunteering on my campaign, we talked about producing an Off-Broadway show based on "Tommy." I had no experience in theater, but rather than deterring me, my ignorance was a spur to try something new. After I lost the election, we organized several workshop performances in 1991 and began production in earnest early in 1992. We wanted to open in June, to coincide with LGBT Pride activities.

David titled the show *The Night Larry Kramer Kissed Me*, a reference to how Larry's play *The Normal Heart* had helped mobilize a generation of gay men, including me, to combat AIDS. Prospective investors, concerned about Larry Kramer's renowned irascibility, feared he would object to the use of his name and sue the production. When I asked Larry for permission, he declined, saying he didn't want anyone to think he was promoting a show with his name in the title. He did agree to attend one of the workshop performances. At an especially emotional point in the play, he got tears in his eyes, and turned to me and said, "There! Are you happy now?" as he daubed his eyes with a handkerchief. Afterward he said he wouldn't bless the use of his name, but he promised not to sue.

The Night Larry Kramer Kissed Me was about the restorative power of activism, telling the story through a series of emotional vignettes in which David recalled his first kiss, the stories of friends who died of AIDS, and Kramer's catalytic work. For young gay men who knew little of what AIDS had done to the gay community in the previous decade, it was an especially valuable message.

We began rehearsals as soon as we signed a lease on the Perry Street

Theatre, in the West Village. I had a lot of fun producing the play; I was lucky to get help from experts, including my friend Tom Viola, who agreed to be the show's associate producer and guide me through the idiosyncrasies of the industry. David's play was perfect for that moment, coinciding with the peak of street activism and the muscular exertion of LGBT political power that helped elect Bill Clinton as president later that year.

The show was a hit, winning Obie and Drama-Logue awards and great reviews. By the time it closed, it was one of the longest-running Off-Broadway one-person shows in the history of New York theater. Later I produced it at the Fort Mason Center in San Francisco—buying signs on the tops of more than a hundred San Francisco taxicabs—and at the Tiffany Theater on Sunset Boulevard in Los Angeles, starring David in both productions.

In the spring of 1992, before the play opened, I had moved my office and residence into an 1840s-era building on West Twelfth Street in Greenwich Village, adjacent to the Meatpacking District. Steep stairs to the third floor opened into a large loft with sandblasted brick walls and a twenty-foot-high ceiling. A giant wooden pulley five feet in diameter hung from the ceiling at one end and a sleeping space was suspended in the middle, accessed by a Victorian cast-iron circular staircase rescued from a firehouse.

The loft became an incubator for all sorts of activism, art, political campaigns, and businesses. My friend Bob Hattoy, who later that year spoke as a gay man with AIDS at the 1992 Democratic convention, described the loft as "like the Warhol Factory, only for activism instead of art." That was a somewhat grandiose appraisal, but I was pleased to accept it, although I never went so far as to wear a white wig.

Just a few weeks after the play opened in June, the Democratic convention was held at Madison Square Garden. For me, it was a far cry from the 1976 convention, when I had been a closeted eighteen-year-old who knew no one, or the 1980 convention, when I thought I knew everyone and everything but had no idea of the pandemic just around the corner.

As disenchanted as I was with partisan politics, having the Democratic convention held in New York that summer—with good friends from around the country attending, including several in key positions—rekindled my interest. In addition to Hattoy's role as a convention speaker, Jean O'Leary and Mario Cooper, respectively, were the chair of the DNC's LGBT caucus and the convention manager.

The four of us, with several others, cohosted a party that gave me a chance to show off the new loft. Four hundred guests, including elected officials, journalists, delegates, and activists mixed in a chaotic, madcap bash, with loud music and dancing, the typical intoxicants, and clusters of conventioneers in every corner. "There are a thousand campaigns under way right now, and that's just in this loft," Jean O'Leary joked.

Having key players from national Democratic politics present underscored how central the LGBT community had become to the national political process. For my part, I was thrilled to see my worlds of LGBT and AIDS activism and Democratic politics coming together. For most of the previous decade, I had felt like I was on two separate tracks that had grown further and further apart. The convention week—and especially that party—brought them together, at least for a while.

Hattoy was a larger-than-life character, politically astute, and outrageously witty, even for a gay man who had a college job working at Disneyland dressed as Donald Duck while sometimes tripping on acid. When he called me, he always began the conversation the same way: "Hey, it's Hattoy, and I was thinking . . ." When it was announced that he had AIDS and would be a speaker at the convention, it was front-page news in every LGBT publication in the country. It felt like a moment of arrival, with someone with AIDS from our community highlighted at a national party convention.

Bob's relationship with the Clintons went back many years. He had been deeply moved by the compassion expressed by the Clintons when he told them he had AIDS. Bill Clinton even promised to make sure Bob would always have health insurance.

Bob's remarks that night left the convention delegates in a frenzy. He was on fire, speaking with passion and authenticity. At one point, he looked into the television cameras and spoke directly to President George Bush: "Mr. President, America has AIDS!" When he closed his comments with the ACT UP anthem, "ACT UP! Fight back! Fight AIDS!," my spirits soared. When Bob arrived at the party at the loft, everyone applauded, as he had, literally overnight, become a symbol of the strength and courage of people with AIDS.

Producers of gay-themed plays seeking commercial success had typically downplayed the gay aspect when marketing to a mainstream audience. Tom Viola and I took a different approach, marketing *The Night Larry Kramer Kissed Me* the same way to mainstream audiences as we did to the LGBT community, without any effort to temper the messaging. All summer long, night after night, leather-jacketed ACT UP boys, Upper East Side socialites, celebrities, and tourists sold out the tiny theater's ninety-nine seats. During the convention, people I knew from Democratic campaigns and friends of friends called to request tickets, which I doled out selectively, as if they were political patronage.

One afternoon I saw two teenage boys standing outside the theatre. I overheard enough of their conversation to realize they wanted to see the show but had enough money for only one ticket. They planned to switch at intermission and were discussing which would see the first half of the show. I offered them a pair of tickets if they would volunteer as ushers that evening.

They were freshmen at Berea College in Kentucky, a progressive school with radical abolitionist roots in a reactionary rural community. They were dating, but not out at school. They had taken the bus to New York as closeted teenagers in love, searching for their community.

They volunteered as ushers for a week and left for Berea and, after having tasted the fruits of New York, they were not only still in love but determined to come out on campus when they got home.

Michael Callen had moved to California—he said he was burnt out after a decade of often-nasty activism of gay men—and never saw the play in New York. But shortly after we opened, he wrote me a note: "I see that you're busy making your boyfriend famous, as I had encouraged you to do. There's nothing quite so erotic as being produced by the one you love!" David and I had gone out only a couple of times, but that was enough for Callen to consider us practically married.

AIDS activism consumed me in the four years after Michael's death and I became stridently intolerant of those I felt were not doing what they could or should. In November 1992, Lou Miano, an advertising executive whom I'd met at a fund-raiser during my congressional campaign, invited me to an elegant dinner party at his apartment on the Upper East Side. When I arrived, a servant took my coat before I was ushered into the living room. There were several men already enjoying drinks; they were older and, I deduced, probably conservative and possibly closeted.

Among the dinner guests was Francis X. Morrissey, Jr., a Harvard-trained attorney who was later disbarred and imprisoned for his role in swindling millions from New York's most prominent socialite philanthropist, Brooke Astor. Then I was introduced to Andrew Napolitano, who had been a judge in New Jersey and later became the senior judicial analyst for FOX News.

A third guest was Robert W. Wilson. I'd never heard of him before that evening; later, I learned he was a billionaire financier. That evening I discovered he was a bigot, offering one ugly comment after another throughout the evening. It started with something anti-Semitic, and Judge Napolitano admonished him, "You can't say things like that!"

Wilson continued to disparage racial minorities and others, even as I and other guests made it clear we were offended. I was so taken aback I wondered if he was drunk or mentally ill.

Over dinner, he started in on people with AIDS. It was a waste to spend so much on AIDS research, he said, because there were more pressing health issues. When he implied people with AIDS deserved what they got, I took the bait and began arguing. It quickly escalated, and his comments became increasingly outrageous. Finally, I lost my temper, slammed my fist down on the table and exploded, saying, "One of these days you'll open *The New York Times* and read that I've died of AIDS. When that happens, I want you to know it is people like you who killed me!"

Everyone at the table froze; the judge's fork stopped halfway between his plate and his mouth. Morrissey stood up and excused himself. The party broke up before we had finished our meal. I was seething. When I left, I went directly to the theater in time to see the end of David Drake's performance. As I listened to the standing ovation, I felt the enormity of the gulf between the youthful, passionate, and creative activism downtown—as in *The Night Larry Kramer Kissed Me*—and the homophobia and denial I frequently encountered uptown. In recent years, Wilson funded an anti-immigration organization the Southern Poverty Law Center labels a "hate group."

I ran into Miano, the host, sometime later and apologized for having ruined his party. He exclaimed, "Ruin it? That was one of the best dinner parties I ever gave! People are still talking about it!"

It wasn't just closeted gay men and homophobes who failed us. With notable exceptions, prominent straight liberals weren't rushing to our side, either. Celebrities who were there early, consistently, and contributed significantly—such as Judith Light, Elizabeth Taylor, Susan Sarandon, and Yoko Ono—earned a revered place in the hearts of people with HIV.

In the fall of 1992, Yoko Ono saw *The Night Larry Kramer Kissed Me*. Sometimes, after an influential person came to the show, I sent him or her a note of thanks, offering complimentary tickets for friends. Yoko wrote back:

> *Dear Sean,*
> *I enjoyed the play tremendously, although "enjoyed" is not quite the word to express my feelings. It was deeply moving and sad as well, even though the wise ending suggested a glimmer of hope. If I could be of any help to promote the play, please feel free to call me. I was going to go backstage to shake hands, pose for a pic, etc., but decided that was too corny, and it might be something you did not want. Meanwhile, you are welcome to pass on the word.*
>
> *Y.*

I responded immediately, asking if she would chair a benefit performance to raise money for the Treatment Action Group, the ACT UP offshoot launched the year before. Her assistant called and we began planning the event. She enlisted Aerosmith's Steven Tyler, *Rolling Stone* magazine's Jann Wenner, and others to join a host committee. I asked Bobby Kennedy and Swen Swenson to join it and both agreed.

The benefit performance sold out quickly. We were already turning people away when ABC started promoting an upcoming episode of *20/20*: Barbara Walters was set to appear with Mark David Chapman in his first television interview since he murdered John Lennon. It was to be broadcast the *same evening* as our benefit. Our phones went crazy with journalists trying to get tickets to the benefit so they could get near enough to Yoko Ono to extract a comment.

I worried that one of those journalists might pick up on the odd coincidence that Yoko was with me, a tangential bystander to her husband's murder, the evening of the broadcast. Afraid she would be caught unaware, I called her assistant to alert him. He was reassuring: "Yoko knows. Don't worry about it, just ignore the press, and we'll have a good event."

The event was a madhouse, with hundreds of people on the street and sidewalk, cameras and autograph books in hand. Yoko was to arrive after the performance, in time for the reception. I opened the door of her black Lincoln Town Car and introduced myself as she got out. She hugged me and clutched my arm while cameras and flashes went off all around us. I escorted her inside and introduced her; she made a few remarks, then I escorted her back to the car. Not an ounce of diva in her. She just wanted to help.

Stumbling upon the shooting of Lennon that December evening in 1980 continued to reverberate through my life in unexpected ways. In the early 2000s, a fanatical conspiracy theorist became convinced that I had been part of a plot to assassinate Lennon. He wrote hundreds of posts on various message boards over the course of several years. Many were crude, anti-Semitic, racist, or homophobic.

At first it was just weird, but then he created web pages for articles he wrote about my supposed role and posted all sorts of personal information, pictures, and other materials related to me, charging that I was an accomplice to Lennon's murder, a CIA plant, and a host of other bizarre claims.

The posts became threatening when he published the addresses of my businesses and incited his readers to "shoot me down in the street" because, according to him, I had shot Lennon. My attorney advised me to file a complaint with the FBI as well as notify the employees at those addresses to be alert to the slim possibility that someone would be inspired by the posts and show up with a gun. Two FBI agents interviewed me and made copies of the posted comments. A few months later, the most inflammatory posts urging harm against me were removed from the web.

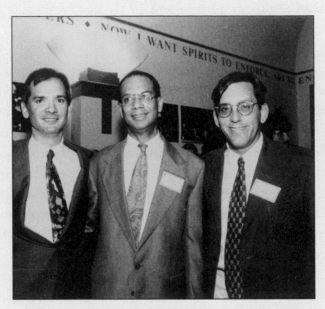

Mario Cooper *(center)* chaired the board of the AIDS Action
Council, the primary lobbying voice on AIDS issues in
Washington, and Bob Hattoy *(right)* was the "Friend of Bill
(Clinton)" with AIDS who spoke at the 1992 Democratic
Convention and worked in the White House. They were our two
best sources inside the Clinton administration.

CHAPTER 23

Ask and Tell

When I was lucky enough to find love, it was usually outside my political and activist circles, with partners who were supportive but whose interests lay elsewhere. After Michael died, I didn't think I had enough of a future to imagine building a new life with someone else. I also felt stigmatized because of my diagnosis; the divide between those who had tested positive and those who were negative was firmly established.

In September 1992, a few months after the play opened, I met Xavier Morales at Zone DK, a gay club in Chelsea. I wasn't looking to date anyone, let alone fall in love. I was just lonely and meandering around late at night, looking for sex. The bar had a dark passageway, and as I walked through, Xavier was leaning against a wall. I didn't know he was there until our bodies brushed and I felt an instant electric attraction. I loved Michael deeply, and it was a love that grew every day we were together. When we met, I thought he was hot, but it wasn't like the magnetic pull and immediate comfort I felt with Xavier even before I saw him in the light. He had a musky, sensual smell and was slender and smoothly muscled. Born and raised in Puerto Rico, he didn't learn his thickly accented English until he was a teenager. He was twenty-nine; I was five years older.

After we ordered beers, I told Xavier that I was HIV-positive, but he didn't seem especially concerned. Later, I found out he didn't know enough about HIV to understand what being positive meant. Xavier was not out of the closet, he lived with his parents in Brooklyn, and English wasn't his native language; it was no surprise that he hadn't learned about HIV.

As we talked at the end of the bar, near the stacks of free publications, I saw a bar magazine, *HX*, which featured a full-page ad for *The Night Larry Kramer Kissed Me* on the back cover. I pointed to the ad and asked Xavier if he had seen the show, thinking I would invite him to a performance. "I didn't like it that much," he said. When I laughed and said I'd produced the play, he was embarrassed. He stammered, telling me that his friend Lawrence, who had taken him, loved it. That gave me an excuse to invite Xavier to my loft: "Would your friend like a copy of the script autographed by David Drake? I've got one at home."

By the time we got into a cab on our way to West Twelfth Street, I was smitten. The sexual attraction was obvious, but on an instinctive level, I was driven to be with Xavier. From almost the instant we met, we felt confident that we could trust the other without question. We were curious about each other's worlds; he knew nothing about politics and had observed gay culture from the distance of the closet. I loved hearing stories of his childhood in rural Puerto Rico, shimmying up trees to pick coconuts and grapefruit, riding a donkey to school, and meeting his father after school at the local cockfights.

Xavier's birthday was the Wednesday after we met, and I sent flowers to his office in the HR department at Bloomingdale's. The next week, I surprised him by dropping by with a voter registration card so that he could cast his first vote ever, for Bill Clinton. Voter registration isn't usually a romantic exercise, but it may have prepared Xavier for what was to come.

*   *   *

When Bill Clinton was elected president in November 1992, many in the LGBT community dared to hope that they and people with HIV would be welcomed into the corridors of power and the government would be responsive to our long-overlooked concerns. Clinton had even mentioned AIDS during his victory speech.

The excitement tanked quickly. Clinton's promise to lift the ban on gay men and lesbians serving in the military turned into the Don't Ask, Don't Tell policy, writing discrimination into law. In 1996, he signed the so-called Defense of Marriage Act, a law he publicly denounced shortly after the Supreme Court overturned it in 2013. Most egregiously in terms of the epidemic, he refused to lift the ban on federal funding of the syringe-exchange programs that dramatically cut HIV transmission among IV drug users.

I felt duped, and I was angry. I knew Clinton was cool with gay people. A decade earlier, I had met him and come out to him. During a break at a 1981 Democratic National Committee meeting in Washington, I was catching up with Tom Higgins, a former Iowa legislator. A handsome man joined our conversation, and Tom introduced us: "Sean, this is Bill Clinton, who was governor of Arkansas until recently."

Clinton held out his hand, and when I shook it, I said something about how he looked too young to be a governor. "Ah'm the youngest *ex*-governor in the country," he quipped back. "Just what I've always wanted."

The three of us talked for a few minutes, gossiping about party politics. I told him about having recently seen Ed Mezvinsky in Denver and shared the news that he was becoming the Pennsylvania Democratic chairman, casually mentioning that I had come out to Mezvinsky as gay. Clinton asked me, "How long have you known?" I told him a little about my past and mentioned how frustrating it had been to keep it a secret when I was working in Kentucky. When we went back to the meeting, Clinton gave me a pat on the back and said, "Don't let the bastards get you down!" When Clinton ran for president, my Community Cardpack was the first LGBT publication to endorse his candidacy.

After the election, there was speculation that Bob Hattoy would be offered a big job in the Interior Department or at EPA. Wanting to work in close proximity to President and Mrs. Clinton, however, he took a lesser job as assistant director of the White House personnel office. It was a great post, and he, as much as anyone other than the president, was responsible for the administration's appointment of so many openly LGBT people. Bob also earned a reputation for speaking his mind to the press, including expressing his disappointment in the administration's poor record on AIDS.

Less than a year into the Clinton presidency, *The New York Times* ran a searing personal essay titled, "Whatever Happened to AIDS?," by Jeffrey Schmalz, an openly gay *Times* reporter who had died of AIDS only three weeks before its publication. Schmalz concluded with bitterness that the issue had quickly disappeared from the national agenda after the election—once it had served its use as a "cause" to attract voters. Hattoy told Schmalz, "I don't think they'll address AIDS until the Perot voters start getting it," referring to the independent swing voters who had given Ross Perot almost 19 percent of the vote in the 1992 presidential election.

This should have been the signal I needed to abandon what little remaining faith I had in party politics. I realize that, not for the first time, my proximity to the powerful—to the center of the action— prevented me from following my conscience and drawing a hard line in the sand like many other AIDS activists. But it wasn't only the seductiveness of power that clouded my judgment. Having worked on campaigns with so many of the political people who came to power in the Clinton administration, I knew them as individuals. Many had suffered their own losses from AIDS and believed they were acting with the best intentions.

*   *   *

Long before we realized what a hit *The Night Larry Kramer Kissed Me* would become, David had accepted a small role in *Philadelphia*, Jonathan Demme's AIDS-themed film starring Tom Hanks and Denzel Washington. We thought the play would be closed by the time the movie was filmed, but we were wrong. The play had been running—and frequently selling out—for over six months when we had to shut it down for a few weeks in January 1993, during the filming of *Philadelphia*.

Reopening a theatrical production after it has gone temporarily dark is high-risk; the momentum can't easily be regained. If we had just shut down, the investors in the play would have recouped their investment, but we decided instead to relaunch the show and see how long we could run. Early in February, David and I were sitting in a diner, talking politics and strategizing about generating publicity for the play's reopening. The gays-in-the-military debate had exploded as one of the first controversies of the Clinton administration, so I suggested we take out a full-page ad in *The New York Times*, urging a repeal of the ban and promoting the reopening of the play. Across the top of a yellow pad, I wrote in big capital letters: "IF YOU'RE STRAIGHT, READ THIS," inspired by a broadsheet distributed at LGBT pride events one year provocatively titled "QUEERS READ THIS."

David and I wrote a demanding argument for repeal, urging readers to contact their members of Congress and engage their family and friends in supporting the National Gay and Lesbian Task Force's effort to lift the ban. The ad copy was forceful:

> Do it for every gay or lesbian soldier sent to the Persian Gulf and then discharged for being gay when they got back . . . Do it for the ⅓ of all teen suicides that are LGBT . . . do it for every gay and lesbian member of your family . . . do it to atone for every fag joke you've ever told . . .

With the word *"fag"* in the text and a headline ordering "straight people" to read it, we weren't sure the *Times* would accept the ad. But they did, and it was a sensation. The phones at my office, home, and the theater box office rang all day with congratulations, press inquiries, and ticket orders. NGLTF received over thirty thousand dollars in donations from about twelve hundred new donors. The ad and our success enraged popular right-wing talk-show host Rush Limbaugh, who waved it in his hand in front of TV cameras and railed against gay activists.

The ad cost about twenty thousand dollars, far more than we could spend for promotion, but the text was so strong that I thought maybe we could recruit others to help pay for it. I faxed it to several people asking for help, and Yoko Ono, David Geffen, Swen Swenson, Marvin Shulman, and several other friends all quickly agreed to contribute a thousand dollars each toward the cost. Most of the ad was the text of our screed, but at the bottom we included a cutout coupon for donations to the National Gay and Lesbian Task Force. We also had the announcement about the reopening of the show and along the very bottom of the ad, in mouse type, we listed the names of the people who had helped pay for it.

Two of the names were Xavier's and mine. In the four months since we met, we had become a couple, without much discussion. We just found that we liked spending time with each other more than with anyone else.

When I asked if he wanted to be listed with me on the ad, I needed to make sure he realized the potential ramifications. "This is *The New York Times*—the whole world will see it," I said. He wasn't out at work or to his family, but he was certain. "I'm ready," he said. That was how Xavier came out to his parents, by showing them his name in *The New York Times*. It could not have been easy for them, but once they knew, they accepted me with love.

Soon afterward, Xavier quit his Bloomingdale's job and began working at my company just as I was starting to launch *POZ*. He started Christopher & Castro, a mail-order business we promoted through the cardpacks, marketing gift items and club wear for gay men that Xavier designed and had manufactured in New York's garment district. The happiest time I had with Michael was during the six months before he died, when he quit his job and we were working on the antiques shop together. I regretted not having encouraged him to do that sooner; with Xavier, and with my own future uncertain, I didn't want to waste any time.

I now had an emotional intimate, someone I trusted without question and believed would be my partner for the rest of my life. Knowing Xavier would care for me if I got sick made me less fearful; in our years together, there has rarely been a time when we weren't each other's first priority. That security enabled me to think optimistically about the future in a way I hadn't been able to since Michael's death.

The fund-raising business, cardpacks, and Community Prescription Service were also doing well, which made it possible for me to think more seriously about the magazine concept. I started talking about it with journalists, publishers, activists, and friends. Few understood what I had in mind, but the process of trying to explain it helped me crystallize the idea and gave me resolve.

I spoke about the magazine to my old friend and mentor Alan Baron, who was as smart and strategic as anyone I knew—about everything except his own life and health. Our conversations took place while he reclined in a hospital bed after having had his leg amputated due to complications from diabetes.

He still had his sense of humor and gave me good advice, even though he pretended to be dismayed that I was "giving up" my short-lived theater-producing career for publishing. He loved musical theater, and I often accompanied him to shows when he was in New York. "I was looking forward to starring in your next show! I can't be a song-and-dance man anymore, but I can be a song man!" he joked.

The last time I saw him was in September 1993, right around the time I started working in earnest on the first issue of *POZ*. He was in George Washington University Hospital in Washington, and when I got to his room, PBS political analyst Mark Shields was visiting as well. Though Alan had introduced me to Mark previously, I felt awkward being in Alan's hospital room at the same time. Mark was a straight, old-line Catholic Democrat who had little inkling of Alan's gay life. We shared great affection for our mutual friend, however, as well as the certainty that as soon as he left the hospital, Alan would probably contact his coke dealer, if he didn't already have a stash under his hospital gown.

At one point, Alan looked from me to Mark and back with a knowing twinkle in his eye. "You Irish Catholics!" he announced. "You never give up on someone, do you? Is it because you believe in redemption, or are you just really good people?" Alan proceeded to detail the long list of friends who had "abandoned" him over the years—sorting them by religious affiliation. Ever the analyst, Alan neatly deduced that his Catholic friends had stuck with him long after his addictions had driven away his friends who were Protestants, Jews, or nonbelievers. "What would I have to do for you to abandon me?" he asked us in all seriousness.

I never abandoned Alan—he died a few weeks later at age fifty, from diabetes-related complications—but his passage marked the death of my first real mentor, as well as of a close friend. It also marked a final severing of my strongest tie to Washington, and to the Democratic Party establishment. I started looking elsewhere—among people who were driven by real causes, rather than by partisanship or politics per se—to satisfy my lifelong political itch.

CHAPTER 24

Launch

As a kid, I plastered my black Schwinn one-speed bike with daisy-shaped blue-and-white "Gene McCarthy for President" stickers. I was as captivated by politics as I was by the half cent my father paid me per mousetrapped mouse.

Most of my life, I have been interested in both business and activism, even when it has been morally and financially tricky navigating between them. The middle space I straddled sometimes left others unsure whether I was fish or fowl, activist or capitalist. Business partners occasionally questioned whether my decisions were in the interest of business or to advance my political agenda. Some activists resented a for-profit business within the movement, and when I was raising money for GMHC and ACT UP I was criticized—generally behind my back—for "exploiting," even "getting rich on," activists and PWAs. Even though that criticism rarely came from people with AIDS, I was sensitive to it. I tried to take pride in what our work made possible, rather than feel the pain of personal criticism

I had to laugh, however, at the perception some had of me as "rich." I bought a restaurant when I was nineteen for $7,500, the contract executed on a paper napkin, and later I got lucky with a few real estate investments.

But I've never been a saver, and after I was diagnosed, I spent what I had accumulated to that date, mostly to launch *POZ*. It was my mortality that gave me the freedom to take financial risks and invest in the LGBT and HIV/AIDS communities. Vito Russo used to tell me that to be a successful lifelong activist, I needed to have some financial security; he said he regretted not having focused more on that goal when he was young.

I've also had friends, including some who are affluent, who have supported the causes and projects I've been involved with over the years, as both donors and investors. In retrospect, I think "campaigning"—whether for myself, others, or a greater good—is my natural mode of being.

I'm proud that many people with HIV and gay men learned practical, detailed information they needed to stay alive from the twelve million fund-raising letters that my firm produced for AIDS-related clients in the late '80s and early '90s. Those fund-raising letters reached more gay men than any gay community publication at the time; for some who didn't read LGBT media, or live in big cities, our fund-raising letters were an important connection to a community.

With the fund-raising business, the cardpacks, producing the play, *POZ,* and other enterprises, I used for-profit endeavors to pursue a political agenda. My life had become consumed with a mission rather than a quest for a career, always shadowed by the likelihood that I would die of AIDS. Once the epidemic had been around me but not of me. Then it became of—and *in*—me, though I fought to keep it from defining me. By the early '90s, it was impossible to separate any part of my life from HIV. There were few distinctions between my personal and professional lives; it is no surprise some found that concerning.

The epidemic, and specter of my own death, was a constant presence, precluding any long-term plans beyond the next demonstration, fund-raiser, or funeral, but at the same time it also energized me with purpose and projects. Ironically, as my health was starting to fail, I was still starting new businesses.

AIDS spawned a "viatical settlement" industry that speculated with the life insurance policies of those who were defined as terminally ill and expected to die soon. Instead of the policy's death benefit going to a designated beneficiary or the deceased's estate, the policyholder could sell it while he or she was alive, at a discount calculated based on expected longevity, and receive the cash to use as they pleased.

I had two policies, one from Chubb and another issued by New York Life, with a combined death benefit of $450,000. The viatical company required my medical records for a doctor to analyze, an extensive questionnaire, and a visit to their doctor before they made me an offer. I sold the policies for $345,000 and used the proceeds, along with my savings and credit card advances, to launch *POZ*. Not everyone close to me thought it was such a great idea; there was even some concern from friends and family that I was suffering AIDS-related dementia.

The idea of a glossy lifestyle magazine for people with AIDS was not universally well received. But I was sure as soon as we produced it, the doubters and naysayers would understand. Before he read the first issue, Leonard Goldstein, a gay neocon political columnist for the *New York Native*, said that people with AIDS starting a magazine called *POZ* was like Holocaust victims starting a magazine called *GAZ*. A joke making the ACT UP rounds was that *POZ* would feature fashion spreads of what to wear at your own funeral.

I initially titled the magazine "Life Plus," but when I received a letter from an attorney for Time-Life claiming that it violated their trademark, we went back to the drawing board. One day I was talking with my friend Matt Levine about someone we'd both recently met; he inquired about the person's HIV status, asking, "Is he a pozzie?" "That's it: *POZ*!" I said. "We'll call the magazine *POZ*!"

Initially, the name required explanation, as people didn't understand that it was a less clinical way of saying "HIV-positive," as well as a double entendre for thinking or acting positively, which was a big part of the magazine's message. The word "poz" has since entered the vernacular.

Our initial business model relied on a mix of subscriptions and advertising; this, too, raised doubts. One trade publication made a crack about readers not living long enough to renew subscriptions. Sam Watters, owner of *The Advocate*, told *Ad Age* that he doubted the prospects for *POZ:* "What advertiser would want to advertise in a magazine on such a grim topic?"

I envisioned *POZ* as a general-interest magazine reflecting the way we lived our lives with AIDS—pursuing careers, falling in love, raising our children, everything life entails—not just the death and dying that defined us in mainstream media. *POZ* would look at the entire world— politics, economics, culture, fashion, and arts—through the prism of the epidemic. We weren't afraid of humor, either, inspired in part by our friends who founded *Diseased Pariah News*, a zine for people with AIDS. We would skip the insider jargon of treatment wonks and the stereotypical victimization of people with HIV. Activist rhetoric had created a vocabulary that mapped out the political dimensions of the epidemic as a function of homophobia and created a language for people with HIV to identify with community, empowerment, resistance, and pride. The urgency of the epidemic had forced an unprecedented level of honesty when talking about sex, within the LGBT community and society at large, which was reflected in *POZ*.

POZ also translated complicated science and factors that affected treatment decision-making into messages our readers could understand, even while that science was changing rapidly. In 1994, the year *POZ* started, the FDA was still approving HIV medications for monotherapy (a single-drug treatment), but within two years, triple-combination therapy (three different anti-retroviral drugs) was the gold standard and monotherapy was considered dangerous.

We tried to tell the story of the epidemic in all its complexities, through the experience of those living with HIV. And we would do so in an attractive, engaging, and hopeful format. On glossy paper.

To launch *POZ,* I knew I needed help. I scoured my Rolodex and reached out to a wide-ranging roster of contributors, especially those who had articulated or depicted the rich and sophisticated discourse the AIDS community had created in the culture to deal with the epidemic. We encouraged them to write about what interested them the most. Some were well established, even famous, others were unknown, and we provided their first byline in a national outlet. Writers such as David Feinberg, Kiki Mason, Scott O'Hara, and others could take uncommon risks and express powerful emotions, as they knew they were approaching the end of their lives.

We never needed surveys or focus groups to figure out what to write about. I discouraged framing an editorial pitch in terms of what our readers "wanted." I was convinced that if we wrote in a truthful way about what was important and interesting, our readers would find us. Many of the best ideas for articles came in over the transom from readers. I read every unsolicited inquiry, because I wanted readers to feel a sense of ownership, and it kept us in better touch with what people with HIV experienced in their daily lives. We told the story of the epidemic through the experience of those who had the disease. Medical and other experts were secondary.

Xavier had moved in with me early in 1993, and he was integral to the magazine's launch in 1994, creating and maintaining the initial database of subscribers and contributing to editorial and marketing discussions. Calls to the magazine rang on our bedside phone after hours, so we took subscription calls late at night, but often there were calls from people newly diagnosed, concerned parents, or frightened partners wanting information or someone to talk to.

We sometimes went to bed while staff members were working late into the night. As the company grew, we took over the entire building—three floors plus the sleeping loft—as well as part of an adjacent building and a small space around the corner on Fourteenth Street.

There was little division in those days between the private lives Xavier and I led and our work with the magazine; the same was true for many of our staff members. There was never any concern about people showing up late or leaving early. For the next several years, nothing else in our lives matched the urgency and importance of what we believed we were doing with *POZ*.

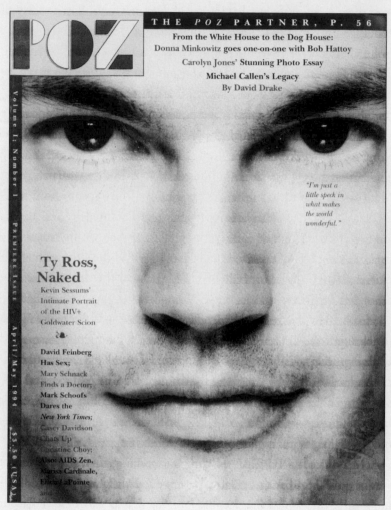

THE *POZ* PARTNER, P. 56

From the White House to the Dog House:
Donna Minkowitz goes one-on-one with Bob Hattoy

Carolyn Jones' Stunning Photo Essay

Michael Callen's Legacy
By David Drake

Volume I; Number I   PREMIERE ISSUE   April/May 1994 $3.50 (USA)

POZ

"I'm just a
little speck in
what makes
the world
wonderful."

Ty Ross,
Naked
Kevin Sessums'
Intimate Portrait
of the HIV+
Goldwater Scion
ࠂ

David Feinberg
Has Sex;
Mary Schnack
Finds a Doctor;
Mark Schoofs
Dares the
New York Times;
Casey Davidson
Chats Up
Christine Choy;
Also: AIDS Zen,
Marisa Cardinale,
Ellen LaPointe
and

The first issue of *POZ* featured an interview Kevin Sessums conducted with Ty
Ross, the HIV-positive grandson of former Republican presidential nominee Barry
Goldwater, photographed by Greg Gorman. Sessums and Gorman both were
important early supporters of (and shareholders in) *POZ*.

CHAPTER 25

Firsts

When the first issue of *POZ* hit newsstands and mailboxes around the country in April 1994, I was sick with a mild case of pneumocystis carinii pneumonia (PCP). The stress leading up to the launch caught up with me, and I was confined to my bed. But that didn't lessen my excitement and pride in our first issue.

Kevin Sessums, *Vanity Fair*'s top celebrity interviewer at the time, wrote the cover story, profiling Ty Ross, a fetching young gay man with HIV. What made Ty a cover candidate was his famous grandfather, Barry Goldwater, the conservative 1964 Republican nominee for U.S. president. We flew Kevin to Los Angeles to spend several days with Ty, and they hit it off so well that they became intimate with each other. Sessums, who was HIV-negative, wrote beautifully about the encounter, using it to explore the common but mostly irrational fear of having sex with people with HIV.

Kevin was already well known, and Ty's famously conservative Republican grandfather was as far removed from the popular impression of AIDS as he could be. That, combined with Kevin's writing and the peculiarity of a magazine for people with a "terminal illness," made for a perfect media storm. Sexy photos of Ty, taken by Hollywood photographer Greg Gorman, only added to the news appeal.

Kevin was criticized from some quarters for sleeping with his interview subject, but the profile was a masterful first-person account that I was proud to present. I wanted *POZ* to directly confront the popular notion that people with HIV should never have sex again after their diagnosis; a profile of someone attractive and detailing his encounter with someone who did not have HIV was perfect.

We also profiled Tom Keane in that first issue, reflecting on his role at the St. Patrick's Cathedral demonstration when he "snapped the cracker." Donna Minkowitz interviewed Bob Hattoy about the Clinton White House. David Feinberg wrote the first sex column, and David Drake contributed a tribute to Callen, who had died a few months earlier. Mark Schoofs contributed a media column about coverage of AIDS in *The New York Times*; he went on to win a Pulitzer Prize for his AIDS coverage in the *Village Voice* and subsequently covered the epidemic for *The Wall Street Journal*. Our first editor, Richard Pérez-Feria, was up-and-coming in the industry and recommended to me by Sessums. Pérez-Feria enlisted veteran magazine designer, J. C. Suares, who created a striking visual identity for the magazine, with lush photography and illustration.

When I got sick as the first issue was coming off-press it marked a new phase in my relationship with Stephen. He was taking an ever growing amount of responsibility in my company, but we had never specifically addressed what would happen in the event that I was incapacitated or died and whether Stephen was a candidate to take over.

When I got PCP, he wrote me an uncharacteristically emotional letter. "I feel as though I've been in shock for the last two hours, and my hands haven't stopped shaking," he began. "I'm very concerned about you and, although I don't often express it, I care for you very much . . . I want to let you know how happy I've been working with you over the last four years. I just can't imagine working anywhere else . . ." His letter meant a lot to me, especially hearing that he was there for the long haul. As his commitment became clear, the dynamic between us became more like a partnership.

I got over the PCP in a few weeks and, by early summer, was again working long hours. I thought it unlikely that I would live to see the magazine to profitability, but I was determined to be around long enough to see it earn respect. I was looking for respect as well: I wanted my work and role as an activist to be as widely recognized as my work as an entrepreneur.

The media response to the launch was overwhelmingly positive. Frank Rich, in his *New York Times* column, said *POZ* was "easily as plush as Vanity Fair" and "against all odds, the only new magazine of the year that leaves me looking forward to the next issue." *POZ* quickly became a player in the national discourse on AIDS, often as a watchdog but sometimes as a provocateur. With our skeptical treatment philosophy, we broke news about drug side effects, the emergence of resistant viruses, and the suppression of those developments by drug companies. With our ear to the ground in the gay community, we were the first national media to use the word and report on the "barebacking" phenomenon, cover prevention strategies beyond condoms, and write about the crystal-meth addiction that was fueling a rise in HIV infections. We exposed the public health message that women could easily pass the virus to men as a myth. Also, by giving visibility to individuals with "star" potential—people with HIV doing groundbreaking work— we helped advance careers in activism, health policy, and the arts, and create a new generation of AIDS leadership.

Some critics argued that *POZ* presented people with HIV in such a positive light—and in such a visually appealing format—that we were "glamorizing" having the disease. Some even accused us of making HIV seem desirable. Others accused us of making the use of condoms less urgent, or leading readers to become less compassionate about people with HIV or less generous in their charitable support. There was admittedly an inherent dichotomy between empowering people with HIV—letting them know they had full lives to lead—and fear-based

...vention messaging, which heightened stigma and depicted HIV as the worst thing that could possibly happen to a person. Every time we profiled someone with HIV who was good-looking, successful, happy, or optimistic, some saw it as undercutting that dire message. But that criticism seldom came from people with HIV. Survey research showed that *POZ* readers trusted the magazine more than they did AIDS organizations, other media, even their own doctors. They recognized the truth in our treatment coverage. We weren't trying to manipulate them to choose one path or another, only to share with them the informed decisions and experiences—successful or not—of other people with HIV.

Our style guidelines helped maintain this trust. The first person we quoted in an article was usually a person with HIV; doctors, scientists, and elected or government officials came later. I also discouraged the use of pseudonyms, because they implied it was shameful for a person with HIV to be identified by name; we also banned the use of stock photography in favor of real people with HIV.

Most important, our approach to the treatment of HIV and other medical conditions was an extension of the principles established in the CPS *InfoPak*: informed skepticism to conventional wisdoms and alertness to alternative options employed by trusted doctors and people with HIV. Give readers all the tools to make treatment decisions with confidence for themselves. We never assumed either the course of the progression of the disease or the course of treatment, if any, a person with HIV might choose.

Editorial meetings were the most rewarding part of running the magazine. I wanted to hear different opinions—to learn about the other side of any issue—and I enjoyed the vigorous back-and-forth as we debated editorial priorities. I was proud when, in 1997, *POZ* was a National Magazine Award finalist for General Excellence.

Walter Armstrong, our editor in chief from 1998 to 2005, had been a member of ACT UP and a veteran of *Outweek* and *QW*, two New York gay newsweekly magazines, and had cofounded AIDS Prevention Action League (APAL) with Stephen. He brought an irreverent yet critical style to the magazine that reflected the rich language that had developed in the culture to cope with AIDS. He invited some of the most daring LGBT writers in San Francisco and New York to write about sex and AIDS, including provocative and thoughtful sex radicals such as Pat Califia and Scott O'Hara. O'Hara died from lymphoma as he and Walter were going over the last corrections for his article on lymphoma treatment ("Out on a Lymphoma"). Walter was moved when Scott's last e-mail to him expressed gratitude to him and *POZ* for providing an opportunity for him to write about issues important to him in the last year of his life.

Walter and I didn't know each other in ACT UP. We met initially through Stephen, who had hired him to write for the CPS *InfoPak* newsletter. We shared similar backgrounds, which strengthened our connection, especially when we discovered that his Haverford college roommate was a childhood friend of mine from Iowa. But it was our differences that created a complementary balance. I was as off-the-cuff and intuitive as he was careful and considered. I am comfortable as a public person; he avoided that kind of visibility. He has a refined literary sensibility and brought fiction and more poetry to the magazine; I wrote fund-raising solicitations and was a news junkie. We worked together closely, but Walter wasn't dependent upon me for ideas or direction. Like Stephen, he relished the independence and autonomy that my company offered. My style is to envision a project, get it started, and then find brilliant people—people I admired and could learn from—to take the reins and run with it. That didn't always work, as sometimes I gave people too much responsibility with too little direction, but with Walter and others at *POZ*, it worked brilliantly.

My monthly SOS columns were made more eloquent and meaningful with Walter's editing and, in the process, he inspired me to think more critically about the epidemic, the magazine's responsibility, and our readers' wants and needs. He has sometimes characterized me as a mentor to him, which I find flattering, but the truth is we had—and continue to have—a mutual mentorship. He rarely has gotten the credit he deserved for the magazine's successes, partly because of his innate modesty and distaste for the spotlight, but also because of his HIV negative status. He made new innovations in prevention emerging from the gay community an important part of the magazine, which helped us establish credibility and an audience beyond just our HIV positive readers. Understanding the relationship between people who had HIV and those who did not was at the core of what many found so meaningful, inspiring, and even disturbing about *POZ*. Suares and a number of the editors—Richard Pérez-Feria, Esther Kaplan, Laura Whitehorn, Lauren Hauptman, Sally Chew, Bob Lederer, and others— and business staff central to the magazine's success, including my sister Megan, were all HIV negative, but profoundly affected by AIDS. One of our staff members was a young woman who had lost both her parents to AIDS, though few in the office knew it.

One of the most popular features of *POZ* in the early years was a monthly column about my own health and treatment. We published my lab test results and solicited opinions from doctors about my treatment choices. My health had been in steady decline, offering a range of interesting predicaments to be covered, including my vanishing CD4 cells and the various opportunistic infections commandeering my body.

I've never been particularly adept with science and, like most PWAs, I always struggle to understand the confusing numbers and odd vocabulary in my medical reports. The column helped demystify the arcana of med-speak for our readers. Experts often disputed the meaning of the numbers on our reports. One doctor would say, "What Sean needs to do is X" and another, "Whatever Sean does, he shouldn't do X." Readers learned a lot about X by being able to listen in on such a conversation and understand how smart, well-informed doctors could disagree with each other. *The New Yorker* called the series "one of the strangest columns in American journalism: a page reproducing, with commentary, the latest lab report analyzing its publisher's blood."

As I grew sicker, the column became a serialized mystery: Is that persistent cough serious? Will they find the cause of Sean's fevers? How will he handle the pancreatitis? How low can his CD4 cells go? Will Sean die?

*   *   *

During these first years of the magazine, Xavier and I hosted a series of dinners to help shape *POZ*'s editorial direction and attract advertiser support. We would invite fifteen to twenty people to our loft: a mix of AIDS activists, contributors to the magazine, pharmaceutical executives, ad agency staff, interesting friends, visiting cousins, anyone we thought might learn from or add to the conversation. We'd usually serve catered lasagna and Caesar salad, and eat with plates on our laps. After a casual conversation during dinner, we'd pass around a plate of homemade brownies, and Stephen or I would lead an after-dinner conversation, encouraging frank discussions of timely and controversial topics.

Sometimes there were arguments, as when Larry Kramer's passionate rhetoric—typically peppered with words such as "genocide," "murder," and "greed"—fueled heated retorts. Guests from ad agencies or pharmaceutical companies, unaccustomed to that kind of direct confrontation, were sometimes shocked or offended, but they were generally eager for a return invitation.

At one of these dinners in the fall of 1994, right after the Republican sweep of the midterm congressional elections, the topic was how Republican control of Congress might result in cutting the research budget at the NIH. Stephen sat next to Larry Kramer, dozing. Every once in a while, Larry's dog, Tiger, would jump up on the couch, and Stephen's eyes would flutter open.

Larry provocatively suggested that if the Republicans slashed the NIH budget, we might be better off, noting that the NIH had never produced a cure for a major disease. That prompted a lively discussion about one of the newer concerns, the potential development of virus that was resistant to all anti-retroviral drugs. When someone suggested we needed to do more research of our own, Stephen perked up.

"I get laughed at about this by people in TAG," he began, referring to the Treatment Action Group. "But I get this sense that if I could have access to every drug that exists right now, and really good virological tests to measure their effects on me, I could significantly improve my immune system. I think there are lots of drugs that have been discarded because they developed resistance too quickly as single-agent uses."

At the time, seven or eight anti-retroviral drugs had been introduced, but each became ineffective after a period of use because the virus mutated and became resistant. Stephen—the math whiz—explained that using several of them at the same time would reduce the statistical likelihood of viral resistance. "If I could take all of them starting tomorrow, a year from now my T-cells [a measure of immune strength] would be back close to normal," Stephen said.

Less than a year later, a new class of drugs used in triple-combination therapy turned an almost certain death sentence into a chronic but manageable illness for those able to access treatment. People who had developed drug-resistant HIV were soon taking combinations of four, five, or six anti-retroviral drugs, just as Stephen envisioned.

Many of the epidemic's most important developments relating to HIV prevention or treatment—including safer sex, prophylaxis against pneumocystis pneumonia, recognition of pharmaceutical side effects, treatment as prevention, pre- and post-exposure prophylaxis—did not come from the scientific and medical establishment but from people with HIV and a handful of community doctors who were also trained as scientists. Their innovations were usually based in some part on anecdotal evidence, but it only makes sense that the people who were taking the drugs, and those who were trying to protect themselves from infection, and their doctors, would be the first to identify problems and experiment with possible solutions.

Michael Callen used to say there was "a special magic in the room" whenever a group of people with AIDS got together. Because our lives were at stake, we generally did our best to share what we were learning without judgment, without personalizing our arguments, without any agenda except to learn.

POZ was a way for people with HIV to get together, in its pages, every month. We did our best to facilitate that special magic.

* * *

The first year of publishing *POZ* was one of the most exciting of my life, despite my failing health. My T-cells should have been around a thousand but were plunging into single digits. But what I lost in T-cells, I made up for in adrenaline. I worked constantly. Even when I was sick for days in bed, I sometimes padded down the iron circular staircase to the office in my slippers and bathrobe. I was never too tired to talk about a good story idea, be interviewed by a reporter, or meet a prospective contributor.

When the early copies of each issue arrived by FedEx direct from the printer, everything in the office stopped. The staff would gather as we tore open the box with the anticipation of six-year-olds on Christmas morning. We each grabbed a copy and settled in to read it even as the deadline for the next issue loomed.

With each passing week, however, climbing the stairs to the loft was more difficult as my balance became uncertain and my strength ebbed; I had to grip the handrail tightly and lift my body slowly from one step to the next. My afternoon naps were more frequent and longer. Sometimes staffers came to my bedroom to discuss matters with me while I was half-dozing.

My glee about publishing *POZ* was tempered by a growing awareness of my mortality. My finances also worried me. I had bankrolled the launch of *POZ* with my savings and proceeds from the sale of my life insurance polices, and now I had put my weekend house on the market, to invest those proceeds in the magazine. I was running out of money and time.

Advertising revenue was far below what we'd expected; after the first couple of issues, most gay community advertisers left us because they weren't interested in paying to market to people with HIV who weren't gay. But we knew some pharmaceutical companies were developing direct-to-consumer advertising campaigns for anti-retroviral drugs. Megan's schedule was packed with meetings with advertising agencies and pharmaceutical marketing staff. She was optimistic that those ads were coming.

They weren't coming fast enough. Something had to be done to avoid a cash crisis, and I thought I had a solution. Richard Pérez-Feria, J. C. Suares, and George Slowik, whom I had hired as the company's chief operating officer, approached me about buying *POZ* and the card-pack business. I negotiated a deal with them privately, saddened to sell the magazine but relieved that it would be in the hands of people who cared deeply about it and could ensure its future beyond my lifetime. The sale was announced at a party commemorating the magazine's first anniversary.

Xavier had designed and sewn a black collarless linen suit for me to wear to the party. I may have been frail and fatigued, but he made sure I looked stylish. After thanking our hosts and the long list of people critical to the magazine's successful first year, I broke the news about the sale, and the crowd gasped in surprise. *The New Yorker*'s "Talk of the Town" column covered the party and noted the intended sale in its May 1, 1995, issue.

A few weeks later, when the deal fell through over a disagreement on terms, I was back at square one. I had already run up over sixty thousand dollars on my credit cards and was struggling to meet each payroll and printing bill.

I finally sat down with Megan, Xavier, and Stephen. I wanted to find a solution, and they needed to weigh in with total honesty, not just a reflexive show of support to please a dying man they loved.

"We've got just enough for a couple more payrolls if we continue as we are now," I told them. "That means we either plan an orderly shutdown—which we can do without shame and with our heads held high—or we need a Plan B." I didn't want to leave the three most important people in my life in the lurch, and I didn't want them to have to deal with shutting down the magazine after I died; I wanted that to happen under my direction and when I could explain the decision to our readers.

Megan's eyes were tearful; her pride in *POZ* equaled my own. She was an amazing salesperson and had become part of her clients' lives, remembering their birthdays and the names of their children while also understanding their marketing objectives, and helping them navigate the complicated AIDS world. She was the first to speak up. "We've got to stick with it," she said. "The advertising is coming. I know it is."

Megan told us that several pharmaceutical companies were developing advertising campaigns created solely for *POZ*. They had to be approved by the advertiser's legal department and then go to the FDA for review.

Stephen spoke next. "There are lots of things we can do around the office to cut costs," he said. "We could save a lot if we don't print as many copies, or we could go to cheaper paper or even skip an issue or two."

Xavier's eyes went back and forth between Megan and Stephen, occasionally glancing my way to judge how I was reacting. In those days, he wasn't as confident with his English or his opinions; he often was silent at meetings, and then shared his thoughts later with me.

I agreed that whatever we decided, we were going to be open with our readers about the financial difficulties the magazine faced. "We know they'll understand a struggle for survival," I said, happy to hear Megan and Stephen speak so passionately about continuing to publish.

Xavier and I talked late that night. When I said I didn't want to leave him destitute after I died, he chastised me: "You have to do what your heart tells you. I got along just fine before we met, and I'll be fine after you're gone."

When the four of us reconvened the next day, we made some rapid-fire decisions. Stephen held a printing bill in his hand. "I looked at these bills, and if we go to forty-pound stock paper, we'll save about six thousand dollars per issue."

"We can cut the press run to a hundred thousand," I chimed in. "And let's see how much we would save if we cut the trim size."

Megan said that an account rep friend at an ad agency, who worked with one of our bigger advertisers, told her that if we could give them a 10 percent discount, she'd ask her client to pay in advance for a year's advertising. "That would bring in some cash quickly," she said.

We slashed the freelance editorial budget and imposed a moratorium on all noncritical expenditures. We made a long list of prospective investors, starting with major publishing companies (Time Warner, Condé Nast, and Rodale), super-rich LGBT people to whom we had connections (David Geffen, Barry Diller), and friends, ex-partners, relatives, and acquaintances we thought might be candidates for modest investment.

In retrospect, it's extraordinary that Stephen, Megan, and I were able to raise any money at all, considering I was emaciated, frail, and starting to sprout lesions that reminded people of Tom Hanks's character in *Philadelphia*. Stephen didn't look as sick as I did, but everyone knew he had HIV and that he and Megan were in their twenties, with little business experience. When I talked to prospective investors about Year 1, Year 2, and Year 3 in our financial projections, I'm sure people were skeptical that I'd live to see them.

We were fortunate to have several friends and strong supporters of *POZ*, including an executive at Johnson & Johnson and Linda Meredith, an ACT UP pal who was a consultant to pharmaceutical companies, who used their positions to direct funding to *POZ* that was instrumental in keeping us in operation.

The new investors were mostly personal friends. One said he figured that if I were to live a normal life span, perhaps another fifty years, he might buy me dinner twice a year. He estimated the cost of dinner twice a year for fifty years and invested that amount.

Megan pushed advertising sales harder than ever. Years later, one advertiser told me, "It was like the magazine became a metaphor for you, Sean. As long as she could keep the magazine alive, it was like she was keeping you alive. It was tough to resist someone's kid sister so passionately pitching pages for her dying brother's magazine."

Stephen and I drafted an updated business plan, and our lawyer created offering documents; our goal was to raise $950,000. The operational savings and prepayment for advertising bought us a little time, but it was a tense three-way race between my dwindling bank account, Megan's advertising sales, and the search for outside investors.

I went through a list of contractors, consultants, and contributors, identifying those with whom we might trade small pieces of equity in the company in exchange for services. Some were friends, such as writers Kevin Sessums and Hal Rubenstein, photographer Greg Gorman, and political consultant Ethan Geto, and they quickly agreed. The owner of the company that managed our database said he had "never seen a group of people work harder or with more dedication to make a company successful"; he took a piece of equity in exchange for a year's worth of services.

We had a lucky break when my house in Piermont sold. I spent the money on the magazine and to buy a smaller house in nearby Palisades. I didn't want Xavier going through the trauma of my death and, at the same time, needing to move; he could afford the smaller house on his own.

Stephen, Megan, and I went on the road to find investors from August 1995 through the end of the year. We started with a dinner for prospective investors at the West Village town house of Enrico Marone Cinzano, heir to the Cinzano aperitif fortune, cohosted by AmFAR's Mathilde Krim. Photographer Greg Gorman hosted a similar event for prospective investors at his stylish studio in Los Angeles. We made presentations in Iowa City, Detroit, Philadelphia, and Washington, D.C.

We drove to Emmaus, Pennsylvania, to make a presentation to Ardeth Rodale, owner of Rodale, Inc., a huge publishing company focused on health and wellness. Their titles include *Men's Health* and *Prevention*.

We knew Ardeth had been affected by the epidemic—her only son had died of AIDS—and she was known to be independent and caring. She greeted us warmly. Stephen and I were men with AIDS who were around the age her son had been when he died. She asked insightful questions, told us about her son, and disclosed that she was a two-time breast cancer survivor.

She told us she loved *POZ* and read every issue. She thought it would be hard to get Rodale to do anything with us, but she was going to give it a shot. A few weeks later, we got an upbeat letter reemphasizing her admiration for *POZ* but saying that Rodale wasn't going to invest. Enclosed was a personal check for five thousand dollars to help pay for free subscriptions for people with HIV. The director of the David Geffen Foundation helped us develop a plan supporting the same free-subscription program, but it fell through. They stopped returning our calls after we published an exposé about a big AIDS gala that was manipulated to promote Calvin Klein, in whose company Geffen had been a major investor, at the expense of the charitable purpose.

Barry Diller sent us a supportive note but declined to hear our pitch. Ironically, years later, he ended up buying the company that owned TheBody.com, an HIV-information source that was one of *POZ*'s online competitors.

In the end, all this moving and shaking was spectacularly unsuccessful. We took in only about $120,000 of our $950,000 goal in cash investments from about a dozen different people. But at a certain point in the process, the determination, passion, and commitment I saw in so many who cared about the magazine made me realize it was going to survive in one form or another, with or without me. Between the advertising paid in advance, trade-outs for services, the proceeds from my house, and cash advances on credit cards, we kept it going until late 1996, when the advertising revenue Megan had foreseen finally started to kick in.

■   ■   ■

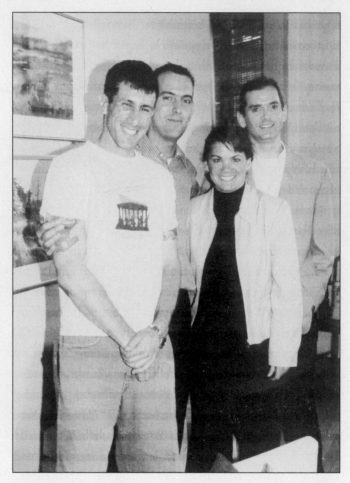

Here's the dream team that kept *POZ* alive during the most difficult period. *From left,* Stephen Gendin, Brad Peebles, my sister Megan Strub, and me.

CHAPTER 26

Pharma Watching

"I could get fired for giving you this," said an ACT UP friend who worked at the PR firm Ogilvy, Adams & Rinehart as he handed me a two-page memo marked "CONFIDENTIAL" in January 1994. "But I think you need to know you're being watched." His firm had prepared the memo for Burroughs Wellcome, then the largest marketer of AIDS drugs in the world, including AZT. Burroughs Wellcome was monitoring our plans for *POZ* before the first issue was even published.

The memo cited Burroughs Wellcome's difficult "history" with me, specifically my note to Community Cardpack readers in 1991 about regretting publication of their awful ad. The PR firm's advice was to take a wait-and-see approach.

In the first year of *POZ*, our advertisers were mostly smaller companies targeting the gay market. We had a host of depressing viatical company ads and a few ads marketing treatments for AIDS-related bacterial and fungal infections, the most unsightly one showing a picture of infected toenails, but we had none for any of the HIV anti-retrovirals. We discounted pages heavily to enlist Perrier, Benetton, and other global brands to make us look more credible and established. But it was a slog to get any significant money in the door.

Many companies didn't want their product or service associated with AIDS. One major vitamin-supplement company told us, "We market our vitamins to well people, not to sick people." A record-company executive said he found *POZ* "disgusting and exploitive." Advertisers to the gay market were initially interested, but after the first few issues—when it was clear that the magazine was for people with HIV, not just gay people—they fell away.

After the introduction of protease inhibitors in 1996, pharmaceutical advertising provided virtually all the magazine's revenue. That wasn't our plan, but we simply weren't able to attract other advertisers. Some critics called *POZ* a shill for pharmaceutical companies, but the charge never stuck. Our readers knew better. No one could read coverage that month after month highlighted side effects, resistant virus, and sharply criticized drug pricing and believe we were anyone's shill.

But having over 90 percent of the magazine's revenue come from half a dozen drug companies was a precarious business model. When a single company got angry and pulled its ad schedule, it was a bad hit to our bottom line. At any given time, it seemed like one or another was canceling, or threatening to cancel, their ads.

Their anger was usually over our reports on side effects of their drugs, sometimes side effects they had sought to hide. So many of us at *POZ* were living with these side effects every day; it was never a consideration to temper coverage in any way. If anything, we were on the alert, knowing that those of us taking the drugs would learn these side effects as soon as or before anyone else. Pharmaceutical companies initially complained that we didn't have "scientific proof" and accused us of "scaring" people with HIV away from treatment.

Eventually, the industry came to view *POZ*'s coverage as a valuable early-warning system. Instead of seeing our coverage as a threat, they saw it as a heads-up alerting them to an issue they eventually would have to address.

After the first few issues, readers and pharmaceutical companies alike could see that while we had a perspective, we were seriously committed to responsible journalism. We didn't take cheap shots, but we were nobody's lapdogs, either. Our staff was hyper-alert to any hint of inappropriate influence or efforts. One of my mantras was that we must always be prepared to shut down the magazine rather than compromise our integrity.

That didn't stop some pharmaceutical advertisers from holding advertising schedules hostage, refusing to commit while they tried to get an explicit or implied commitment to cover a topic in a certain way. Megan was an impenetrable shield, deflecting efforts to influence our editorial staff and protecting them from pressure. She also became friends with many of her business contacts. When a product manager from one our largest pharmaceutical advertisers suggested to a competitor, also one of our largest advertisers, that they both pull their *POZ* ads and force us out of business, the competitor not only refused but also told Megan about the conversation.

We did have some influence over the way the pharmaceutical industry chose to engage its potential customers. The first drug ads in the magazine were boilerplate and science-oriented, similar to what they ran in professional journals, perhaps illustrated with a drawing of a molecular structure. When the ads started including people, they usually looked forlorn, staring at the moon or walking alone on a beach. In mouse type in the corner was typically a disclaimer: "Person depicted is a professional model, not an actual person with AIDS."

That disclaimer drove me crazy. It played right into the stigma of having HIV. Megan encouraged advertisers to use people with HIV as models and even offered to find them. We put a notice in the magazine, got dozens of inquiries from readers, and turned them over to a modeling agency that launched a division specializing in HIV-positive models. Eventually ads were created showing a diversity of real people with HIV, including women, people of color, and male couples looking vaguely lovey-dovey.

Stephen and I sometimes accompanied Megan on visits to her clients. We were curiosities: Real Live People with AIDS! At a meeting at Hoffman–La Roche's headquarters in New Jersey, Stephen mentioned casually that he had been there before. One of the executives gave an expectant smile and asked, "Oh, whom did you meet with?" Stephen told the man calmly, "We didn't really meet with anyone; I was with ACT UP, and we chained ourselves to your front gates and got arrested."

Another time, Stephen and I went with Megan to a meeting with half a dozen midlevel male executives and their young female assistants at Ortho Pharmaceutical, a division of Johnson & Johnson. I was in a suit, and Stephen was wearing red pants with a bulky, brightly colored sweater. Some of the women were eager to convey how comfortable they were with us and casually referred to their gay friends or HIV knowledge.

Not long before that meeting, the first transdermal patch, Testo-derm, had been introduced to combat low testosterone, which was common in men with HIV. Stephen, ever on the pharmaceutical front-lines, was one of the first to get a prescription. It was an imperfect product because the patch had to be stuck to a man's scrotum, and if he got sweaty, it would fall off.

At lunchtime, when we were walking down the hall to the buffet, we heard one young woman from the meeting calling after us. "Stephen! I think you dropped this," she said, trotting toward us with something in her hand. She handed Stephen a small round piece of white gauzy fabric with a shiny adhesive on one side. "What is it, anyway?" she asked as she held it in front of her face peering at it closely. Stephen said only, "You don't really want to know, I promise you!"

I started using testosterone replacement therapy as well because my T-cells were plummeting and I was losing weight. When strange fevers and bouts of sickness became frequent, I started taking anti-retroviral drugs and treatments to prevent opportunistic infections: Bactrim to prevent PCP; Biaxin to prevent mycobacterium avium-intracellulare (MAI); Marinol, a synthetic form of THC, to get the munchies so I could hold or gain weight; antidepressants; and sometimes an anti-anxiety or sleeping pill.

On occasion, before Megan took me to meetings with pharmaceuti-cal companies, we reviewed my meds if they included any of that com-pany's products. It could change the dynamic of a meeting when I said, "I'm not just trying to sell you advertising. I'm your customer, too."

CHAPTER 27

Creating Communities

For a large part of our gay white male readership, AIDS was their number one challenge. Before AIDS, many of us had seldom felt like we were served inadequately by "the system." Yet while we were so angry at being ignored and neglected by the government and others, we were ignorant and neglectful of how the epidemic affected other communities, including a fast-rising number of African-American women. In communities of color, AIDS activism had to find its place in a hierarchy of burdens that included racism, addiction, mental health issues, homelessness and poverty. They were less often addressed in isolation; activism was typically integrated into a broader agenda. This interconnected approach is one of the most important contributions black AIDS organizations—especially those led by women—have contributed to combating the epidemic.

As *POZ*'s staff became more knowledgeable about (and interested in) the diversity of the epidemic, we had to reconcile sometimes difficult or conflicting values, including racism in the white gay community and homophobia in the black community.

Our approach was to expand and deepen coverage of issues important to other communities rather than downplay the gay dimension that we knew so well. The most visible measure of diversity was found in whose stories we told. We put a range of faces on the cover from the start: After Ty Ross came dancer Bill T. Jones, Republican activist Mary Fisher, and MTV's *Real World* star Pedro Zamora. But those depictions didn't overcome the fact that the dominant editorial influence in the magazine was from gay, white, college-educated AIDS activist males. Hiring and nurturing a more diverse staff and gaining critical insight into the role race plays in the epidemic was an ongoing challenge. We took it seriously and made progress over the years, but never entirely escaped the criticism, nor should we have.

Nothing we did would matter if we couldn't get the magazine into people's hands, so we provided a free subscription to anyone with HIV who requested one. I didn't want the cost of a subscription to stand in the way of someone getting much-needed information. Because many people were uncomfortable putting their name on an HIV-related mailing list, even if the magazine was mailed in a discreet wrapper, we established free distribution sites around the country at several hundred clinics, community centers, and other venues. I remember a *POZ* reader in Alabama wanting to know what day the next box of magazines was scheduled to arrive at her local clinic. "I have to coordinate my next appointment," she said. "If I'm not there within a few days after *POZ* arrives, they're all out of them."

When the advertising revenue picked up in 1996, we launched *POZ en Español*, at Xavier's urging, to reach native Spanish speakers in the United States, the Caribbean, and Mexico. At first I was reluctant because I spoke little Spanish, but Xavier agreed to take on the role of associate publisher.

POZ en Español featured original content, it wasn't a translation of English-language *POZ*. We knew that in Spanish-speaking households, the primary health care decision-maker was typically a mother. Our editor, Gonzalo Aburto, who was Mexican, built a voice for the magazine that spoke not just to individuals with HIV but also to their families. He recruited writers and editors from Spain, the Caribbean, and Latin America. Xavier and Gonzalo sometimes had to negotiate the language in the articles word by word to make sure the magazine spoke as clearly to Puerto Ricans as it did to Mexicans or Venezuelans.

It was a coup when we were able to distribute *POZ* magazine to a network of African-American churches through a list provided by the AIDS Interfaith Alliance. We were connecting with a deeply affected community that couldn't be reached through LGBT community centers, clinics, or mailing lists. When a congregation in Tennessee significantly cut back the monthly order, I asked the pastor what had happened. "At first my parishioners didn't know what *POZ* was," he said, "and they were glad to pick it up. But once everyone in the congregation knew the magazine was about AIDS, they were reluctant because it was stigmatizing."

Eventually we started a new magazine, *Real Health*, specifically to address a range of health issues of particular concern to the African-American community, such as diabetes and heart disease. Around 40 percent of the content was about HIV, but we mixed it in with other articles to reduce the stigma and ultimately restore distribution through African-American churches.

That wasn't the only distribution challenge. In September 1998, our decision to shrink-wrap three condoms with each magazine, with the cover line "FREE BACK-TO-SCHOOL CONDOM INSIDE," cost us one of our largest newsstand outlets, Barnes & Noble.

Condoms were controversial, and schools around the country were instituting abstinence-only sex education. New York had banned the distribution of condoms through school nurses, and in some circumstances, it was illegal to send them through the mail. Barnes & Noble's CEO, Len Riggio, was a devout Catholic.

When we sent out a press release blasting their decision, we were invited to meet with Riggio at his huge office on lower Fifth Avenue. He agreed to reinstate our distribution, but within a few months they cut their order back to almost nothing.

*   *   *

We sent the first issue of the magazine, unsolicited, to four thousand prison addresses (identified by zip code) selected from my company's database of LGBT community members and supporters. But some prisons considered *POZ* a gay publication or pornography and therefore prohibited its distribution. Dan Johnston, a friend who was an activist lawyer, volunteered to write to prison officials and politicians to get the prison bans overturned. Sometimes Dan had to threaten litigation to get officials' attention.

There were activists working on prison and AIDS issues in ACT UP, but I didn't pay much attention to their work until I started *POZ* and had more direct contact with those who were incarcerated and had HIV. When I learned that one in four people with HIV in the United States did time, I realized how inadequate our coverage was. When we got letters from prisoners, describing horrific conditions, it reminded me of *Andersonville*, a novel by MacKinlay Kantor about a notorious Confederate prisoner-of-war camp that I read when I was in fifth grade. It was shocking to realize how in some ways prison conditions hadn't changed much.

Several people at the company had served time in prison. Laura Whitehorn, who coordinated and improved our coverage of prison issues, was imprisoned for fourteen years stemming from her involvement with the Resistance Conspiracy case, when a radical leftist group carried out a series of bombings against U.S. military and government targets. While in prison, she was one of several political prisoners who pioneered HIV education and empowerment programs for other inmates and brought attention to the poor quality of care for people with HIV. Her commitment to the needs of prisoners was responsible for *POZ* improving our coverage of this most-ignored group of PWAs. She edited or wrote a number of feature stories about HIV in prisons, including one by Rachel Maddow before she became known as an MSNBC host. Laura also diligently corresponded with every prisoner who contacted us about poor conditions or discriminatory actions.

One particularly powerful letter, signed by about twenty prisoners with HIV, came from the Stiles Unit at a prison in Beaumont, Texas. Retribution against prisoners who filed complaints or contacted the media was common and could be severe, yet these prisoners requested that their names be printed, regardless of the risk. I was moved by their courage and solidarity in bringing attention to the prison's terrible medical care. HIV drugs were casually substituted, dosing was inconsistent and the doctors were trained minimally, if at all, in HIV. Meanwhile, prisons failed to make condoms available, which contributed to the spread of the virus.

The Texas letter prompted me to write a column that began, "There is a factory in Texas that manufactures vast amounts of multiple drug resistant (MDR) strains of HIV in a population at extraordinary risk of transmitting these strains to others . . . This 'factory' is the Texas Department of Corrections, and it's hard to imagine how MDR HIV could be any more efficiently created and spread."

Corrections-system officials were upset at the public scrutiny, especially after a member of the state House of Representatives quoted my column, waving a copy of *POZ* in the air during a legislative debate. The prisoners were thrilled, and several wrote to us later, reporting an improvement in care.

Not all prisoner letters were about medical care or prison conditions. One man began his letter by effusively complimenting *POZ* and assuring me that *POZ* was widely read by his fellow inmates. He said he was scheduled for release in a few months and wondered if I might be looking for a partner. He found me very attractive, he wrote, and had clipped the tiny photograph that accompanied my column and taped it to the wall of his cell. He went on to so say he thought of me every night and promised, in elaborate detail, to take care of my every sexual need. In closing, he said he was looking forward to becoming my "bitch."

My inflated ego was punctured, however, when I got to the P.S.: "In case you're already taken, can you give this letter to your friend Stephen Gendin? He is a FINE LOOKING young man!"

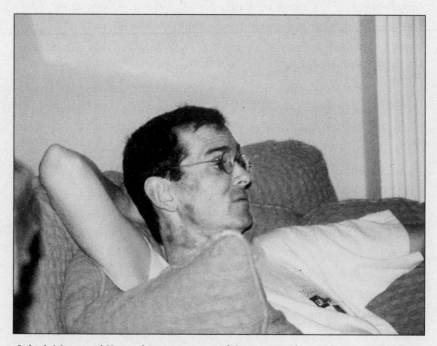

I think Megan and Xavier threw away most of the pictures of me with Kaposi's Sarcoma. This one was taken in the fall of 1995 while my lesions were still worsening, a few months before combination therapy was introduced and the lesions began to fade. Some lesions on my torso and legs became almost the size of my hand, with a thick, waxy dark necrotic crust; the ones on my face and neck never got that bad.

CHAPTER 28

Dark Mark

When I got KS in 1994, it changed my social experience of AIDS. KS's scarlet mark—with its eerie evocation of a stigmatic's holy wound—announced my illness to all; I no longer had any control over when and to whom it was disclosed.

Red or dark purple KS lesions inspired the same visceral dread as buboes, the blisterlike lymph nodes heralding the bubonic plague in the fourteenth century. The only difference was that with KS, people on the street stopped short of running from you. Instead, you were considered the walking dead. Frequently, your presence evoked fear and anger, whether you were seated in a restaurant, sniffing a cantaloupe at the grocery, or reaching to press a button on an elevator.

Even before the discovery of the virus, before the HIV test and CD4 cell counts and viral load measurements ruled our lives, legions of gay men routinely scrutinized their bodies with dread: "Was this red mark on my arm yesterday, or did it show up overnight? Is it getting darker or lighter?" From the early 1980s to the mid-1990s, I was KS-terrified, obsessing over every pimple, blemish, freckle, and bruise. Until they arrived, I would repeat a common refrain among people with HIV: "I can deal with anything but KS."

At the gym, bodies were surreptitiously surveyed, no longer just in appreciation of cobblestone abs but in apprehension of telltale spots. Performing a snap assessment of one another for signs of the disease became second nature. The bold gaze of desire had to make way for subtler inspections.

I never had a gym body; my skinny frame was a source of shame. Ironically, my resulting detachment helped me manage the psychological impact of KS. The lesion-peppered landscape of the carnal body that carried "me" around did not translate, in my mind, to a diseased soul.

Still, it wasn't easy when I spotted my first lesion. I was staying at a friend's pool house in Los Angeles in August 1994 when I stepped out of the shower and saw it while drying off in front of the mirror. An oval-shaped reddish spot, about an inch long and half an inch wide, sat horizontally on the right side of my torso, halfway between my armpit and the top of my hip.

The spot had fuzzy edges and didn't hurt or change color when I touched it—two signs pointing toward KS. My initial alarm was tempered by the memory of every previous mysterious blemish or mark that faded away within a few days. "You've done this before, don't get all worked up," I told myself.

There were so many mirrors and lights in the pool house that I couldn't help scrutinizing my body for more spots. No crevice went unchecked, but I found only that one spot on my torso. I showed it to my host, who happened to be a medical pathologist. He looked at it carefully and palpated it gently between his fingers, suggesting a biopsy when I was back in New York. Although he feigned unconcern, I could tell he was disturbed by what he saw.

I acted blasé as well. If it heralded the arrival of what I had dreaded for so long, so be it; that was the attitude I copped. I thought of the KS lesions as long-expected guests, their arrival overdue, even if I had hoped they would never show up.

*   *   *

A few weeks later, I was in the backseat of a taxi with Megan on our way to a meeting at an ad agency. I told her about the spot on my torso. When I lifted my shirt to show it to her, her response sent a chill through me: "I wonder if that is what is on the back of your ear."

Not knowing what else to say, Megan opened her purse and handed me her compact mirror. By holding the mirror in front of and slightly above my head and folding my ear forward, I could just barely see the edge of a dark, almost black, spot.

In an instant, any doubt or denial was gone. With KS, I'd reached the stage where the virus was literally popping out of my skin. The pale spot on my side had looked so temporary; the one behind my ear was dark and insistent, like ink. I was especially concerned that it was so close to my brain.

But I knew the lesions that I could see wouldn't kill me; it was only once they spread internally that I had to really worry. It was then that I decided to change doctors. Now that I had KS, I was entering a new and more serious phase of the disease; I was battling more frequent fevers, skin rashes, and persistent fatigue. I wanted someone whose perspective on treatment, including skepticism concerning AZT, was more in line with my own.

So in the fall of 1994, I made an appointment with Dr. Joseph Sonnabend. I had known of him since the first days of the epidemic, but we did not meet in person until Michael got sick. I always knew I might see Sonnabend if I became very sick, but to go to him before then felt like I would be acknowledging I was sicker than I felt. I thought of Sonnabend as the doctor for people with HIV who were extremely ill; I frequently heard of him working miracles, bringing someone back to life after other doctors had given up. When I was feeling okay to take his time for my problems would have felt selfish, like I was denying his service to those in greater need. The lesion on my ear changed the equation.

Sonnabend conducted his practice in a one-bedroom apartment transformed into a cramped two-room office—one for waiting and one for examining—on the parlor floor of a crumbling brownstone far west on Seventeenth Street. It was crowded floor to ceiling with filing cabinets, magazines, books, posters, and medical supplies, amid garage-sale furniture. After accompanying me to an appointment, Xavier proclaimed the office a dump and was suspicious of whatever medical care might be delivered there.

Sonnabend's patients helped one another, creating their own micro-community. Those of us in the waiting room would sometimes do our own triage, rearranging appointments based on a collective assessment of who was in the most immediate need.

Before I arrived at his office, I knew the options for KS: slash, burn, poison, or cover. The lesions could be cut out surgically, radiated into oblivion, injected with powerful chemotherapy, or masked with makeup. But none of these strategies had been shown to reduce the proliferation of lesions or extend life. Treating them cosmetically was important to many people but not me. Sonnabend and I agreed to do nothing other than regular X-rays to monitor for internal growth.

As the lesions crept up my neck and across my face, many people couldn't understand my approach, especially if they knew others with KS who treated their lesions cosmetically.

But I made a decision that the KS so visible to everyone else was not going to bother me. My life was rich and vibrant, but dealing with advanced AIDS was no party. The last thing I wanted was the added psychological burden of having to worry about hiding the spots.

I did sometimes feel guilty when I went to a restaurant or somewhere public with Xavier or Megan and people stared. They had to have been embarrassed, but never showed it. The only time I questioned my decision not to disguise or remove them was when we were fund-raising for the magazine. In retrospect, it was probably ridiculous to have even tried. Not many lenders or investors were interested in financing a dead man walking.

*   *   *

I thought I had reached a sort of psychological equilibrium with the lesions, but that didn't mean I wasn't vulnerable to embarrassment or humiliation. As the publisher of *POZ*, I was an exceptionally public person with AIDS. Every health issue that arose for me—both physical and mental—was documented in the pages of the magazine. I was so determined not to hide the KS that when Greg Gorman took pictures of me with clearly visible lesions on my neck, I chose one to run with my monthly *POZ* column. I thought I was already as AIDS-stigmatized as was possible. Former friends who were in deep denial or embarrassed by my illness had long since left my circle. I figured it couldn't get worse.

The visible evidence of disease made people uncomfortable. Long-time friends became tense when talking to me, their eyes darting around as if not sure where to look. When I walked on the street, small children sometimes pointed at me. I saw parents reach out to take their child's hands protectively if I was walking nearby. I love dogs and often greet them on the street, but it seemed like even they knew something was wrong; sometimes they barked at me or became agitated. During television interviews, makeup artists gave the lesions a wide berth while dusting powder on my face for the cameras; the brushes were often then thrown away. News producers would adjust lighting to highlight the lesions on my neck for dramatic effect. This didn't offend me; it was a natural fearful reaction to something they didn't know much about and found horrifying.

Some people assumed I had declined to have the lesions removed as a political statement. That wasn't unheard of: Vito Russo, Bob Rafsky, Mark Fotopoulos, and other ACT UP colleagues wore their KS as a badge of courage, reveling in how it forced others to confront the ugly reality of AIDS in their midst. That was a nice side benefit of my decision not to treat the lesions. At the time, Fotopoulos, a successful actor, was appearing in *The Loves of Anatol*, the play about which theater critic John Simon made the infamous comment, "Homosexuals in the theater! My God, I can't wait till AIDS gets all of them."

The most painful responses sometimes came from other gay men. My lesions made cruising on the street or meeting people in gay bars for sex almost impossible. On a visit to Los Angeles, I went to the Meat Rack, a popular sex venue. The Meat Rack was cozy, with a clublike atmosphere. I had been there before, but this was my first time with visible lesions. The club was in a warehouse way east on Santa Monica Boulevard. At the entrance, a clerk in a small vestibule with a Plexiglas window checked ID and collected a fee. When I arrived, he glanced toward me and then looked away. I figured he was busy, and I stood at the window for several minutes until I realized he was ignoring me. I tapped on the window.

Without looking up, he said, "I'm sorry, they won't let me."

"Let you what?" I asked.

"Let you in," he finally said, briefly meeting my gaze.

It dawned on me why he was refusing entry. I decided to make him say it.

"Why not?" I asked, and when he pretended not to hear me, I repeated it.

"Because of this," he said, gesturing to his own face. "I'm sorry, but they won't let me. I could lose my job."

I had become accustomed to the lesions alienating me from people who didn't know much about AIDS. But being rejected by a gay men's sex club, where I assumed everyone was better informed about HIV, was startling and depressing. It reminded me that our most insidious opposition is sometimes found within our own community.

It was an early warning for me about what, in time, would become a profound divide between gay men and gay men with HIV/AIDS. My rejection at the Meat Rack was far from my only experience with gay-on-gay HIV stigma. When I started getting lesions, I tried to book a tour to Africa for Xavier and me through Hanns Ebenstein Travel, a well-known upscale tour operator based in Key West that catered to gay men. Xavier had always longed to visit the African savannah, and I wanted to have this once-in-a-lifetime experience with him before I became too sick to travel.

Hanns was an advertiser in our cardpacks, and I called him to confirm that there were no travel restrictions because of my HIV. He assured me there were not, but when he found out I had KS, he asked, "Is it visible?" When I said yes, he asked, "Are you sure you would be comfortable, Sean? Are you sure you want to travel if you have lesions that can be seen?" I said I was fine with it and did so all the time. He said, "Maybe you shouldn't join us. Even if you are comfortable, I'm afraid some of the others in the group wouldn't be. They're not as sophisticated about these things as you and I are."

As KS progressively laid claim to more of my body, I thought often of Michael Callen, who had died at the end of 1993. When fulminating KS ravaged his body in 1991, he had explored all sorts of treatments, including powdered shark-cartilage slurry administered anally. He joked about the experiment expanding erotic horizons between man and fish. At first, the shark cartilage seemed to be effective, and the size and number of his lesions lessened. The success was short-lived. Within a few months, the lesions had returned, and the shark slurry joined the long list of other exotic treatments that had disappointed dying people with AIDS.

Callen shared his battle with rare wit and detail in the gay and AIDS press, but of all his pithy observations, one in particular was seared into my brain: When his Kaposi's sarcoma spread to his internal organs, he cited research showing that 90 percent of those diagnosed with KS in their lungs died within nine months: "90 in Nine" was what he called the phenomenon. He beat that average, but not by much.

I also thought often of a children's book my mother and her sister had written and illustrated in the early 1960s, called *The Polka-Dot Dilly*. It was about a boy who had a mysterious illness and became covered with spots; no doctor was able to find the cure. My mother always claimed to have psychic abilities; whether that was the case or it was a spectacular coincidence, I do not know. But my mother and aunt were pleased when we acknowledged their prescience by publishing excerpts from their book in the June 1995 issue of *POZ*:

Poor Willy! It's silly, and yet it is true
That instead of contracting the measles or flu
He came down with the Polka-Dot Dilly.
His father was worried. His mother was sad.

"My heavens, what's happened to Willy, poor lad?
He's covered with dots from his heels to his head.
We surely will have to keep Willy in bed.
He's splattered with spots willy-nilly!"

The medical specialists all gathered round
To see if a pill or a drink could be found
That would cure Willy's Dilly and make his spots fade,
And many a sober suggestion was made
On how to heal polka-dot Willy.

The cure for Willy's affliction is found in the ordinary—pickle relish—and worked like magic, with no side effects, no reference to its cost, and no accounting for any effect from the disease on society. No one shuns Willy, flees from his presence, or does anything other than shower him with love and affection and search for a treatment for what ails him.

My KS lesions spread widely and at a quickening pace. The very first one I had noticed in August 1994—the small reddish mark on my torso that was barely the diameter of a dime—within a year became nearly the size of my hand and developed a waxy black surface of necrotizing tissue. It was only a matter of time, I knew, before they would grow on my internal organs and I would enter the nine-month countdown phase.

■　　　■　　　■

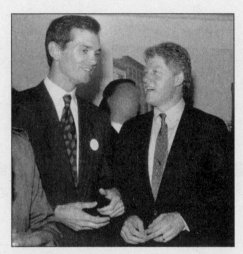

I was proud to be the first LGBT community publisher who endorsed Clinton's 1992 campaign for president, but that pride turned to anger when his administration was such a disappointment and failed to show the leadership we expected.

CHAPTER 29

Feeling Our Pain

POZ did its best to be a thorn in the side of the Clinton administration, and hold the president accountable for promises he'd made during his campaign. They could not entirely ignore us because our criticism was on target.

Like many other people with HIV, I felt betrayed by Clinton, because I'd believed him during his campaign when he told my ACT UP colleague Bob Rafsky, "I feel your pain." The pride I once felt at having been the first LGBT community publisher to endorse his campaign turned to regret when it became apparent that his promises were empty.

In our third issue, in August 1994, we published a feature on the fifty most important AIDS policy leaders in the United States. Kristine Gebbie, Clinton's rubber-stamp AIDS czar, had recently resigned after accomplishing virtually nothing. "There was near unanimity among people we consulted that Gebbie should not be on the list," I wrote in my column. "The board chairperson of one AIDS research group told me 'including her would totally invalidate the credibility

of this project. She is a laughingstock and not taken seriously by anyone working in AIDS whose judgment I respect.' "

Bob Hattoy was working in the White House, and we spoke several
times a week. When *POZ* had inside information on the Clinton
administration, it was usually Hattoy who had given us the tip. After
the column on Gebbie came out, he cackled with glee, telling me,
"Copies of *POZ* are sitting on every desk in the West Wing. They. Are.
Pissed. I told them I couldn't control what you write. But this is good;
now they're paying attention."

That was the issue featuring Pedro Zamora on the cover. He was a
handsome young Cuban-American who publicly chronicled his battle
with AIDS on *The Real World*. When Pedro died, the White House
revealed that President Clinton had personally telephoned Pedro in his
last days. Donna Shalala, whose record on AIDS as Clinton's health and
human services secretary was especially egregious, was quoted as saying,
"I love Pedro."

Most of the media, including the LGBT media, dutifully published
the spin, but in my December 1994 column, I wrote, "If Shalala really
'loves Pedro' as she claims, she will kick some butt at the FDA, CDC,
and NIH—all agencies under her supervision—to cut the red tape,
expedite new treatments, dramatically increase anonymous testing, re-
empower the Office on Alternative Health and increase funding for
prevention and care."

Hattoy said their political cowardice stemmed in part from the gays-
in-the-military debacle. It made Clinton's top advisers skittish about
anything to do with gay issues—as AIDS was then seen—so inaction
was the default strategy.

After the December column, Hattoy asked that I use Xavier's name
instead of my own when calling him at the White House. If his coworkers knew he was communicating with *POZ*, it could jeopardize his job.

Though Clinton's top aides were looking for an excuse to fire Hattoy, his personal friendship with the Clintons protected him, as well as his AIDS diagnosis. "The White House boys all thought I was going to die and nobody wanted to be the guy who fired the dying guy with AIDS," Hattoy said.

After Bob committed several well-publicized gaffes ("gaffe" is Washingtonspeak for when a politician tells the truth), he was pushed out of the White House to a liaison position at the Department of the Interior. He was prohibited from providing quotes to any member of media without prior approval.

Hiding Hattoy didn't change anything concerning the administration's response to AIDS. Vincent Gagliostro, part of the art collective that created the "Silence=Death" image, created a poster for the inside back cover of the April 1995 issue that expressed the community's dismay over Washington's response to the epidemic. It was a black-and-white photograph of Clinton and Newt Gingrich with big guffawing smiles on their faces, two good old boys sharing a big joke. Vincent added a transparent red stripe across their smiles; the caption above read, "WIPE THAT SMILE OFF YOUR FACE," and below, "AIDS IS A NATIONAL EMERGENCY."

There was no AIDS issue during the Clinton years that was more pressing than lifting the ban on the use of federal money to fund needle-exchange programs. There was ample proof that such programs dramatically reduced HIV transmission; conversely, there was no evidence showing that they increased drug use. They were a key part of HIV-prevention strategies in many countries.

Early in the Clinton administration, Secretary Shalala passed the authority to lift the ban to Jocelyn Elders, the fearless surgeon general who later was forced to resign when she spoke frankly about sex education in schools. After the Republicans swept the 1994 congressional elections, Elders's authority to take unilateral action reverted back to Shalala, who refused to lift the ban. When research showed a dramatic increase in young girls and women acquiring HIV through sex with older drug-injecting men, we laid the blame at Shalala's feet. These were infections that might have been prevented with needle-exchange programs. We started keeping track of "Shalala Infections," running a box in every issue tallying the climbing number of new infections that we calculated had resulted from her failure to lift the ban.

Shalala downplayed reports from the CDC that supported lifting the ban, misrepresented research findings, and questioned whether needle-exchange reduced transmission or increased drug use, contrary to the evidence. I called her out in harsh terms, labeling her failure to lift the ban an "act of genocidal neglect . . . pathetic, if not criminal," and quoted Elizabeth Taylor, who said the U.S. government's failure to fund needle-exchange programs amounted to "a measured act of premeditated murder."

Our needle-exchange campaign benefited from Larry Kramer's brash rhetoric. *POZ*'s first anniversary issue, in May 1995, featured Kramer on the cover, interviewed by Andrew Sullivan, then the editor of *The New Republic* and a prominent gay Catholic leader of the neo-conservative movement.

I had a hunch that Andrew was HIV-positive—which was why I wanted him to interview Kramer—but he didn't disclose his HIV-positive status to Larry, me, or our readers. In the interview, he and Kramer discussed the nature of evil. Larry said, "I think that because he [Anthony Fauci] has not done what he was capable of doing, [it] opens him up to very acceptable charges of evil. I certainly think Donna Shalala is evil. Evil, evil, evil." Larry's comment was a perfect pull quote and we ran it on the center spread, in stark white type, against an ominous Albert Watson portrait of Kramer.

It got the attention of C-SPAN when they invited me to their studio to discuss the magazine's first anniversary. At the time, KS lesions were starting to appear on my neck and face. When I was in the green-room, the producer asked if I wanted makeup. "No, I'm fine," I said. It was a small black-box studio, with the interviewer and me seated at a table surrounded by black curtains. I didn't notice the cameras, nearly invisible in the folds of the curtains.

When the interviewer held up the page with Larry's quote and asked about his comment, I explained Shalala's various failures and argued that part of her reluctance was "because . . . as a closeted lesbian, she goes that extra mile to say 'my personal life isn't impacting these decisions.' " Then I caught myself and said, "You probably won't air this."

After the interview, I said to the producer, "You can edit that out," explaining that I'd forgotten about the camera and hadn't intended to out Shalala (who denied she was a lesbian). He replied, "This is C-SPAN. We run interviews as they are, we don't edit them. This will air on Thursday." My heart started pounding in anticipation of the broadcast. I was worried that Jean O'Leary, who told me Shalala was a lesbian, would be upset with me. Before I left the studio, they gave me a VCR tape of the interview. When I met Xavier in the greenroom, I said, "We've got to get out of here. You'll never believe what I just said on camera."

Later that day, I told Hattoy what had happened. He laughed and said, "I'm glad I don't know you anymore." That evening we spoke again, and he said, "I couldn't wait to tell Victor [Zonana, Shalala's openly gay press secretary], and boy, was he freaked out!"

The show didn't run on Thursday. In fact it never aired, and later, Hattoy apologized for spilling the beans to Zonana, who, Hattoy said, stopped C-SPAN from running the interview. I shared the copy I had—complete with the network's captioning chiron and logo—with friends, including a manager at Uncle Charlie's gay bar. He ran the clip in a rotation on the video monitor for a few weeks. When it got to the point where I outed Shalala, the patrons of the bar sometimes would cheer. In retrospect, Shalala's consideration of a 1998 gubernatorial run in Wisconsin, which was a secret at the time, may have contributed as much to her reluctance to lift the ban as anything else.

The disappointment with Clinton's record on AIDS was widespread, even among campaign donors and supporters he appointed to his advisory commission on AIDS. Scott Hitt, a gay physician from Los Angeles with a big HIV practice, chaired the Presidential Advisory Council on HIV/AIDS (PACHA) and had been an early supporter of and important fund-raiser for Clinton's presidential campaign. He thanked me for *POZ*'s coverage: "You're a great 'bad cop'; keep up the pressure."

The community anger was a concern for Clinton's plan for reelection, prompting the White House to hold a conference on AIDS in December 1995. But it was so scripted toward a predetermined "isn't it all wonderful" message that it became a farce. When Hattoy was told that he wouldn't be allowed to attend the conference because "there aren't enough chairs," he went ballistic. A senior White House staffer, afraid of having to explain to the press why the president's friend with AIDS—who'd spoken at the nominating convention—wasn't at the conference, had the president call Hattoy to invite him. "Bob, my friend, I understand you're frustrated," Clinton said.

Hattoy responded, "Frustrated? I speak out about AIDS, and your staff blames me as the problem. I am not the problem. AIDS is the problem." Hattoy said Clinton wasn't aware that of the six people with AIDS whom he knew personally from his campaign team, five were dead; only Hattoy was still alive. This was during the fateful period when Monica Lewinsky was spending time in the Oval Office.

Criticism wasn't tolerated at the White House conference, and Richard Socarides, an openly gay presidential appointee involved in organizing it, told me that I was "too controversial" to be invited. *POZ* was granted one pass with the caveat that we not ask the president any questions. White House staffer Marcia Scott told Mario Cooper, who chaired the board of the AIDS Action Council, that "political calculus" wouldn't allow the Clinton administration to have a meaningful discussion of needle-exchange programs.

NAMES Project founder Cleve Jones was part of a prevention breakout group. He told me, "The group was great, and we agreed, using the strongest language possible, that needle-exchange programs were the prevention priority. But when the report came out, the language was watered down, to the point where needle exchange was just one on a long list of appropriate prevention measures.

A few months before Clinton's reelection in 1996, PACHA, led by Scott Hitt, issued a progress report on the Clinton administration's AIDS record. It was surprisingly frank. They called Clinton's effort "insufficient," said it "lacks focus and is overly timid," and noted that "the time for increased commitment, along with moral and political courage, is now."

I eventually endorsed Clinton's reelection in 1996. As poor as he was on AIDS, there was no reason to think Bob Dole or Ross Perot would do any better and on many issues it was certain they would be worse. But I lamented the disappearance of the Clinton we had elected in 1992, the Clinton we'd believed cared and would make a difference. I hoped that after he was reelected he would show more leadership, since he didn't have to worry about running again, but little changed. I had been proud of a photograph of Clinton and me taken during the 1992 campaign, and I had it on display in my office. But as his cowardice worsened the epidemic, and as he implemented the welfare "reform" that hurt so many, formulated "Don't Ask, Don't Tell," and signed the Defense of Marriage Act, seeing that picture every day only made me angry. I took it down, ashamed that I had been conned again.

By March 1998, the PACHA appointees, including Hitt, had had enough. They issued an extraordinary statement announcing their vote of no confidence in the administration because of its failure to lift the ban on needle-exchange funding: "Tragically, we must conclude it is a lack of political will, not scientific evidence, that is creating this failure to act." Hitt also sent a letter from PACHA directly to Shalala. "At best this is hypocrisy," he wrote, "at worst it's a lie. And no matter what, it's immoral."

At one point, after she had decided to forgo a run for Wisconsin governor, Shalala was apparently willing to lift the ban and may have even urged the president to do so. But Clinton's top aides, Hattoy told *POZ*, were opposed. When the administration's drug czar, General Barry McCaffrey, came out publicly in opposition and reportedly threatened to resign over the matter, it was a death knell. Clinton, who famously "did not inhale," was loath to cross McCaffrey.

The Clinton administration sabotaged HIV prevention and treatment efforts in other ways. One concerned intellectual property rights controlling the use of generic medications around the world. Near the end of Clinton's presidency, we learned from a leaked State Department memo that former vice president Al Gore had exerted pressure on South Africa to rescind legislation allowing use of generic antiretrovirals at a vastly lower cost, rather than paying U.S. companies their huge markups. Gore's senior campaign staff included several people who had been lobbyists for the pharmaceutical industry.

Gore's role broke in *The Washington Post*, but the gay establishment, which by then had been coopted by the Clinton administration and the Democratic Party, quickly acquiesced, selling out people with HIV in Africa and elsewhere. The LGBT community was no longer the AIDS movement's backbone of support, as it had incrementally moved away from AIDS issues since Clinton's election. The administration had hired many openly LGBT community leaders and campaign volunteers. Many big LGBT donors to the Clinton campaign enjoyed access to the president, prestigious appointments, overnight stays in the Lincoln Bedroom, and other perquisites of access that earlier in my career I would have been delighted to enjoy. Hattoy was disgusted with how the gay community's major donors and leadership had rolled over for the administration, "The religious right is organizing pew by pew by pew, and we're going to cocktail parties in Washington trying to get a picture with Hillary." Those same major LGBT donors to Clinton's campaign also funded the community organizations that became so timid once Clinton was elected.

After ACT UP and others bird-dogged Gore on the generics issue, picketing or interrupting his presidential campaign appearances, spokesperson for the Human Rights Campaign David Smith responded, "To single out the vice president is not fair." Daniel Zingale, director of the AIDS Action Council, expressed similar go-along-to-get-along sentiments.

"This 'feeling your pain' business," Hattoy said, referring to Clinton's famous comment, "there's something evil about it. It doesn't sit well with me—it's the banal evil. Until these people [Clinton and Shalala] change their behavior, words don't count. It's behavior that counts."

CHAPTER 30

Barebacking

We celebrated sex in *POZ* to help our readers get past the sense that they were damaged, tainted, or undesirable after a diagnosis. We rejected the popular belief that because we had the virus, we should no longer have sex. Ending AIDS wasn't going to happen by scolding people with HIV or trying to prohibit them from having sex.

We concurred with what Sonnabend said early in the epidemic, that we wouldn't defeat AIDS until we acknowledged that "the rectum is a sexual organ, and it deserves the respect a penis gets and a vagina gets."

In the mid-'90s, HIV prevention had little nuance. It was basically: "Use a condom every time!" That phrase had become white noise, about as effective as Nancy Reagan's "Just say no to drugs!" It was palatable to the politicians and reassuring to those who already used condoms but didn't do much to change the behaviors of those who were putting themselves and others at risk. There was little respect or support for gay male sexuality, and media campaigns promoting "safe hot sex!" couldn't erase the reality that many men had an underlying desire for natural, skin-to-skin, condomless sex. At no point in the epidemic have more than about half of sexually active gay men used condoms consistently, and after combination therapy was introduced in 1996, the meaning of an HIV diagnosis changed dramatically. The risk/reward equation got more complicated when we learned that anti-retroviral therapy could reduce the virus to undetectable levels and make people with HIV vastly less infectious.

Gay men had been devising prevention and risk reduction strategies since *How to Have Sex in an Epidemic* proposed the use of condoms in 1983. We "discovered" sero-sorting (having sex only with partners of the same status) and sero-positioning (topping only if negative, bottoming if positive) and struggled to find ways to expand the sexual safety zone for people with HIV, including where condoms might not be as necessary.

While new risk reduction measures were being discovered and popularized, the Internet took off and changed the way gay men met for casual sex. In October 1996, when the fledgling America Online began offering unlimited access for a $19.95 monthly subscription, many gay men started using chat rooms to meet prospective partners. Not long after I became an AOL member in 1995, I searched the member database to see how frequently members disclosed their HIV-positive status in online profiles. The first time I searched (using various keywords), I found fewer than ten, but every few months I searched again and saw the count rise quickly. By early 1997, the number of members acknowledging that they were HIV-positive had grown to several thousand.

When I noticed the phrase "riding bareback" on a handful of AOL profiles, I walked down the hall to Stephen's office, as he was more tuned in to the online cruising scene. I asked if he knew what it meant to ride bareback. He looked up from his computer screen, nonchalant. "Yeah, that's fucking without a condom," he said, "skin-to-skin sex." I asked him to write a column about it for *POZ*. I knew the word "barebacking" would make a provocative cover line.

Having sex without condoms was hardly new, but acknowledging it publicly as an intentional choice was radical, even transgressive. The gay community had worked hard to normalize condom use, so someone saying he did not use them was almost blasphemous.

Our June 1997 issue was the first time the term "barebacking" (in a sexual context) was used in any national media. Stephen's column was an honest and humorous analysis of why he sometimes had sex without a condom—on purpose (gasp!)—and what it meant to him. He wrote about having bareback sex with activist and writer Tony Valenzuela at a conference a year earlier after Valenzuela, speaking on a panel, came out about his preference for condomless sex. I got the cover line I envisioned: "BAREBACK SEX: Let the Debate Begin."

Stephen wrote, "I can't comment on a negative guy's decision to go raw, but for us positive men, the benefits are obvious. The physical sensation is much better. The connection feels closer and more intimate. The sharing of cum on the physical level heightens the sense of sharing on the emotional and spiritual planes . . . Then there's the satisfaction of knowing that seroconverting has its advantages (or, to use American Express–speak, 'Membership has its privileges'). It's a tasty revenge."

When journalist and ACT UP member Michelangelo Signorile wrote that *POZ* "sometimes seems to eerily glamorize AIDS," cultural critic Douglas Crimp fired back. "Puffed up with moral indignation, Signorile . . . now feigns utter incomprehension that there could be a 'significant number' of gay men 'willfully and sometimes angrily defying safer sex efforts, rebelling against the rest of us, and thereby keeping HIV transmission thriving, affecting adversely the entire gay world . . . the divide Signorile now enforces is that between the 'responsible' and the 'irresponsible.' "

Many shared Signorile's view and joined him in criticizing us and, in particular, Stephen. One reader attacked the "selfish, specious musings Stephen Gendin passes off as ideas that rationalize his flirtation with skin-to-skin sex stunts." Others said he was "oblivious to his own hypocrisy" and "preaching a kamikaze sex code."

When we ran a follow-up cover story on Valenzuela, interviewed by Stephen, along with an analysis of the phenomenon by Michael Scarce that included a set of safer barebacking tips, there was more dissent. Even members of our staff had a heated argument about publishing the risk-reduction tips.

The photograph we ran on the cover, of Valenzuela naked on the back of a horse along with the headline "They Shoot Barebackers, Don't They?," was attention-getting, but I regretted it. The clever wordplay and image fed the accusation that we were being sensationalistic rather than leading a serious community discussion.

Two years later, we ran a sobering follow-up when Stephen's partner, Kyle "Hush" McDowell, got HIV from Stephen after they stopped using condoms consistently. This made for an irresistible target: Stephen, who was HIV-positive, sex-positive, cofounder of the AIDS Prevention Action League and Sex Panic!, and now a barebacking provocateur, had infected his partner.

It was humiliating for Stephen, worse for Hush, and important for *POZ* to address. For several years we had led the community's discussion about those who intentionally have sex without a condom in various risk scenarios. Now we had to explain to our readers, as best as we could, what had happened in this one circumstance.

Fortunately, Stephen and Hush wanted to understand as well and agreed to each write a version of what happened in November 1999. "Both Sides Now" detailed the history of their relationship, their erotic and sexual obsessions, and how they came to have the unprotected sex that had resulted in Hush's seroconversion.

Josef Astor photographed them as a couple, with Stephen standing in his undershorts and a sleeveless undershirt and Hush, bare-chested and blindfolded, kneeling before him, hands behind his back. Stephen is holding a ripe red strawberry right in front of Hush's mouth.

Stephen made his own confusion clear:

I have struggled to comprehend my role in our unsafe sex, but many months of discussion in therapy, in my HIV support group, and with my friends have brought little clarity. It terrifies me to realize that if I can't understand why it happened with someone I love as much as Hush, I might not be able to prevent it with other men. And given all the talk of the "second wave" of infections among gay men, I also feel a communal duty to pass along what, if anything, I've learned . . . Hush's seroconversion is one of the few things in my life that I'm deeply ashamed of.

Hush's was just as honest:

Call this the seroconversion of a codependent. I'm writing it because of my sense of frustration with the HIV-prevention discussion and because of how I lost my way. I didn't feel I could talk to anyone about some frightening tendencies in my relationship. I hope that what I have to say may open up a space for others to deal with their difficulties, and maybe even prevent infections.

The fury directed at Stephen, Valenzuela, Scarce, and *POZ* over the barebacking coverage reminded me of how Callen, Berkowitz, and Sonnabend were treated when they told the truth about the dangers of unprotected promiscuity fifteen years earlier. It's easy to shoot the messenger.

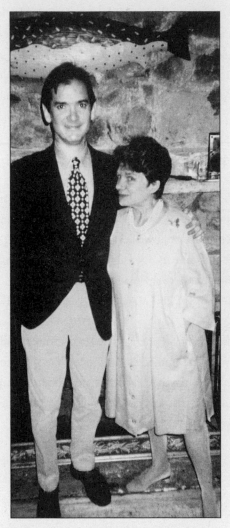

No wedding cake, thrown rice, or cheesy rendition of "Here Comes the Bride," just two friends helping each other. Doris O'Donnell and I got married in 1996 at my sister's house in Grandview-on-Hudson, New York, so Doris could qualify for Medicare, and my disability benefits, after my expected death, could pass through Doris to Xavier. I'm lucky things didn't work out as we had planned.

CHAPTER 31

Eugene and Angel

During the summer of 1995, when I was very sick and covered in KS lesions, my friend Doris O'Donnell asked me to marry her.

Doris was a close friend, mentor, and twenty-five years older. Her entire life was steeped in politics, journalism, and social-justice movements, from anti-McCarthyism through the civil rights and peace movements, feminism, and AIDS.

Getting married wasn't a bad idea. She lived off a small inheritance but had never worked anywhere long enough to qualify for Social Security or Medicare; if we married, she would immediately be eligible for those benefits. Also, as my legal spouse, she could inherit my private disability benefits, which otherwise would terminate upon my death. Our plan was for Doris to pass the disability benefits on to Xavier.

Xavier, having more respect for the institution of marriage, hated the idea and didn't care that he stood to benefit financially. If he and I couldn't get married, he wasn't enthusiastic about me marrying anyone else, no matter the reason.

When Doris and I did marry, in the summer of 1996 at Megan's house, in Grandview-on-Hudson, just north of New York City, Xavier declined to attend. We wrote our own vows and hosted a luncheon afterward for a handful of close friends. A woman sporting a bright amethyst crystal on a leather thong around her neck performed the service. The next day, Doris wrote about the wedding in her diary, listing the names of the guests—including several dogs, Beekman, Ernie, and Ollie—and the lunch menu. Her final note recalled her disastrous first wedding forty years before: "I remembered how I shook all through wedding No. 1 . . . unlike yesterday." Later, when people asked her why we got married, Doris would say, "Sean and I got married for the only good reason to get married: money!"

A few weeks after the ceremony, Doris and I traveled to Italy on what we jokingly referred to as "our honeymoon." The KS lesions were growing daily, and I knew my body was weakening. I expected it to be my last trip to Europe, possibly my last time on an airplane. When we checked in at the airport, we found that our seats weren't together. As we were boarding the plane, Doris asked to be reseated but was told, "The flight is overbooked, and we're now boarding; we can't rearrange the seating." She argued with the flight attendant, holding up the line, and I thought we might get kicked off the flight. Finally, in an authoritative and elevated voice, Doris insisted, "We must sit together! My friend has AIDS, and I must be with him at all times!"

Hearing the word *AIDS* spoken loudly and with a touch of defiance was almost as shocking to me as it was to everyone else. In a few minutes, we were shown to adjacent seats in an emergency-exit row, with extra legroom. The third seat in our row remained unoccupied during the "overbooked" flight.

We were on our way to Italy to see Gore Vidal in Ravello, a picturesque medieval village overlooking the Gulf of Salerno from a bluff above the Amalfi Coast. Gore and Doris had grown up together in Washington, D.C., and they shared a sibling-like friendship that revealed to me a gentle, sentimental side of the notoriously sharp-tongued writer. Doris had a photograph Gore gave her in 1937, when he was twelve years old and she was five, signed "Eugene," his given name. Doris had wanted to introduce me to Gore since 1990, when I ran for Congress in the same lower Hudson River Valley region where Gore had run thirty years before. He lost his race by about the same margin as I lost mine. In the care packages Doris regularly sent Gore, she always included the latest issue of *POZ*, and she had told him about me.

After we checked in at the Palumbo Hotel, just off the village square, Doris called Gore at Villa La Rondinaia ("the bird's nest"); his home was a short walk from the hotel. "I'll be right over, but go on down to the bar and ask for Marco," he told us. "He runs the place. Tell him you're meeting me, and he'll put you at my table."

When Gore arrived, everyone in the bar acknowledged him as though he were royalty. His first words to Doris were "And how is my angel doing?" as he kissed her on each cheek. With mock formality and an arched eyebrow, he turned to me and inquired sternly, "And this is the young man who failed to first come and ask me for your hand in marriage?"

As I shook his hand, I saw his eyes catch the KS lesions on my neck. I recognized the anxiety I so often saw in people's faces, even though his voice sounded jocular. I felt the weight of my lesions on his mind as we had a drink and then another, watching the sun set on the watery horizon from the Palumbo's plush lounge. Later, he admitted that mine were the first Kaposi's sarcoma lesions he had seen up close.

The next day, Gore and his partner, Howard Austen, gave us a tour of La Rondinaia's several levels clinging to the side of a cliff, at the end of a long garden path leading from the village piazza. Gore's library was lined with bookshelves packed from floor to ceiling, a huge partner's desk, tables covered with books, manuscripts, framed photographs, objets d'art, and sculpture. The villa was partially furnished with cast-offs from movie sets; the dining table chairs, covered in silver gilt, were made for a scene in *Ben Hur*, which Gore helped write.

Gore and Howard took us to one of their favorite restaurants on the edge of the sea for lunch. Doris brought a copy of the column I had been working on the night before, about proposed reparations for people with HIV because of the government's negligence. She asked Gore to read it, and he did so with pen in hand. "If you're going to say it, just go ahead and say it!" he said, striking out modifying clauses and statements that he felt were too tentative, making the sentences declarative. My Gore Vidal–edited column ran in our December 1996 edition.

After lunch, Gore told me about his nephew Hugh Steers, a talented painter who had died of AIDS the year before at 32. With tears in his eyes, he said he regretted not understanding how sick Hugh had been at the end of his life. I asked if he wanted to write a tribute to be published in *POZ*. When Gore sent it, he included a note to me: "A pity Hugh lived in such a fifth-rate era for the arts . . . He was a latter-day Goya with an even harsher subject. I hope posterity goes better than his terity—he was luckless on the grand scale." Steers's haunting paintings of men with AIDS now hang in the Whitney and the Walker art museums.

■   ■   ■

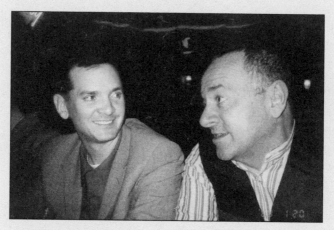

A *POZ* Life Expo held at New York's Javits Convention Center. That's artist Barton Benes with me at a dinner party.

CHAPTER 32

Memento Mori

By the time Doris and I returned to New York in November 1995, my health had deteriorated noticeably. My right eyelid was so swollen, it looked like I had a serious case of pinkeye. When reading a newspaper or magazine, I had to hold the pages up close and squint.

I started having breathing problems, so at night I was often restless and squirmed in bed, trying to find a position that allowed me to breathe comfortably. Xavier propped pillows under and around my body so my lungs would hang inside my rib cage relatively unobstructed, permitting intermittent sleep and fewer panicky gasps for air. Sometimes I was incontinent, but my night sweats so thoroughly soaked the sheets that at times Xavier and I couldn't tell what was sweat and what was urine. My visits to the *POZ* office became fewer and shorter, frequently sandwiched between naps.

When my HIV viral load hit 3.3 million late in 1995, it indicated an extremely aggressive rate of viral replication. From a high of around five hundred when I was diagnosed a decade earlier, my T-cell count had fallen consistently, dropping below one hundred around the time I launched *POZ*, then below ten to a single digit and, now, a T-cell count of one.

I started to see events in my life as "last times": the last time I would visit my parents in Iowa, the last time I would fly on an airplane, the last time I would enjoy a meal at a favorite restaurant. Once, when I made love to Xavier, I thought it might be the last time. When a postcard arrived to remind me of an upcoming dental checkup, I threw it away.

I couldn't imagine my future, but I thought about a future without me. I wondered how Megan, Xavier, and Stephen would deal with my death, who would attend my funeral, and what would happen to the magazine. I worried about Xavier and hoped he would find someone to love and not cut himself off from the world, as was his tendency.

That fall, there was a contentious debate in Oregon over a citizens' initiative to allow physician-assisted death; it ultimately passed with 51 percent of the vote. I followed the campaign closely, because many times I wondered how much suffering I would be able to endure. I did not keep a lethal stockpile of pills, although I thought about it. I worried that if I tried to do it on my own, I might screw it up and end up in a permanent coma. Asking for help was too large a burden to place on Xavier or Megan. But I could ask Stephen and knew he would understand and be willing to assist.

We all had become accustomed to having friends end their own lives. Most did so quietly and without notice, sometimes with a friendly physician who would note a cause of death other than suicide on the death certificate, to protect it as a secret. An exception was my friend Stephen Patrick, who alerted his friends and family of his decision by letter:

> *To My Family and Friends:*
> *I'm writing to all of you to say farewell. By the time you receive this letter, unless something goes terribly wrong, I will be dead . . . I've come to realize that I must exit life now, if I want to be in control of events at the end . . .*
> *Please don't grieve for me. I'm not depressed or sad about the decision I've made. I had a long and happy life that included an enrich-*

*ing long-term relationship, a satisfying career, and considerable world
travel undertaken when I was young enough to fully enjoy it. Instead
of grieving for me, please be happy that I was able to be in charge of
my final days . . .*

I found his letter oddly comforting, although I couldn't have written such a letter. But on the toughest days, I did think back to that conversation with Ken Dawson, as he lay dying, about his changing definition of quality of life. "A little erosion every day" was how he described it. Even as he passed milestones he once thought he would not be willing to endure, he continued to have good days and valued living over dying.

When I realized that my mental capacity was diminishing, I felt it more keenly than any of the physical limitations. My mind slowed down; making decisions, processing information, and sometimes communicating became more difficult. Once when I had a terrible fever, I heard Xavier and Megan talking about me a few feet from my bed. They thought I was too far out of it to understand what was going on, but I could hear them, even though I felt like there was a gauzy barrier between us. When I tried to speak, it was as if they were somewhere distant and couldn't hear me. While they worried about me, I was thinking, I'm not that sick, I'm not dying right now. Then I wondered if I was sicker than I realized; perhaps that inability to communicate was what dying felt like.

Several years later, I found a draft of a letter Xavier had written to my parents in Iowa, a plea for them to come to New York to see me. "This looks like it might be the end," he wrote. I didn't see that letter at the time Xavier wrote it, but his dire prognosis was a logical conclusion. The development we had been dreading for eighteen months was now at hand: X-rays showed flimsy, fibrous patches of KS growing inside my lungs. Callen's "90 in Nine" warning haunted me.

*   *   *

When the pulmonary KS was diagnosed in October 1995, Sonnabend sent me to see an oncologist who was enrolling patients in a clinical trial testing DaunoXome, a new chemotherapeutic agent that had shown some efficacy against KS. At first weekly, then every other week, Xavier took me to the New York University Medical Center for infusions.

At each visit, I spent an hour in a big La-Z-Boy-style chair with a needle in my arm, infusing DaunoXome from a hanging IV bag. The other gay patients and I called it "the beauty parlor," a reference to both the salon-style chairs and the chatter among the other patrons, mostly Orthodox Jewish women with breast cancer.

If my white blood-cell count was too low to tolerate the treatment, I was turned away. I learned to inject myself with Neupogen every other day to increase the white blood cells count: when it wasn't enough, I doubled up on the injections.

After the infusions, I would get an energy rush for several hours caused by a steroid mixed with the DaunoXome to reduce nausea. Then I would crash, suffering immobilizing fatigue and vomiting, wondering whether it was worth it. The chemo gave me a horrible metallic taste in my mouth that nothing could mask. My hair became dull and thin, my skin sallow and gray. I developed a constant ringing in my ears that I had to train my mind to ignore.

One weekend Max Westerman and I went to a friend's house in the Catskills. I thought I would be okay, as I had the chemo midday Thursday. By Friday evening, I was horribly nauseated and feverish. I spent the weekend on a couch, vomiting into a casserole dish, while my friends were trying to enjoy themselves, pretending that my heaving and the smell of my vomit weren't a bother.

It was hardest when I knew I was a burden on others; it became a struggle every time I had to go back for another infusion. I knew that if I didn't go, I would probably die. But it made me feel so miserable, far sicker than anything AIDS had done to me to date. I constantly weighed whether survival was worth it. It wasn't about despondency or depression; it was a question of quality of life, mine and that of those I loved.

*   *   *

One friend I loved deeply was Barton Benes, whom I'd met in 1990, not long after both of us lost our partners. He was particularly knowledgeable about KS because his partner, Howard Meyer, had it severely in his last years before he died.

Barton was an artist who lived alone in Westbeth, the artists' colony in the West Village, in a loft he and Howard had shared since 1973. It was filled with the exotic souvenirs of an artistic life: paintings, primitive and tribal art, relics, mummies (including a human arm), Turkish rugs, ancient tapestries, and curiosities in every corner. The taxidermy collection included the foot of an elephant, a giraffe's head and neck, and the mounted heads of a water buffalo, deer, and various animals with sculptural horns and antlers.

Barton used relics—including bodily fluids and the ashes of cremated friends—to make powerful, provocative art, often relating to the epidemic. One piece was a giant hourglass filled with the cremated remains of two lovers who both died of AIDS. When the sister of a friend of Barton's died of AIDS, he made from her ashes two hundred AIDS ribbons—a symbol he despised—and mounted them starkly on the wall. The piece was titled *Brenda*.

Even when Barton was telling stories about Howard's last months— during which KS turned large sections of his body nearly black with thick, waxy, foul-smelling lesions and dead skin—he maintained his macabre sense of humor. One day Barton was getting Howard out of bed and dressed, preparing to go to the doctor, when he found something black in the sheets: a piece of dark organic matter about the size of a flattened walnut. Thinking it was a piece of dead tissue that had fallen off of Howard, Barton put it in his pocket to show their doctor. The doctor held it up to the light, put it under a microscope, and confirmed that it was decaying flesh. He examined Howard but couldn't find where it might have come from.

When they got back to their loft, as Barton was helping Howard into bed, he looked up at the stuffed deer head hanging on the wall above their bed and saw that it was missing its nose.

Although Barton was plagued by his own health problems for years before his death in 2012, he never lost his compulsion to create. My favorite memento mori he made was a small pile of pottery shards that sat on the corner of the dining table. Each shard had a photograph glued to it, torn from snapshots of deceased friends. Whenever I visited Barton, I couldn't help but sift through the pile, noting any new additions. It was like going through the pages of a photo album, each image prompting a memory or anecdote: "Oh, that's Seth. Now, *he* was something . . ." Barton loved his shards almost as much as he loved the friends who inspired them.

Years later, after my health improved, a friend told me that Barton had made a shard for me in anticipation of my death. When I asked Barton, he first denied it and feigned shock at the mere suggestion. When pressed, he admitted he had selected both the image and the shard. "But they were just on my workbench loose," he protested. "I never glued them together!"

■   ■   ■

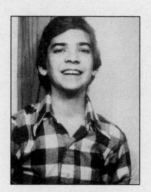

This was when I was in
seventh grade, before I
was sexually abused by a
teacher.

CHAPTER 33

Recall

During those sickest days, when I was heavily medicated, suffering high fevers, and thinking my time was running out, my mind involuntarily Ping-Ponged through thirty-seven years of memory. I began to recall long-suppressed physical, psychological, and sexual abuse from my childhood.

As my external life became smaller—I wasn't traveling, didn't interact with as many people on a daily basis, and was less concerned about the business or anything beyond my immediate circumstance—it was as if my brain finally had the time and capacity to explore closets I had kept closed for many years.

First it was glimpses, images of me naked and being used sexually by an older man. They would flit in and out of focus as though I were watching from afar. As a young adult, I had considered the possibility that I was sexually abused. There had been clues: I remembered hearing students at my Jesuit boarding school gossip about faculty members who "played with" students. When an upperclassman once asked if a teacher had "committed sodomy" on me, I didn't know what sodomy was. I could tell it was something bad, so I said no.

In my sickbed, I returned again and again to those conversations and other clues, searching for something hidden that I felt compelled to uncover. I remembered my pale prepubescent body at twelve or thirteen, its skin clean, fresh, and firm. Then I saw that body naked and vulnerable, trembling in fear while it was pressed against the hairy, flabby body of a middle-aged man stinking of alcohol and cigarettes.

I remembered the spooky after-hours silence of the nineteenth-century redbrick junior high school building. I was in the basketball coach's office. My parents had pushed me to join the team as the water boy. The office had a heavy old-fashioned wooden door with a frosted window and a lock that made a loud click when turned. Dusty venetian blinds made a scratchy, shuffling sound as they were pulled down. The coach was giving me a physical, which he said was required by law. I remember his heavy, excited breathing and acrid breath as he smeared K-Y jelly on my anus. It would make the exam "go faster," he said. I'd always despised the smell of K-Y, and now I realized why.

A couple of years later, at boarding school, I sprained my arm and was badly bruised in a softball game. The school clinic had closed for the day, so one of the senior administrators took me to his home to tend to my injuries. Even though I was almost fifteen, I had no pubic hair and was humiliated when he told me to take off my clothes and stand on a white towel he had placed on the floor of his bedroom so he could "examine" the damage. He sat on the bed with a glass of Scotch in one hand, marveling at my smooth pubic area. He emitted a sort of mirthful chuckle, then ran a finger around the nearly bare base of my penis and my pubescent testicles. "I can't believe it," he slurred.

It was Catholicism that taught me to hate homosexuality and fear and repress desire. This self-hatred separated me from my body and made me ashamed of it. Neither of the abusers was a Catholic priest, but one was an usher in my home parish and the other a senior faculty member at the Jesuit boarding school I attended. These men were imbued with the Church's unassailable authority.

I began to connect the dots between the sexual abuse I suffered and Catholicism's psychological torment of me as a child, and the unhealthy sexual relationships, behaviors, and promiscuity I'd engaged in as an adult. I don't disclaim responsibility, but I now believe that the sexual and psychological abuse I suffered as a child laid the groundwork for the behaviors I engaged in as an adult that led to acquiring HIV. If gay men as a whole had less shame and self-hatred imposed upon them by society when they were children, I wonder if we might have been more moderate in our sexual behaviors as adults when we finally found communities of our own where we could escape society's torment and be with each other.

I didn't learn to respect my body when I was young—how could I when it wasn't being respected by important adults in my life?—and I was well into adulthood before I took ownership of my body, let alone took any pride in it.

I had long since resolved my feelings about the Catholic Church, most dramatically that day in St. Patrick's Cathedral. But recalling painful suppressed sexual abuse memories was something I had subconsciously avoided. As I searched my memory and thought back to those times, I was afraid of what I would discover. I had always feared the abuse was really my fault, that I could have stopped it, or could have told other adults about it.

I was bullied in school because my interests were suspect (antiques, reading, art), I was small (I grew to six-one as an adult but was nearly the shortest kid in my high school class), and I'd been tagged with the epithet "faggot" off and on since the fourth grade. When I was so frightened that I talked to a school principal or teacher about it, I was usually told to "be a man" and fight back. I didn't have adults in my life that I could have talked to about something so personal, that brought me so much shame, and for which I felt responsibility.

I finally realized how at the time I thought of the men who sexually abused me as protectors and how important that was to me. I had felt indebted to them; their friendship was a survival strategy. It was this dependency that made me vulnerable to their abuse. As I read and learned more about sexual abuse, I also realized they were probably victims of abuse when they were children too and, of course, they too were steeped in Catholicism and hadn't escaped it as I did. Understanding this enabled me to release anger I had clenched and suppressed for years.

The men who abused me may have helped keep bullies away from me, but it came with the high price of tolerating their assaults. Now, in my sickbed, I was breaking that contract.

I put together these pieces over a period of several years, getting in touch with classmates who confirmed that they also had damaging experiences with these men. As I learned more and processed the memories flooding back, I wanted to know more about what had happened to the two abusers and whether they were still working with children. I was thinking about exposing them, but was reluctant to go public, fearing both the stigma and potentially having to testify against them.

One day while visiting my great-aunt Helen at Oaknoll, a retirement community in Iowa City, I passed a room bearing the name of the junior high teacher/coach/usher. I impulsively knocked and stood waiting, not sure what I felt or what I might say. A stooped, scowling, unshaved man opened the door and said curtly, "Yes?"

When I said, "It's Sean Strub. Do you remember me?," his eyes instantly widened, as though becoming aware of danger. He stepped back and said, "What do you want?," his voice slightly tremulous, his expression a mixture of annoyance and fear. I looked at him for a moment, and my anger dissipated into pity. "Nothing, just saying hello as I passed by," I said.

I telephoned the other abuser at his home in the Midwest one evening. Although he sounded drunk or high, as soon as he heard my name, he became alert and solicitous. I found out he was no longer working in a school and was semi-retired. He asked about my brother and my parents and wanted to know how I was and what I was doing. When I told him I had AIDS, he said he would pray for me.

"You're the one who needs prayers," I replied.

He was silent for a minute and then said softly, "Yes, I guess you're right."

We didn't speak explicitly about what he had done to me, but it was the unspoken theme of our brief exchange. He tried to be apologetic without saying he was sorry, contrite without acknowledging the infliction of any harm. As we were ending the conversation, he said, "If you ever need any help, financial or whatever, please let me know." It sounded to me like a well-practiced offer he had made to others.

Emotionally excavating these experiences was immensely important for me. The advent of combination protease therapy in 1996 may have treated my HIV successfully, but I am certain I owe my full recovery to the process of self-examination, prompted by my illness, that helped me understand and reconcile the sexual abuse I suffered as a child.

CHAPTER 34

Lazarus

While the DaunoXome infusions at the "beauty parlor" were no cure for my KS, they did slow the growth of new lesions. After a few weeks of treatment in late 1995 and early 1996, X-rays showed that the lesions in my lungs had stabilized, and a few of the spots on my skin had faded slightly.

I knew there was a new class of drugs, protease inhibitors, on the horizon, and preliminary trial results were encouraging. I was hopeful, but I was always hopeful even as one new drug after another fell short of its promise. In any case, my main focus wasn't so much on future treatments as it was with coping with how sick I felt from the chemo and making sure I could breathe properly.

The rumor that protease inhibitors were interrupting viral replication in a different and dramatically more effective manner was enticing. The idea Stephen brought up at our *POZ* dinner a year before, that using drugs in combination might stop the virus from mutating and developing resistance, was now the buzz. "Combination therapy" with a drug "cocktail," with components from each of the three classes of AIDS drugs, might be what we had been fighting and hoping for.

Ever since AZT's approval process, there was always talk about the next great drug in the pipeline; this was the next chapter in that ongoing story. I wasn't going to get excited and put my hopes in preliminary trial results. Even if the drugs did work against HIV, my most life-threatening concern, KS, was caused by an entirely different virus, HHV-8, and no one was suggesting the new drugs would be effective against it.

The first protease inhibitor to hit the market, Roche's Invirase, was approved for sale in December 1995, but the Treatment Action Group, *POZ*, and others were critical because it was poorly absorbed in the bloodstream and facilitated development of a resistant virus. We didn't think anyone should take it unless they were on the brink of death; we debated at the magazine whether or not we should accept their advertising (we did). Roche had rushed the approval, knowing it was an inferior product and could limit future treatment options for those who took it. Two superior protease inhibitors, Merck's Crixivan and Abbott's Norvir, were approved in March 1996.

I started taking Norvir when it came out in March. In combination with the chemotherapy, it made me even more miserable. I was taking thirty pills a day, including swallowing six gelatinous Norvir pills three times a day, each about the size of a large jellybean. Sometimes I debated whether to continue the treatment. Among Norvir's side effects was what we dubbed "projectile diarrhea." It would come on with little warning—sometimes as little as fifteen seconds—and rocket out of the rectum, comparable to the convulsive action of a sneeze. Worse than the physical discomfort and mess was the limitation it placed on my mobility. A friend said the prescribing instructions should include "Carry an extra pair of underwear at all times." Once I had to threaten to defecate in the aisle of the D'Agostino supermarket in the West Village to get access to the bathroom.

Nonetheless, after only a few weeks on my "PI," I knew I was getting better and was convinced my viral load was dropping. When the KS lesions started to fade, I was certain it was from the protease inhibitor, not the chemotherapy. The oncologist was annoyed when I stopped the chemo; later, I learned he was compensated for every patient he enrolled in the clinical trial. As soon as I stopped the chemo, my energy increased and I started to gain weight.

My planning window, which for years had been steadily shrinking, started to expand. I had a renewed sense of energy and expectation. I felt confident making plans a few weeks and, soon, a few months into the future. Eventually, I could think about the following spring or summer. It was exciting but tentative. Every day I wondered, Is this the day my treatment will stop working?

The stress of recovery was peculiar. Many of my relationships were shaped by the expectation that I wouldn't be around much longer. As my expectations for the future grew, the perspective of others changed on the same schedule. In February 1997, *The New York Times* profiled what had come to be called the "Lazarus Syndrome," the experience of people with HIV who had been "brought back from the dead" by the new treatments. Many who had been confined to bed could walk; others were returning to work. It was spectacular.

Those who had died in the months prior to the release of the new treatments were mourned with a special sadness. "If he only could have held on a few more months," we would say, guilty relief that we had made it.

I knew my own health was improving, but it was incremental, with good days and bad. On bad days, it seemed I had traded the side effects of chemo for a slew of new side effects. Some people taking Crixivan were developing large potbellies, a side effect we referred to in *POZ* as "Crix-belly." Crixivan's manufacturer, Merck, complained that the phrase unfairly maligned the product and pointed out a similar phenomenon with those taking other protease inhibitors; we started calling it "protease paunch" instead. Outside the pages of the magazine or gatherings of people with HIV, to dwell on side effects was considered almost ungrateful, with an implication that the mind-set was trapped in an earlier time in the epidemic.

There were also the renewed obligations of a more "normal" life to contend with, even though life was far from normal. It took time to adjust to the prospect of having a future. Something as simple as buying new clothes felt like an expression of optimism about my future that I may or may not have felt in that moment. I had the dental checkup that just a few months before hadn't seemed worth the effort. I began to sort out my finances, which were neglected while I was coasting toward my demise. And I started seeing old friends and acquaintances I had not been in touch with for years. Sometimes those reunions were awkward because they, too, had to adjust to the fact that I was no longer within sight of death.

The smaller house Xavier and I bought in Palisades in 1995 was a 1920s Cape Cod–style cottage with two bedrooms and a fenced backyard. It was charming, but once my health started to return, I found it too small, too close to the road. I missed the space and grandeur of the larger house in Piermont, and the homophobic next-door neighbor did not help matters. Mostly, though, we had moved into that house expecting that I would die in it, and now that I had a future again, I wanted to get out of there.

In October 1996, barely six months after starting protease therapy, I leafed through the back pages of *The New York Times* Sunday magazine, fantasizing about the beautiful properties listed for sale. I noticed a simple ad without a picture: "600 Acre Hunting Camp on Trout Stream. Perfect Executive Retreat 75 miles from Manhattan." The phrase "owner financing available" grabbed me, too.

The property was in Pike County, a heavily forested, culturally conservative corner of northeast Pennsylvania. Xavier and I drove up that afternoon with our dog, Willy. We met the owner at his house in the nearby picturesque village of Milford to drive to the property together. As we approached, he pulled over, saying, "I'll let you out here. Just follow this stream for about half a mile, until you pass a small dam. Then look for the waterfall. I'll meet you at the main lodge. You'll see it as you hike downstream."

Pike County has a sharp and craggy terrain, with thick plates of bluestone and shale smashed together by glaciers tens of thousands of years ago. It's almost entirely covered by dense forests of hemlock, pine, shagbark hickory, maple, and oak. The branches of the deciduous species were mostly bare. Tufts of snow were scattered through the woods.

The Dwarfskill stream is a small, pristine tributary of the Raymondskill, which feeds the Delaware River between Milford and Dingmans Ferry. We followed the stream as it flowed into a narrowing glen with increasingly steep sides. The air was brisk, and we had no idea how long we would walk before finding the owner. Six hundred acres sounded huge; Xavier was concerned about my stamina. Just a few months before, such a trek would have been unthinkable.

After about twenty-five minutes, we heard the waterfall, but at first didn't see it, only the stream meandering slowly ahead of us through dense woods. Then we realized we were standing practically on top of it, twenty-five feet above the deep pool at its base. We were surrounded by wilderness and no noise except water crashing into water. No cars, no sirens in the distance, no planes in the sky, just clean water rushing through a bluestone cataract, as it had for thousands of years, with misty clouds bubbling from its base.

When we got out of the car, I was conscious of how clean and fresh the air was. By the time we hiked to the waterfall, that sensation had intensified. Pneumonias, bronchial infections, and cancerous KS tumors had battered my lungs for years. Now I felt like I was in an oxygen factory and breathing deeply for the first time, almost like a joyous hyperventilation. Standing there with Xavier, entranced by the waterfall's unstoppable flow, was as close as I have ever come to a spiritual awakening. I felt like a new part of my life had opened up before me.

We didn't close on the property until the following summer. Several years later, we donated the development rights for several hundred acres of the property to the Delaware Highlands Conservancy, a local land trust. The conservation easement reduced the value of the property dramatically, but protected the land in perpetuity. Knowing that that land and waterfall will still be there, protected forever from development, long after Xavier and I are gone, gives me a sense of pride and satisfaction.

By 1998, I was spending most of my time in Pennsylvania, giving up activism and city life to live "off the grid" in a knotty-pine cabin in the middle of a hemlock forest. Xavier and I created a country life, complete with chickens, geese, turkeys, ducks, guinea hens, and rabbits. Our dog Willy loved living in the woods, even more so after we adopted another dog, Olive, and he had a companion. Walking to the henhouse in the morning was one of my favorite rituals; Willy would trot along at my side, carrying the egg basket in his teeth. The woods were thick with deer; sometimes we saw a black bear, and a flock of wild turkeys ambled by the lodge almost every day.

Feeling close to nature helped center me in a new life, one that wasn't defined by my expected impending death. Xavier and I went days at a time without leaving the property or seeing anyone. I loved the serenity and solitude, hearing the rush of the stream and a breeze whistling through the trees.

Several times evangelicals ventured down the half-mile driveway to knock on our door and proselytize. When they woke us up early one Sunday morning, Xavier, annoyed at their frequent visits, swung open the front door wearing only his underwear and told them, "We're militant homosexuals and not interested!" We didn't see them again.

The village of Milford was six miles away, with beautifully landscaped streetscapes, eclectic architecture, a rich history, and rapidly rising real estate values. The hunting camp appreciated enough to enable me to start buying and restoring historic buildings, turning a ramshackle boardinghouse into a restaurant and an old lumberyard into an antique center operated by my older sister, Missi. With my characteristic compulsive activity greased by some good old grandiosity, I launched businesses, including a monthly regional magazine, and began various projects that extended indefinitely into the future.

I met Dick Snyder, a corporate executive from New York who had retired in Milford to raise and breed llamas. He got me involved with a community-enhancement project in Milford. In fifteen years, from 1997 to 2012, we raised more than $4 million to improve public spaces in Milford, install new granite curbing, bluestone sidewalks, historic-style pedestrian lighting and benches, and renovate landscaping. We helped launch film and music festivals and joined the boards of directors of several regional nonprofit organizations. It was a creative collaboration to revitalize Milford's quintessential small-town American charm while welcoming the community's growing diversity.

Dick and I became friends and business partners. We restored the historic Hotel Fauchère, which had been run by the same family from 1852 until it closed in 1976. Louis Fauchère, the founder, was a master chef at Delmonico's in New York in the mid-nineteenth century; when he opened the Hotel Fauchère in Milford as a summer destination and restaurant, he brought a city clientele to the town, establishing it as a favored destination during the Gilded Era.

As absorbing as all this activity was for me, and as helpful as it was to the local economy, not everyone cheered an outsider from the big city moving in. As my high profile projects gave me a growing influence in the community, some feared I was "taking over the town." That I was an outspoken gay activist with AIDS didn't help. After I bought the old lumberyard, one elderly member of the borough council told people he heard I was going to open an adult bookstore and that I was part of a homosexual plot to turn Milford into "Gayford." He claimed there was a takeover plan, "It's written out, I've seen it!" he told one person.

I immersed myself in local community activities, organizing efforts in Milford as I once had run political campaigns. I was convinced every critic was just someone who didn't understand me or never had met anyone gay before.

I love the film *Mr. Smith Goes to Washington*, and sometimes saw my rebirth in Milford as a reversal of its plot. In the movie, an earnest and naive small-town community leader goes to Washington to battle cynicism in the nation's capital. I brought a world-weary cynicism from my years in politics and the epidemic to a small rural community, where I found renewal in small-town life that I compared to living in a Norman Rockwell painting. My New York friends were only vaguely aware of what was happening in Pennsylvania; all they knew was that I was no longer in the city or at *POZ* very much. "Sean's burnt out on AIDS," some said.

In reality, I was pursuing interests I had shelved fifteen years earlier. Had the epidemic not hijacked my life, I might have become a small-town newspaper publisher, historic preservationist, antique dealer, or galleryist, or run for local office. All those paths I now felt free to pursue. My life "planning window," that had steadily shrunk through the '80s and early '90s, was now going in the other direction, eventually extending to the future with no expectation that AIDS would interrupt it. Like a lot of people with AIDS who had expected to die, I had to spend time putting my life back together and trying to figure out what to do next.

But I could never have put AIDS behind me, even if I had wanted to.

■   ■   ■

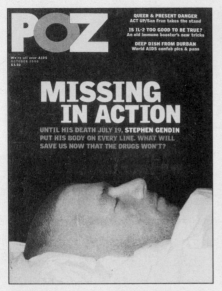

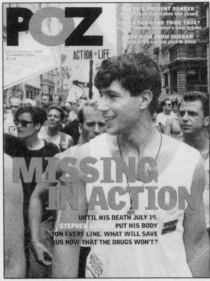

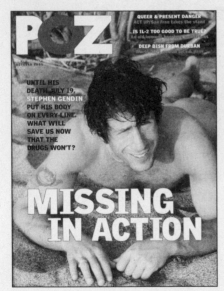

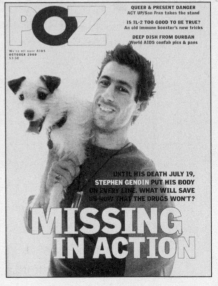

When Stephen died, we stopped the issue we were working on and hastily put together a memorial tribute to him, with four different covers, each depicting a different time in his life.

CHAPTER 35

Stephen

During the decade of my friendship with Stephen, I felt like I was sharing something important, but intangible, with him that had been shared with me, by Vito Russo and other older activists. That made me feel good, like I was honoring my mentors by sharing their wisdom with a new generation; it broadened the sense of brotherhood and my chosen family that I cherished.

For most of that time, we both assumed that I would die before Stephen. I was older, had been infected longer, and had more symptoms. I thought of Stephen as my activist and entrepreneurial heir. But in the late '90s, our roles reversed. I was getting better, while he was getting sicker.

When Hush called around two A.M. on July 19, 2000, with the terrible news that Stephen had died, it was a shock. We knew he was very ill—he had just started treatment for lymphoma—but he was still in the office regularly. I did not recognize that he was so close to death.

A week earlier I had given Stephen a ride to his apartment on Forty-fifth Street, and we sat in my Prius outside his building for half an hour, talking and reminiscing. I put my arm across the back of the seat and softly stroked his hair; he was fragile and seemed to appreciate the affection.

I don't think I understood the depth of my love for Stephen until the moment I learned of his death. I was alone in Pennsylvania; Xavier was in the city. I was devastated, selfishly angry about my own pain, and furious at the personal attacks Stephen had suffered due to Hush's seroconversion, which were fresh in my memory.

I went to my computer around three A.M. and sent an e-mail to *POZ* staff and friends with the news:

> I have never met a man I admired more; his death slams the very worst pain and loss in my heart. I hate this fucking disease. No one deserves the agony we have endured for two decades. Activism, in the absence of Stephen's integrity, honesty, and deep drive for meaning, now feels impossible. I check my anger—momentarily— with the memory of Stephen's extraordinarily gentle nature and awesome intellect. He is, was, and will always be my beloved hero. I want so desperately to believe in a hereafter, one without disease, where Stephen and so many other friends can play and cuddle and love one another.

Then I drove into New York. I needed to be with Xavier, and I wanted to be at the office when the staff arrived for work and learned the news. It was somber and silent, quiet weeping and soft voices. Redden's Funeral Home was a five-minute walk from the loft, and a group of us walked there together. It was a familiar ritual; Redden's was where, over the years, I last saw the bodies of Michael Misove and many other friends.

Stephen was laid out in the same room where I last saw Michael in 1988. Hush had shaved Stephen's head a few days before, in preparation for the expected hair loss from the chemo regimen Stephen had just begun. Seeing Stephen's head shorn was a shock; I had become accustomed to the constantly changing colors of his outrageous hairstyles. I awkwardly hugged his body. As my head bent close to his and kissed him, my tears formed puddles on his eyes. I wished his mouth would break into that marvelous Stephen smile. I struggled to find deeper meaning in his death, but I could not. I wanted to assign blame or make a dramatic vow—fulfill Stephen's old fantasy of killing Jesse Helms?—but I couldn't do that, either.

Near the end of his life, Stephen realized he might have hastened his own death by making aggressive and experimental treatment choices. He had turned his body into a virtual lab experiment testing every new treatment, but not even the protease inhibitors were able to keep his resistant virus at bay for long. At one point he was taking five—or was it seven?—HIV drugs at the same time. I regret not having pushed harder with him for a more cautious approach. It hurts me to acknowledge that, had he managed his treatment differently, he might still be alive.

In Stephen's quest for survival he demonstrated great independence and original thinking. His curiosity and brilliance led to his taking risks with his body that expanded our knowledge about the benefits and limitations of anti-retroviral therapies.

He had physical beauty, and an eccentric combination of sexy geek and a shy, sly charisma. Many men and women alike became infatuated with him from afar; a few found his distracted air arrogant or unfriendly.

When I first met him, I thought his aloof manner masked insecurity; he didn't know how to engage in chitchat or the murmurs of assent of routine conversation. Over time I learned that it was not insecurity at all but something much deeper. His brain worked differently.

In Stephen's last years, he came to accept that he was missing out on some essential aspect of human experience. Summoning his great resources of intellect and determination, he set about trying to "fix" himself through therapy, courses, and reading about spirituality and self-actualization. He wanted to use the time he had left to grow as much as possible.

Some people fell into AIDS activism as a matter of circumstance, because they or someone they loved got sick. With Stephen, it was a decision from the beginning. He was fifteen when the epidemic was recognized, and he was acutely conscious of his sexuality, so AIDS was always part of the equation. I don't think he had moments when he felt resentful, that the epidemic had diverted his life from some other path. Activism was his primary passion, from when he started an ACT UP group in college while at Brown University in 1988 until his death twelve years later, and activism became the outlet for his longing to spiritually minister to other gay men with whom he felt a profound bond. He never knew adult ambitions in the absence of AIDS.

Stephen's death came at a time of precipitous decline in AIDS activism, especially among white men, following the introduction of protease inhibitors. When the threat of death was no longer imminent, many tried to go back to their previous lives or attempted to forge new ones. Stephen had been one of a few powerful voices remaining from what had once been a mighty chorus.

When he died, we at *POZ* put aside the issue we were working on in favor of one devoted to his memory. We included his last column— he had turned it in right before he died—along with reflections from friends on his exceptional life and legacy. We created four different covers, each with a different picture of Stephen. In one he was at a demonstration, wearing a sleeveless T-shirt, his hair neatly cropped—an ACT UP "poster boy," as Larry Kramer described him. Another showed him on the beach at Fire Island Pines, looking up at the camera with mischievous and youthful sexiness, his bare callipygous buttocks visible. The third showed him in colorful clothes and playing with Zoom, his Jack Russell terrier whose tail was often dyed to match Stephen's hair color of the moment. The final image was of his shorn head. Walter had suggested to Ronnilyn Pustil, one of our editors, that she take the photograph the morning we saw his body at Redden's.

Each cover reflected a theme from Stephen's life. Together, they were intended to represent the four seasons of an adulthood, cruelly reduced to a single decade for Stephen, as for so many young gay men with AIDS. Subscribers randomly received one of the four different covers, though many requested copies of the other three so they could have a complete set.

Stephen's memorial became a de facto ACT UP reunion, with over a hundred people crowding the Gay and Lesbian Community Services Center. There were many speakers—including Ann Northrop, Larry Kramer, and Michael Warner among others—as well as Hush and Stephen's former partner, Mark Aurigemma.

I tried to convey what he had meant to me and shared anecdotes that illustrated his hyper-rationality. One of my favorite "Stephen stories" highlighted his practical approach to sexual pleasure. Stephen was involved with Sex Panic!, a direct action group that campaigned for sexual freedom in the age of AIDS and opposed political measures to control sex. He was invited to be a guest on the *Rolonda* show, a daytime cable program in the mid-'90s era of "trash television." The episode was titled "Why Do People Go to Sex Clubs?" Of the four guests, three wore slinky clothes, black leather, chains, or stud collars, and two were dramatically made up, all sitting on stools on a stage. Stephen sat on the stool farthest to the left, wearing a suit and tie with a white shirt, pretending to be exactly what he was not: a clean-cut young preppy. The host was on her feet with a microphone, guiding the discussion.

While the other three guests tried to outdo one another with "shocking" tales of their supposed sex-club exploits, Stephen listened quietly. Several times, Rolonda looked toward Stephen with her eyebrows arched, as if saying, "You want to jump in here?" Finally, she put her hand up to stop the others from talking and said, "I want to hear from Stephen. He hasn't said a word yet."

As she walked toward Stephen, she slowly looked him up and down. Stopping in front of him, she smiled and looked at the audience, then back at Stephen, saying, "Stephen, you are a good looking young man.

Mmm-mmm, you are *good*-looking. I'll bet you could have sex all the time, with just about anyone you wanted to. Why, oh why would you *ever* go to a sex club?"

Stephen paused as if conducting a quick mental review to make sure he had the right answer. Then, with an earnest look, he said, "Because it's efficient!" He looked slightly mystified as Rolonda and the audience howled with laughter.

Stephen's memorial service was one of the last in what had become a tradition of dramatic memorials for prominent former ACT UP members. Stephen had come to the conclusion that AIDS activism, as we knew it, was over. His last column described with great bitterness the glitzy meetings that TAG and other treatment activists routinely attended on pharma's tab.

> These days, my friends and I often mourn the loss of activism. Everyone we know is still doing AIDS work, but our involvement has become institutionalized. We aren't volunteers anymore: we're professionals. AIDS is a 9-to-5 JOB. It disgusts me to see what I've become. Ten years ago, we would never have accepted such gifts and graft from drug companies. Now we've come to count on it. But nothing's free, and whether we know it or not, we're paying the price with our lives.

Stephen's death triggered grieving I had shelved for years. Depressed, I withdrew even further from New York City and from *POZ*. Every problem, decision, or triumph in the business reminded me of how much I missed him.

I was grieving other losses as well. Xavier and I had come to the difficult decision to break up; Stephen's death accentuated pressures that had built over time. When we met in 1992, Xavier was living with his family in Brooklyn; he moved directly from there into my loft. When I started getting sicker, he quit his job to care for me, never really having the opportunity to become independently established. His ambitions became secondary to my fragile health. The assumption was that he would get to his own life, after my demise.

Our lives changed dramatically as my health returned. Our breakup hurt, but we remained kind to each other. He took over the lease on the West Twelfth Street loft, and I relished the quiet and solitude of the cabin in Pennsylvania.

Megan had gotten married and was settling into a new life with her husband, so we didn't see each other as much. Doris was having mobility problems and seldom left her apartment; we had gotten divorced when I didn't die, but that was, like the marriage, a legal measure driven by financial convenience. Max Westerman, my closest friend since we met at the Ninth Circle in 1979, had moved to Brazil. Of my other friends who had survived, many had moved away or invented new lives. Sometimes we discovered that our bond had been our sickness; what we had shared when we were so ill was stronger than what we shared when our health returned.

At the same time, I was increasingly resentful of the incessant stress from trying to keep *POZ* afloat. I determined to stop taking cash advances on my credit cards and juggling short-term loans to meet *POZ*'s payroll. After I'd come so close to death and then recovered, my values had changed.

For several years, Brad Peebles had been running the overall company, while Walter was editor-in-chief and Megan was the publisher of *POZ*. It wasn't easy with the company undercapitalized, me in Pennsylvania most of the time, and, now, Stephen's death. Megan and I appointed Brad to take Stephen's place on the company's board of directors, and I gradually turned more responsibility over to the two of them. Brad, armed with an MBA and previous experience at Condé Nast, tried to professionalize the company and lead it to profitability; Megan became a buffer between us. It was difficult; I wanted to maintain the same level of pride and ownership I always had, while offloading the stress and responsibility, a textbook example of "founder's syndrome." I floated in and out of engagement with the company and sometimes questioned whether I was withdrawing voluntarily or being pushed out. I found myself sniping from the sidelines, compelled to criticize and complain but not willing to return to my previous role. Brad and Megan were annoyed with my loss of interest and sometimes became angry at my meddling in the company's day-to-day management.

The truth is, I love starting organizations and tend to put so much of myself into them that I have a hard time letting others take over. I've always been a better creator and instigator than operator or manager, but it took me decades to learn that lesson.

In July 2001, a year after Stephen's death, I more formally stepped back from the magazine. In a message to readers, I noted the pain of Stephen's death, my struggle with depression, and the company's difficult financial situation. At the end of the column, I wrote:

> No matter what brickbats are thrown our way, nothing can diminish the pride I take on behalf of everyone living or dead who has helped *POZ* accomplish so much. For a bunch of diseased queers, junkies, and ex-cons, I think we've done a pretty good job . . . We searched for truth and campaigned for justice. We learned that it all starts in our own hearts, in how we live our lives and treat others. No amount of activism will change the world until enough of us change ourselves.

CHAPTER 36

Postpartum

In that farewell column, I wrote that without Stephen, I felt adrift running *POZ*; it seemed like my enthusiasm and sometimes my hope were gone. I told readers that, during the previous winter, I had suffered the most serious episode of depression I'd ever experienced. "Many friends find it easy to empathize with you when you are wasting or sprouting KS. Fewer understand the debilitating effects of depression, which can make it the loneliest and most frightening disease," I wrote.

Like a lot of people, I had suffered from undiagnosed mild to moderate depression off and on throughout my adult life. Ironically, when I was most sick with AIDS, I wasn't particularly depressed. But when my health returned, so did the depression.

In the several years following Stephen's death, I lacked a larger purpose in my life even as I launched more projects in Milford. Indeed, a burst of activity did not ward off a serious episode of depression that ultimately left me suicidal. It wasn't like the deliberative contemplation about ending my life when I was ill; I was overwhelmed instead by hopelessness.

My solitude exacerbated the problem. "Dr. Sonnabend" had become "Joe," and a close friend. He had retired and moved back to London but was generous with his time, and when we were Skyping about my treatment, I finally confided in him about the persistent depression and suicidal ideation.

He urged me to stop taking Sustiva, a powerful new anti-retroviral drug I'd started in 2003. Though Sustiva is known for causing disturbing dreams and restless sleep in the first few weeks of ramping up, the company's promotional material—noted in advertisements in *POZ*—promised those side effects were brief. Since I had made it through those initial few weeks, I thought any risk had passed. Long-term depression wasn't noted as a risk on the required prescribing information.

I searched online and discovered that many people with HIV were having similar problems attributed to Sustiva; some had attempted to kill themselves while on the drug. Three days after I quit Sustiva, the dark clouds began to lift. The depression wasn't gone, but it had returned to the level I had managed for years. Today Sustiva is considered dangerous for people with a history of depression and includes such a warning label on its prescribing information.

In his speech at Stephen's memorial service, Larry Kramer had spoken specifically about this drug, but I either wasn't paying attention or chalked it up to Larry's dramatic rhetoric. "Sustiva is one of the most inhumane medicines ever launched into the bloodstream of man," he said. "[DuPont executives need to] start behaving like scientists and not like Nazi experimenters."

My suicidal feelings had frightened me, shattered my newly emergent sense of self-esteem, and made me skittish. Dick Snyder and I took on new restorations and projects, and from the outside, it looked like I was "accomplishing" a lot. On the inside, I was a mess. I began to see my frenetic efforts in Milford as driven as much by pathology as passion.

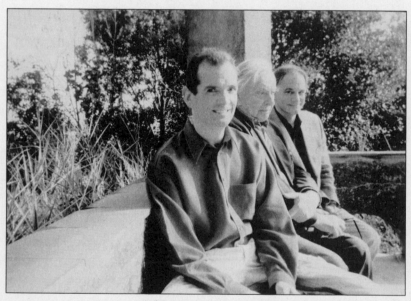

Howard Austen, Gore Vidal's partner, took this picture of me and John Berendt, with Gore in the center, at La Rondinaia, their palazzo in Ravello, Italy, in 2000. (Photo courtesy of Howard Austen.)

CHAPTER 37

Naked to the World

For years, *POZ*'s creative director, J. C. Suares, had told me I should meet his friend John Berendt, who wrote *Midnight in the Garden of Good and Evil*. In one of life's serendipitous moments, John and I finally met through my artist friend Barton Benes, who had met him at a dinner party in 1999 at the Dakota (the building where John Lennon lived). Barton had brought a gift for the host, a small reliquary he had made with sixteen tiny relics mounted and labeled in a frame, including Sharon Stone's powder puff, a piece of celluloid from an Andy Warhol film, a fragment from Hitler's hideaway in Berchtesgaden, and other curiosities.

Early in John's career, he had worked on *The David Frost Show*, and one night Roy Rogers and Dale Evans were guests. They left behind a glass medicine bottle filled with a clear solution that had little bits of matter floating in it that John described as "tiny, feathery white fragments." The label was from a pharmacy in Palm Desert, California. It was a prescription for "Mr. Roy Rogers" for a "nasal douche."

When John told this to Barton, his eyes lit up, and he offered to trade a piece of his art for Roy Rogers's "boogers bottle," as Barton called it. I met John at Barton's studio the night they were to have the exchange.

While Barton cooked us dinner, John and I created our own contribution to Barton's reliquary work by spitting into a glass. Our "conjoined spit" became part of Barton's art.

After we'd been brought together by Roy Rogers's snot and consummated our new friendship with spit, I wasn't surprised to read later that *Time* magazine referred to John as "a weirdo magnet." He became one of my closest friends and strongest sources of emotional support. We shared a background in magazines—he as an editor at *Esquire* and then editor in chief of *New York* magazine—and he had followed *POZ* from its launch.

We traveled together, attended book festivals, and spent weekends at my house in Milford. John helped me reenter a world beyond one defined by AIDS, creating a new life after Stephen died and my relationships with Megan and Xavier had changed in important ways.

Once, when I was visiting John in Venice, where he was writing *The City of Falling Angels*, we went to the Amalfi Coast to introduce him to Gore Vidal. I was a little nervous, because Doris had warned me that Gore wasn't known for his friendliness toward other writers. But when we got to La Rondinaia, Gore was warm and welcoming; he had even reread *Midnight in the Garden of Good and Evil* in anticipation of our visit.

Gore's partner, Howard Austen, joined us for a lunch at a nearby trattoria. After lunch, Gore, John, and I had a drink in the piazza in Ravello's center, and we talked about how the epidemic had changed since the introduction of combination therapy. Gore marveled at how my lesions had faded away. He recalled that when he'd seen them, he didn't expect me to survive much longer. "*Fronti nulla fides,*" he said to me, testing my Latin. When he saw the blank look on my face, he translated: "Appearances can't be trusted."

After several more stops for cocktails, we ended up back at La Rondinaia later that evening, after Howard had gone to bed. Gore sliced some cheese, served us a holiday panna cotta and fixed more drinks, then we settled in for a marathon conversation in front of a crackling fireplace.

There were several books about Lincoln on the coffee table. A few weeks before our trip, Larry Kramer had given a speech in Wisconsin, claiming that correspondence between Lincoln and his onetime bedmate, Joshua Speed, evidenced Lincoln's likely homosexuality.

"What do you think about Larry Kramer's claim that Abraham Lincoln was gay?" I asked Gore, who had written an historical novel about Lincoln. "Kramer ruined it," he said. "No one will take it seriously, no matter how convincing the case, because he made Lincoln's homosexuality the claim of gay activists with an agenda rather than the scholarship of serious historians."

Gore added that Lincoln's predecessor, President James Buchanan, the country's only bachelor president, was homosexual. Buchanan had lived for fifteen years with William Rufus DeVane King, the country's only bachelor vice president (under Buchanan's predecessor, Franklin Pierce). I pointed out that meant there had been a gay president or vice president across three consecutive administrations, and Gore's eyes lit up. "Yes, a cabal!" he said.

We watched *Gore Vidal's American Presidency*, which he wrote and appeared in, detailing the rise and abuse of executive powers from Washington through to the then-current occupant of the White House, George W. Bush. Gore claimed the History Channel was so "appalled" by his depiction of an imperial presidency that they'd aired it only once rather than in the usual broadcast rotation. They prefaced the broadcast with a disclaimer by Roger Mudd and had a panel of historians at the end to critique Gore's analysis.

At one point, I got up to go to the bathroom, but Gore said, "No, no, no, the flush will wake up Howard. Just go ahead and piss out the window," gesturing toward the French doors in his library that faced the Gulf of Salerno. As I stood on the wrought-iron Juliet balcony outside the window, John joined me and unzipped. Then Gore came over, and the three of us stood shoulder to shoulder, peeing over the balcony into a dark night sky, our urine splashing on a skylight on the villa's lower-level roof.

With his free hand, Gore pointed out an island off the coast where Rudolph Nureyev lived for a while before his death from AIDS in 1993. As we walked back to sit in front of the fire, Gore showed us a standing telescope that he'd focused on the chaise longue next to Nureyev's swimming pool, where the dancer liked to sunbathe nude.

John and I stayed late into the night. We drank a lot, but couldn't begin to keep pace with Gore, whose capacity for alcohol seemed to be unlimited. His eyes became moist several times while he talked about men he had loved in the 1950s, including Dick York, famous for his role as Darrin Stephens on the 1960s television program *Bewitched*; he had a part in *Visit to a Small Planet*, a play that Gore wrote for television in 1955. We spent most of the evening talking about politics, from our losing campaigns for Congress in the Hudson River Valley (his in 1960, mine in 1990) to the abysmal state of America's global standing, the buffoonery of the Bush administration, and the erosion of civil liberties and democratic ideals. When the topic of LGBT activism came up, I asked him, "How much of an effect do you think your homosexuality has had on your career?"

"Well, it kept me from getting elected president," he said. After a quiet pause, he added, "If not for that, it would have all been so different."

"You mean your career would have been different?" I asked.

"No, I've had a wonderful *career*," he said, making the word sound pathetically inappropriate for his monumental body of work. "I mean the *country*! The *world*! If I had been elected president, it *all* would have been different."

Two years after Stephen died, I sold Community Prescription Service, using the proceeds to pay off debt that had accrued over the years I was financing *POZ*. In 2004, I sold *POZ*, right after the magazine's tenth anniversary. Walter and his staff had prepared a great anniversary issue, reviewing the highlights, triumphs, and controversies of the "*POZ* decade." I saw that issue as a swan song for my involvement. While discussing ideas for the cover, I reminisced about the magazine's launch and the early media coverage that described *POZ* as "putting a face on AIDS." That was when it occurred to me that the anniversary issue could take the mission a step further: I thought of artist Spencer Tunick, who photographs large groups of naked people in public spaces.

Tunick's enthusiastic response to my request that he photograph a group of naked people with HIV thrilled me until my horrifying realization that I, too, would have to get naked. Though I had made progress with my body shame over the years, getting naked with a group of others in the cold, hard daylight was a daunting prospect. But it was my idea, so I had to do it.

With only a few days' notice, we sent out e-mails encouraging people to show up and participate in the shoot at Restaurant Florent, a popular eatery in the Meatpacking district owned by my friend Florent Morellet. At seven A.M. on a cold March morning in 2004, more than a hundred people gathered outside the restaurant. They were filmed by HBO for a short documentary about the shoot called *Positively Naked* as everyone huddled together, drinking coffee and trying to stay warm.

We hadn't limited the shoot to people with HIV, so many HIV-negative people, including Megan and other colleagues from *POZ*, showed up prepared to strip naked. I nervously worked my way through the crowd, trying to get as far from my sister as possible. We were close, but not *that* close.

Tunick asked everyone but HIV positive people to leave; he wanted only positive people in the picture. I piped up, "Finally, it's the neggies who are getting kicked out of something!," and everyone laughed. Then Tunick gave the command, "You may now disrobe!" Restaurant Florent was not a large space; we were already close to one another, so it was like undressing in a crowded locker room while Tunick and his assistants took pictures and the HBO crew filmed. The whirring and clicking of shutters, coming from seemingly every angle, was disconcerting as we stuffed our clothes in plastic bags and stashed them behind the luncheonette-style counter.

Then Tunick instructed us to sprawl all over the floor, encouraging us to interact, put our arms around each other, our heads in the laps of strangers. He also placed some participants on the banquette or on the counter stools. A few of us, following Tunick's direction, stood on the countertop. Everyone was naked.

Bodies that were variously gym-perfect, voluptuous, elderly, emaciated, or showing "protease paunches" all became equal. I found it liberating and felt a layer of the body shame melt away. After the first few awkward minutes, we all seemed to transcend our individual bodies and became a communion of spirit, flesh, destiny, and art. Every kind of division disappeared and I became more conscious of feeling kindness and at one with the others than I was self-conscious of the cameras.

Tunick took a number of different shots, and we narrowed down the cover choices to two. In one, everybody was close together, with heads in laps, arms around shoulders, and groupings of two or three or four hugging and another that was more staid, with everyone looking at the camera like members of an Elks Club posed for their annual portrait. Spencer preferred the first image, which was a stronger artistic statement. But it was also a pile of intertwined naked bodies that could be misread: some staff saw bodies at an orgy, while others were reminded of bodies piled at a concentration camp. We went with AIDS Elks Club.

All of us at *POZ* were pleased not only by the inspired cover image but by the equally inspired event. We got media attention for our usual "edgy" style. But more important, we closed the "*POZ* decade"—and an indescribably tumultuous ten years of deaths and rebirths, losses and gains in both AIDS and activism—on a high that fulfilled our mission. Stephen was missing—and many others I could name—but in great gay style, we left our audience laughing.

■   ■   ■

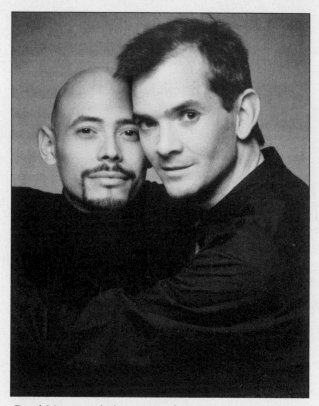

David Morgan took this picture of Xavier and me in the early '90s. I once thought that was going to be the last good picture taken of me, before I lost more weight and my face was marred by Kaposi's sarcoma lesions.

CHAPTER 38

HIV Is Not a Crime

By the start of 2000, I had arrived at that stage in my AIDS-activist "career" when I was being given awards and honors—the community's equivalent of a gold watch at retirement. Vito Russo used to say we must be careful that our community doesn't just honor "living conformists and dead troublemakers." I wondered if I was now a living conformist. I did know I was one of the "old" face of AIDS—a gay white man in his forties or fifties, who was part of what the ad agencies for the HIV drug makers were calling "an oversaturated market."

As welcome as honors are, their real value is that they have provided me the opportunity to give my signature speech about empowerment and activism. That always includes a plug for the Denver Principles, for which I gain a deeper appreciation with each passing year—especially as I see AIDS, Inc., paying only lip service to the ideals expressed in that document. But I am uncomfortable hearing myself described in flowery introductions as a "hero," because I'm not as altruistic as the term implies. I did not put my life at risk as heroes typically do. My activism was tempered by a fear of stigmatizing myself; sometimes the challenge of fighting AIDS—which meant fighting the system itself—

seemed too daunting. More selfish ambitions took precedence as well, like concerns about conformity, my reputation in the community, or financial security.

What ultimately drove me to devote so much of my life to the epidemic was my own sense of mortality, and a desire to leave a legacy that transcended my entrepreneurial successes, as much as it was the AIDS crisis per se. Nor do I believe I did enough soon enough, especially in the earliest years of the crisis.

I've had it much easier than most people with HIV. I have never gone hungry or homeless, I received a good education, always had healthcare and always felt loved. Even at my sickest, I was only occasionally in serious pain and was never hospitalized.

I have to acknowledge that AIDS, as horrific as it has been, has shaped my character, centered my values, and taught me important lessons. I've learned that life has the most meaning when I advocate or care for others, and that activism itself is most powerful when the voices of those at the center of the suffering and injustice are heard most clearly. That's what led me to focus on what is commonly referred to as "HIV criminalization."

The inappropriate use of one's HIV status in criminal prosecutions, most notably through criminal statutes that apply only to people with HIV, is something I had been aware of for many years. In February 1998, I wrote in *POZ*:

> The pieces are rapidly falling into place for the further criminalization of people with HIV. The [mandatory] name-reporting campaign has come to fruition, with some of the traditionally strongest allies of people with HIV essentially giving up the fight.

And it has only gotten worse, as HIV criminalization prosecutions have increased dramatically since that time. Throughout the '80s and '90s, most of those criminalized were heterosexual, African-American men, usually charged with not disclosing their HIV-positive status to a sex partner or with spitting or biting during an assault or arrest. Rarely has actual HIV transmission, or even *the risk of* transmission, been a factor in these charges. Cases involving sexual contact most often turn on whether the accused can prove having disclosed; in cases involving assault or interactions with law enforcement, it is typically just a question of whether the accused knew he or she had HIV. Such charges are rarely brought against people with *other* sexually transmitted infections. Human papillomavirus, for example. More women in the United States died last year from cervical cancer caused by HPV than died of AIDS, but there are no HPV-specific criminal statutes, nor is there an HPV criminalization phenomenon. The difference has everything to do with HIV's association with an "outlaw" sexuality, anal intercourse, gay men, people of color, and people who use drugs.

When I re-engaged in AIDS work a few years ago, I concentrated on reviving the empowerment movement, as embodied in the Denver Principles. Then I heard about Nick Rhoades, who was sentenced by an Iowa court to twenty-five years in prison and lifetime sex offender registration for not disclosing his status to an adult sex partner he met online. Nick and his accuser agreed that he had used a condom and had an undetectable viral count. Even though he posed virtually no risk to his partner—there's never been a confirmed documented sexual HIV transmission from someone with an undetectable viral load—the court did not consider that information relevant. Nick's case shocked me to a degree that I have rarely experienced, in thirty years of this shocking epidemic.

Nick was raised near my hometown in Iowa and he is white. When I read Nick's story, I realized it could have just as easily been mine. There have been times when I, like most HIV-positive gay men I know, did not disclose my HIV status to a sex partner, particularly when I knew the risk of transmission was nil or nonexistent. Whether negative or positive, everyone was told to "use a condom to protect yourself," because one's claimed HIV-negative status was never a sure thing. This was the norm in the gay community, but now it is not only illegal but even in the absence of transmission risk, punishable with draconian sentencing. As I learned more, I became outraged at the injustice and embarrassed that my home state was among the most aggressive in prosecuting these cases.

There is no more extreme manifestation of stigma than when government enshrines it in the law. Sadly, the United States leads the world in HIV criminalization prosecutions. I knew I needed to do something. Creating different laws for people based on immutable characteristics, such as race, ethnicity, sexual orientation, gender or gender identity, physical ability, or genetic makeup is wrong. But that's what two-thirds of the states have done, creating a viral underclass in the law based on HIV status.

While I identified with Nick's case in particular, I found there were people with HIV serving decades in prison all over the country for similar offenses. I learned that criminalization is terrible public health policy because it discourages people from getting tested: ignorance of one's HIV status is the best defense. Yet it has been shown that those who don't get tested are far more likely to transmit HIV than those who know they have it. Criminalization punishes responsible behavior—being tested to know your HIV status—and privileges the irresponsibility of not getting tested. No one should knowingly put another person at risk of harm without that person's knowledge, a principle included in the Denver Principles. But HIV criminalization isn't about harm or risk. It is about stigma, period.

I'm not proud to admit it took the case of someone like me—a white Iowa man—to make criminalization a priority in my activism. It puts in stark relief the racism, conscious or unconscious, in me and in much social justice activism.

I began to seek out people with HIV who had been criminalized. I videotaped Nick telling his story. I went to South Carolina to videotape Monique Moree, an African-American woman who was prosecuted by the U.S. army, even though her partner did not want her charged and testified that she had told him to use a condom.

A Louisiana man, Robert Suttle, who read online an article I had written about HIV criminalization, called me two days after he was released from prison. "My grandfather always said 'your misery is your ministry,'" he told me. "So I started thinking that I might find a new life in advocacy."

Robert knew he couldn't be rehired at his old job in the local Shreveport courts system. "Now I'm not just a gay African-American man with HIV, I'm a convicted felon and registered sex offender. What sort of future do I have? I think HIV criminalization is just one more way to lock up black men."

I knew from the start that by combating HIV criminalization, I was taking on a cause that was highly unpopular, even among gay men. But I believed most people hadn't been educated on the issue and didn't understand how it makes the epidemic worse and how unjustly the criminal statues have been applied.

So Robert and I, with the support of Nick, Monique, and others formed the Sero Project, which is a network of people with HIV, and their allies, fighting for freedom from stigma and injustice. The challenge is daunting. The issues—public health, legal and personal freedom—are complicated. But we have helped launch a nationwide anti-criminalization movement that has already achieved a number of successes. In 2013, the U.S. House passed legislation requiring federal review of military statutes related to HIV; legislation requiring a similar review of state statutes is pending. Professional and community organizations have spoken out in favor of reform and we've mobilized advocates across the country.

Sero has provided opportunities for Nick, Monique, Robert, and others who have been criminalized to share their stories globally at UNAIDS meetings in Geneva, Oslo, and New York, as well as at scores of venues across the U.S. What began with outrage has turned into a movement. People with HIV in Iowa, for example, with the support of their Republican-led Iowa Department of Health, nearly got bi-partisan criminalization reform legislation through the Iowa State Senate in 2013. They'll be back until they get it done.

Sero has helped rekindle the people with HIV self-empowerment movement, begun more than three decades ago, bringing young people and those who have been criminalized or are incarcerated, as well as transgender women, into policy debates and activism, shining a spotlight on stigma. Years ago, combating stigma was a primary focus of AIDS activism, but since the introduction of combination therapy it became sidelined as an issue, rather than addressed as a fundamental obstacle to ending the epidemic.

Effective treatment for HIV has also contributed to the stubborn persistence of stigma. Until 1996, it was widely assumed that all of us with AIDS were going to die. The "general public," no matter how they felt about homosexuality, injection drug use, or other contentious issues, had come a long way toward compassion for people with HIV. Our community showed that we were fighters rather than victims, creating services, demanding resources and respect, taking care of our sick, dying with dignity.

Yet, as it became widely understood that new treatments enable us to live much longer, we increasingly became defined not by our expected death but by our potential to infect others, as "viral vectors." As we lived longer, the criminal justice and public health systems have come to view us, even define us, as inherently dangerous.

Many of the men of my generation got HIV before the virus was discovered and before it was known how to avoid infection. Today most people who get HIV do know how to avoid it, but simply having the knowledge isn't enough. Prevention strategies based on rationality have never been sufficient when it comes to sex, a drive that lives deep beneath the rational. The newly infected today are often denied the sympathy extended to those of us who got it so many years ago, making us the new "innocent victims." Sadly, many of us long-term survivors are the first to cast stones against the younger generation who "should have known better."

*   *   *

Letters to the judge presiding over Nick's case convinced him to reconsider the sentencing and he released Nick after a year in prison, but Nick must still register as a sex offender. He can't travel without permission, he is forbidden from using any social networking sites, he can't be unsupervised around children, is required to wear an ankle-monitoring bracelet and he must regularly undergo humiliating lie detector tests administered by the state about every sexual thought, behavior, or contact he has. He's even been threatened with "phallometric testing," which, Nick says, he "thinks has something to do with putting a device on my penis." Dan Johnston, the civil rights attorney who as a volunteer helped get *POZ* distributed in prisons, agreed to represent Nick to try to set aside his conviction. Then Lambda Legal joined the effort to pursue an appeal. The army dropped the charges against Monique, but kicked her out. She fell in love and is now remarried, raising three boys, while she has become a popular HIV-awareness motivational speaker.

Robert Suttle moved from Shreveport, Louisiana, into a small apartment in Milford, Pennsylvania, where I live, to help me launch the Sero Project. Right after he arrived, I went with him to the state police barracks for the obligatory transfer of his sex offender registration. A week later, our local police chief printed up "warning" flyers with Robert's picture, as he was required to do by law, and distributed them door-to-door, including to the businesses in the small commercial district in our village, telling the owners to warn their employees. Milford is a town of only 1,100 and word gets around fast. Understandably, Robert felt extremely uncomfortable. As a person of color, he already stood out in a rural community that was almost entirely white.

He decided to put this humiliating experience to good use and wrote an essay for our local weekly newspaper, detailing what happened to him and why he moved to Milford. In the following days, I noticed people staring at us while we ate lunch at the Milford diner. But the more common reaction was support. Milford's mayor—who is conservative, Catholic, Republican—called me and said he believed Robert had suffered an injustice. He wanted to meet him, "so I can tell anyone who asks that I've looked him in the eye and know he is a good person doing important work." After meeting Robert he told me, "If you ever need a letter of support or anything, I'll be glad to write one on my official letterhead."

My work with the Sero Project has brought me back to the grass-roots community activism I enjoy most and has made me more aware of those who have been left behind by the mainstream LGBT and HIV movements. The progress the LGBT community has made since the mid-1990s in gaining acceptance by, and assimilation into, straight society has admittedly been remarkable. I'm glad that today I am invited to attend same-sex marriage ceremonies as often as I once attended memorial services. But while the "equality" mantra has begun to be realized in the law, little has changed for the most disenfranchised, especially those with HIV and those at greatest risk, like transgender women and young African-American men who have sex with men. That is a challenge the LGBT and HIV communities have yet to fully face.

Sero's goals won't be met in my lifetime and, given my past history of creating projects and then moving on, I'm pretty sure Sero won't occupy me for the rest of my life. But seeing people with HIV assuming leadership and overcoming stigma is a heartening part of the enduring legacy of Michael Callen, Richard Berkowitz, Joseph Sonnabend, and others whose early work has enabled so many of us to be alive today.

Those who have died remain with us in ways that are sometimes surprising. Two decades after Michael Misove died, one of his nieces—who was a small child when he died—Googled her uncle's name and found only two references, both in *POZ* columns by me. She contacted me, having recognized my name as the "special friend" her grandmother had once referenced on a rare occasion when Michael's name was mentioned. When he died, his name largely disappeared, even from his own family's lore. It was as if this remarkable human being had never walked the earth.

To his niece, he was a blank, a mystery, at most three labels strung together by the simplest of verbs: "Michael was gay, lived in New York, and died of AIDS." To her credit, she wanted to unpack the sentence. I tried, to the best of my limited abilities, to bring Michael back to life for her in words—which he loved more than anything else—as I have tried here in these pages, for Michael and others.

In 2008, Xavier returned to the United States from Denmark, where he had been earning an MBA. He was going to stay with me for a few weeks until he found a place of his own, but we realized almost immediately that we wanted to be together again. It was probably healthy for both of us that we had split up for a while, but the several years since we got back together have been more joyful and renewing than any other time in any relationship I have ever had. We both are also fortunate to enjoy close relationships with our families. Xavier's father sometimes sends us letters addressed to *"Mis dos hijos"* (My two sons). A few years ago, my father told me he thought that my coming out had made us a better family and him a better person.

One of the lessons of Catholicism that stuck with me, even through the periods when I was most furious with the Church, was that life's meaning is found in contemplation, penance, and service. Of these three, my only real talent is in service. I've always been more interested in action than reflection—I sometimes wonder if my propensity to take on one project after another is a way to escape reflection.

Sometimes that service is simply a matter of being present with no other action necessary. Joe Sonnabend once let me look at a box of letters and cards he received over the years from the surviving partners and parents of patients of his who had died. One is more moving and emotional than the next; I can't imagine anyone reading them without getting tears in their eyes. They all thank Joe for his care and kindness, but I was struck by how many simply thanked him for "being there" for the person they loved. When I see someone very ill or hospitalized and feel helpless, not knowing what I can do to help alleviate their pain, I remember those cards and remind myself that even when all I can do is "be there," that is enough.

I have tried to be there, for one person or cause or another since elementary school. I expect to do the same for the rest of my life. And when that time comes, I still want to die as a fighter.

ACKNOWLEDGMENTS

Of the many good friends and advisers who helped me in the process of writing *Body Counts*, none deserve more appreciation than Walter Armstrong, who helped me from the first word of the initial proposal to the last word of the manuscript. For nearly twenty years, he has listened patiently to my ramblings and rants, deciphered my scribbles and screeds, and helped make sense of and give context to what I am trying to say with a kindness and patience that is almost superhuman.

I also owe a particular debt to Bob Levine, without whose encouragement and support I would not have written this book, and to Nan Graham, whose faith and confidence in me sometimes exceeded my own. Nan's colleague, Paul Whitlatch, ably shepherded me through the editing process with patience and professionalism.

John Berendt, Jonathan Boorstein, Beverly Dyer, Elliott Millenson, Hillary Needleman, and Ken Siman went above and beyond the requirements of friendship in commenting and providing valuable suggestions on my many drafts, frequently on short notice or at odd hours. Several former *POZ* colleagues provided comments or advice that improved the manuscript significantly, including Sally Chew, Shawn Decker, Lauren Hauptman, Doug Ireland, Matt Levine, Manjula Martin, Ronnilyn Pustil, and Laura Whitehorn.

I'm also grateful to Donald Baxter, Chip Beam, Edwin Bernard, Fred Bernstein, Richard Berkowitz, Jay Blotcher, John Catlett, Cindy Cesnalis, Cecilia Chung, Mario Cooper, Claudia Copquin, Chris Cormier, David Drake, Matt Ebert, Forest Evashevski, Annie Flanders, Greg Gorman, Krista Gromalski, Julia Gruen, Judy Harris, Alan Klein, James Krellenstein, Tami Haught, Carter Hooper, Vanessa Johnson, Dan Johnston, Ted Kerr, Christopher King, Mark King, Emily LaFond, Suzanne Levine, Christopher Makos, Bill Malson, Linda Meredith, Monique Moree, Liz Morten, Tim Murphy, Jim Nathan, Hillary Needleman, Gloria Nieto, Maya North, Janet Oliver, Torie Osborn, Nancy Pinchot, Richard Pleasants, Billy Reue, Nick Rhoades, Mike Rogers, Marilyn Rosenthal, Nelson Santos, Josh Sapan, Dick Scanlan, Stephen Schlanser, Linda Shankweiler, Aiden Shaw, Sara Simon, Laurel Sprague, Dick Snyder, Nathan Snyder, Cindy Stine, Missi Strub, Gilbey Strub, Robert Suttle, Kerry Thomas, Matt Vitemb, Jay Vithalani, Reed Vreeland, Max Westerman, Peter Wise, Bob Witeck, Bob Wykoff, and Angus Whyte for their support, comments, and friendship.

My appreciation to Xavier, Megan, my family, and other close friends cannot be adequately conveyed in an acknowledgment sentence at the back of a book. They, as much as any pill or potion, are what have pulled me through the last thirty years, enduring my lowest and weakest moments, and always at my side to celebrate the triumphant ones. AIDS has taught me a lot about love.

To Joe Sonnabend, and in more recent years, Paul Bellman, I only wish every person could enjoy the quality of doctoring I have received from each of you. Throughout an era when afflictions became commodities, bought and sold as profit opportunities, you have maintained the humanity, compassion, skepticism, and individualized care that is a credit to your profession.

The criminalization reform work I have undertaken through the Sero Project would not be possible without the support of John Swaner and Gregory Whiting, Tom Viola and his amazing team at Broadway Cares/Equity Fights AIDS; Henry van Ameringen, who recognizes injustice long before it is visible to others; and Scott Anderson and Matt Blinstrubas at the Elton John AIDS Foundation. Sir Elton's partner, David Furnish, saw the short film *HIV Is Not a Crime*, and met Nick Rhoades and Robert Suttle at my sister Gilbey's home in London. He was outraged and shared it with Sir Elton; they then provided funding that greatly expanded the Sero Project's work.

Finally, to everyone with HIV, especially those who have read *POZ* and followed or supported my work over the years, I am proud to be one of you. Not because having a virus is something to be proud of; that is perhaps an unfortunate accident or tragedy, but it is no accomplishment. But because those of us with HIV have learned something unique about society, survival, and ourselves that only we understand.

INDEX

Page numbers in italic type indicate illustrations.

Abbott, 362
Aburto, Gonzalo, 310–11
Abzug, Bella, 100, 128
Achtenberg, Roberta, 20
acquired immune deficiency syndrome,
     see AIDS
ACT UP (AIDS Coalition to Unleash Power),
     178, 195–205, 269, 272, 292–93, 300,
     312, 319, 325
   demonstrations and, 2–3, 70, 195–97,
     199–200, 202–3, 220, 223, 225, *226,*
     227–32, 242, 244, 255–56, 308
   fund–raising of, 199, 201–5, *218,* 219,
     221–25, 227–28, 241, 255, 283
   Gendin and, 203–4, 241, 252, 308,
     374–75
   generic medications and, 332–33
   Haring and, 220–25, *226,* 227
   POZ and, 285, 305, 337
   Silence=Death logo and, 3, 196, 220, 230,
     241
   Strub's attendance at meetings of, 200–203,
     205, 219, 242
   Strub's congressional campaign and,
     242–43, 245
   Strub's work for, 201–5, 219, 222–24,
     228–29, 255, 265, 283, 293
   and survival of people with AIDS, 235–36
   talent contest of, 265–66
Advocate, The, 245, 286
African Americans, 25, 101, 248
   AIDS and, 171, 309, 311

HIV criminalization and, 392–95,
     397–98
   POZ and, 309, 311
AIDS (acquired immune deficiency syndrome),
     124–53, 155–60, 169–81, 183–92, 225,
     228, 265, 312, 341
   African Americans and, 171, 309
   call to action on, 132–33
   causes of, 116, 125–27, 129–32, 134–38,
     142, 144–45, 147, 170
   chance in, 126–27, 129
   Clinton and, 245, 277–78, 325–27,
     329–32
   of Cohn, 57, 164
   as conversation topic, 133–34, 147
   cure for, 119, 128, 133–34, 146
   deaths due to, 40–41, 56–58, 68, 109,
     113–14, 116, 118–20, 124–25, 131–35,
     138, 146, 149–51, 153, 156, 159, 162,
     170, 173–74, 177, 188–92, 196, 198,
     203, 207–8, 210, 212–15, 223, 235, 237,
     239, 241, 245, 259–61, 266, 270–71,
     278, 285–86, 294, 301–2, 321, 330, 344,
     351, 363, *370,* 371–76, 384, 386, 393,
     396, 398–99
   demonstrations and, 41, 155–56, 166,
     169–71, 186, *194,* 195–200, 220–21,
     231
   diagnoses of, 144, 151, 173, 175, 184,
     220, 327
   education on, 144–45, 152
   empowerment and, 157, 222, 237

AIDS (*cont.*)
  as epidemic, 115–16, 118–20, 128–30,
    133, 135–36, 146–47, 158, *168*,
    169–70, 172, 176, 180–81, 184–85,
    196, 200, 240–41, 251, 255, 260, 262,
    268, 284, 286–87, 290, 293, 296, 301,
    317, 327, 335, 351, 363, 368, 374, 384,
    392–93, 396
  films based on, 279, 300
  first cases of, *108*, 109, 113, 115
  funding for, 119, 137, 145, 148–49, 157,
    171, 175, 178, 188–90, 196–203, 208,
    244, 255–56, 260, 271, 283–84, 326
  gays and, 20, 68, *108*, 109, 113–16,
    118–20, 124–29, 131–39, 141–53, 162,
    169–75, 181, 197, 200, 237, 373–76,
    391, 396
  Gendin and, 301–2, 373–76
  Haring and, 170, 220–21
  Helms and, 149, 255–56, 258
  HIV testing and, 164–66, 253–54
  KS and, 315, 318–21
  lobbying for, 196–97, *274*
  naming of, 119
  New York and, 119–20, 126–27, 130, 132,
    134–36, 138–39, 141–42, 144, 147,
    150–52, 155–56, 159, 165, 169–72,
    174–75, 184, 186, 203, 207
  New York Post on, 170–71
  politicians and, 100, 116, 144–45, 151,
    158, 197–98, 245, 267–69, *274*,
    277–78, 325–27, 329–32
  POZ and, 285–87, 289–91, 293–95, 299,
    301–2, 305–7, 309–11, 319, 325–27,
    330, 335, 337, 387–88
  prevention of, 127, 136–38, 142–43,
    147–49, 158, 326
  prognoses for people with, 235–36
  reactions of people with, 172–73
  reluctance to talk about, *96*, 129–30,
    133–34
  research on, 137, 145, 175–76, 180–81,
    198, 236, 255–56, 271, 325–26
  sex with, 137–38, 147, 175, 375
  stigmatizing of, 155–56, 159, 171, 179,
    275, 311, 319
  of Strub, 3, 146–47, 153, 240, 247, 271,
    301–2, 315, 318–19, 342, 350, 359,
    367–68, 379
  Strub's activism and, 185–87, 192, 196–97,
    391–96
  Strub's businesses and, 155–57, 252

  Strub's congressional campaign and,
    240–44
  support and networks for, 120, 139–44,
    148, 172–75, 178, 197, 237, 326
  survival of people with, 235–37, 239, 262
  symptoms of, 113–14, 119–20, 131–32,
    141–42, 147, 149–52, 155, 160, 259
  transmission of, 68, 114–15, 125, 137,
    144–45, 152, 157–59
  treatments for, 130, 142, 151, 158, 175–81,
    183, 203, 211, 235–37, 254–56, 305,
    326, 361, 374, 376, 384
  viatical settlement industry and, 284–85
  visiting people with, 190–91, 207–8,
    259–60
  women with, 186–87, 309
AIDS Action Council, 208, *274*, 330, 333
AIDS Coalition to Unleash Power, *see* ACT
  UP
AIDS Interfaith Alliance, 311
AIDS Prevention Action League (APAL),
  292, 338
AIDS–related complex (ARC), 165–67, 179, 275
  of Strub, 165–66, 169–70, 172, 176–77,
    183, 185, 235, 284
Allen, Woody, 208
Almanac of American Politics, 11
AL721, 178–80
alternative therapies, 237
American Foundation for AIDS Research
  (AmFAR), 198, 211, 301
America Online (AOL), 336
American Psychiatric Association, 45, 100,
  128
Americans for Democratic Action, 11
amphotericin B, 211
Andalusia, 92–94, *96*, 133–34
Andersonville (Kantor), 312
Andy, 31–32
Annual Gay and Lesbian Health Conference,
  141, 143
anti–retroviral drugs, 237, 253, 286, 295–97,
  308, 336, 373, 380
  generic, 332–33
  POZ and, 297, 305
Anvil, 55, 67
Armstrong, Walter, 292–94, 374, 377, 387
Associated Press, 247
Auction for Action, 223–25, 227
Austen, Howard, 343–44, *382*, 384
AZT, 182, 261–62, 317, 361–62
  BW and, 253–54, 305

pros and cons of, 176–77, 253, 261
Strub's use of, 176–78, 183

Bactrim, 181–82, 308
Baker, Dan, 241, 257, 265
barebacking, 291, 335–39
Barnes & Noble, 311
Baron, Alan, 49–54, 58–61, 97, 99–104,
    151, 163
    cocaine used by, 51–52, 78–79, 282
    gay politics and, 100–104, 106–7, 122
    hospitalization and death of, 281–82
    newsletter of, 50–52, 78
    Strub's relationship with, 52–54, 60–61,
        78, 282
Barrios, Bobby, 207–8
Barry, 36–37, 48
Basquiat, Jean–Michel, 222
bathhouses, 57, 71–72, 85, 109, 115, 134, 148
    AIDS and, 120, 126, 129, 152
    sexually transmitted infections and, 117–18
Bauman, Bob, 56–57
Baxter, Barbara, 87
Bayh, Birch, 24
Beatty, Warren, 103
Benes, Barton, 223, *346*
    Berendt and, 383–84
    creativity of, 351–52, 383–84
    Meyer's KS and, 351–52
Bennett, Michael, 223
Berea College, 269–70
Berendt, John, *382,* 383–86
Berger, Ira, 156–57
Berkowitz, Richard, 124–27, 136–38, 174,
    336, 398
    AIDS causes and, 125–27, 129–30, 132,
        137
    AIDS prevention and, 127, 137–38, 147
    People With Aids Caucus and, 141–42
    on safe sex, 137–38, 147, 175, 339
Biaxin, 308
Biddle, James, 92–93, *96,* 133–34
Book Study Group, 197
Boswell, John, 75–76
Bowers v. Hardwick, 187–88, 196
Brasserie, 67
Brenda (Benes), 351
Briggs Initiative, 103
Britt, Harry, 70
Broder, David, 59
Broder, Samuel, 181–82
Brown, Jerry, 6–7, 121–22

Brown, John Y., 97–99
Bruno, Joseph, 57
Bryant, Anita, 40, 128
bubonic plague, 115–17, 315
Buchanan, James, 385
Buchanan, Pat, 144–45
Buckley, Pat, 244
Bucks County, Pa., 58, 248
    gay scene in, 131, 169–70
    Strub's home in, 131, 144, 164, 167, 196,
        208, 211
Burger, Warren, 187
Burroughs Wellcome (BW), 180, 253–54,
    305
Burton, John, 52
Bush, George W., 385–86
Byckiewicz, Steve, 244
Byrd, Robert C., 17–18

Callen, Michael, 124–27, 136, 172, 198, 252,
    270, 296, 336, 398
    AIDS causes and, 125–27, 129–30, 132,
        142
    AIDS prevention and, 127, 137–38, 142,
        147
    AZT and, 177, 253
    death of, 290, 321
    KS of, 222, 321, 349
    PCP prophylaxis and, 181–82
    People With Aids Caucus and, 141–42
    PWAC and, *168,* 174–75, 178, 235
    on safe sex, 137–38, 147, 175, 339
    and survival of people with AIDS, 235–37
Campbell, Bobbi, 120
Campion Jesuit High School, 26–27, 30
Camus, Albert, 117
cancer, 57, 114, 131–32, 135, 181, 213, 393
    of breasts, 9, 302, 350
    lymphoma and, 293, 371
    survival of, 236–37
    see also Kaposi's sarcoma
Capote, Truman, 84
cardpack business, 241, 247, 251–52, 266,
    278, 281, 284, 298, 305, 321
Carter, Jimmy, 52, 240
    presidential campaigns of, 8, 24, 50, 78,
        85, 87–88
    and White House meeting of gay and
        lesbian leaders, *22,* 40
Catholics, Catholicism, 9, 84, 121–22,
    160–61, 241–42, 247, 282, 311, 328,
    397

Catholics, Catholicism (*cont.*)
 demonstrations and, 220, 228–31, 242
 gays and, 10, 56, 227
 Misove's mother and, 213–14
 in New York, 204, 227
 Strub's education and, 26–27
 Strub's religious beliefs and, 1–2, 10, 13–14,
  16, 26, 76–77, 80, 165, 177, 183, 202,
  221, 229–33, 242, 356–58, 399
 Strub's sexual abuse and, 356–58
CD4 cells, 184, 220, 294, 315
Celluloid Closet (Russo), 109–10, 113
Centers for Disease Control and Prevention
  (CDC), 144, 326, 328
 on first AIDS cases, *108*, 113
Central Junior High School, 232–33
Central Park, 67–68
Chapman, Mark David, *264*, 272
chemotherapy, 254, 318, 350, 361–63, 273
Christianity, Social Tolerance, and Homosexuality
  (Boswell), 75–76
Christopher & Castro, 280–81
Cisco, 151–52
civil disobedience:
 ACT UP and, 70, 200
 demonstrations and, 70, 186, *194*,
  197–200, 255–56
 TAG and, 255–56
civil rights, 19, 26, 75, 100–101, 103, 341, 397
Clark, Dick, 6, 11, 15, 18, 23, 26
Clinton, Bill, 20, 267–69, 329–33
 AIDS and, 245, 277–78, 325–27, 329–32
 gays and, 277–79, *324*, 325–26, 331–32
 Hattoy and, 268–69, *274*, 278, 326–27,
  330, 332–33
 needle–exchange programs and, 327, 330–32
 POZ and, 290, 325–27, 330, 332
 presidential campaigns of, 276–78, *324*,
  325, 329–32
Clinton, Hillary, 268–69, 278, 327, 332
Cohn, Roy, 57, 163–64
Collins, Todd, 155–56, 158, 162, 167, 185
Columbia University, 92, 161
 Strub's enrollment at, 68, 79, 81, 86–87, 121
combination therapy, 237, 286, 296, *314*,
  336, 359, 361–62, 384, 396
Community Prescription Service (CPS),
  252–54, 261, 281, 292–93, 386
Congress, U.S., 52–53, 145, 279, 295, 327
 Strub's elevator operator job and, 11–12
 see also House of Representatives, U.S.;
  Senate, U.S.

Continental Baths, 72
Cooke, Terence Cardinal, 77
Cooper, Mario, 268, *274*, 330
Corti, Jim, 179–80
Costanza, Midge, 40–41
 Strub's congressional campaign and,
  240–41, 243, 247
 and White House meeting of gay and
  lesbian leaders, *22*, 40
Council on Economic Priorities (CEP), 135,
  164
Crangle, Joseph, 58–60
 jobs offered to Strub by, 58–59, 62, 77
 Strub's relationship with, 62, 76–78
Craver, Roger, 53–54, 99
Crimp, Douglas, 337
Crixivan, 362–63
Cruising, 74
cryptococcal meningitis, 3, 210–12,
  214–15
C–SPAN, 328–29
Culver, John, 11, 13
cytomegalovirus (CMV), 118, 138, 146

Daily Iowan, The, 8, 14
Dakota, 88, 90–91, 383
Daniel, Dennis, *346*
DaunoXome, 350, 361
David Frost Show, The, 383
David's Front Page, 59–61
Dawson, Ken, 259–61, 349
ddC, 261–62
ddI, 261–62
Deagle, Richard, 220, *226*
DeBolt, Don, 92
Defense of Marriage Act, 277, 331
Democratic Midterm Convention, 58–59
Democratic National Committee (DNC), 23,
  110–12, 240, 268, 277
Democratic National Conventions, 23–25,
  84–85
 Hattoy's speech at, 267–69, *274*
 Strub's attendance at, 23–24, 55, 185,
  267–68
Democrats, Democratic Party, 52, 63, 103
 closeted gays and, 55–56, 58–59
 in Denver, 109, 111–12
 in Kentucky, 97–100, 104, 110
 in Pennsylvania, 110, 119, 277
 presidential campaigns of, 6–8, 18, 24,
  50, 78, 85, 87–88, 276–78, *324*, 325,
  329–33

Strub's political ambitions and, 17–18, 240, 243, 246
Strub's political beliefs and, 23–24, 49, 76, 84–85, 87–88, 94, 97, 109–10, 119, 121, 185, 277, 282
Denver, Colo.:
  People With Aids Caucus and, 141–44
  Strub's trip to, *108*, 109–14
Denver Principles, 142–43, *168*, 172, 391, 393–94
Dessel, Hal, 27
dextran sulfate, 179–80
Diflucan, 211–12
Diller, Barry, 300, 302
direct mailing, 156–58, 180, 240–41, 251
  ACT UP and, 199–201, 203, 205, 222–23
  gays and, 57, 101–3, 106, 122
  GMHC and, 157–58, 185
  PWAC and, 185–87
  Strub's mentoring on, 53–54, 99
Dlugos, Tim, 122, 124, 131, 191, 197
Doderer, Minnette, 16
Dolan, Terry, 57
Domenici, Pete, 12
Donghia, Angelo, 133
Don't Ask, Don't Tell, 277, 331
Dow, John, 246–47
Downey, Jeanne, *82*, 91
Drake, David, 265–67, 290
  ACT UP talent contest and, 265–66
  The Night Larry Kramer Kissed Me and, *264*, 266–67, 269–73, 276, 279–80, 284
Dunne, Richard, 157

Ebenstein, Hanns, 320–21
Elders, Jocelyn, 327
Elizabeth, Queen of England, 19
Endean, Steve, 100–106, 198
Engle, Paul, 47
Engstrom, Ev, *108*, 109–10, 112
Equal Rights Amendment (ERA), 8, 16, 85
Eric, 37–38
Erlenbach, Mike, 252
Everard, 72

Factory, 86, 150, 267
Falwell, Jerry, 10, 101–2, 105, 128
Fauchère, Louis, 367
Fauci, Anthony, 145, 235–36, 328
  PCP prophylaxis and, 181–82
Feinberg, David, 287, 290

feminists, feminism, 8, 16, 71, 101, 103, 119, 143, 341
Fierstein, Harvey, 201
Fink, Stanley, 58, 62
Flannery, Bill, 14–16, 26, 53, 111
Florida, 40, 101, 119
Food and Drug Administration (FDA), 286, 299, 326
  AL721 and, 178–80
  and ddC and ddI, 261
Forbes, Malcolm, 225
Ford, Gerald, 8, 24
Fotopoulos, Mark, 319–20
Foulon, Joe, 173–75
Frank, Barney, 58, 240
fund–raising, 94, 124, 163, 169, 180, 259–60, 277, 281, 284, 293, 318
  of ACT UP, 199, 201–5, *218*, 219, 221–25, 227–28, 241, 255, 283
  for AIDS, 119, 137, 148–49, 157, 171, 175, 188–90, 196–97, 199–202, 208, 244, 260
  gays and, 57, 101–3, 105, 107, 122, 188–90, 201
  of GMHC, 119–20, 156–58, 175, 185, 283
  in Kentucky, 98–100
  NGLTF and, 189, 201, 280
  of PWAC, 171, 185–87
  Strub's congressional campaign and, 241–46, 270
  Strub's copywriting and, 122, 131
  Strub's mentoring on, 53–54
  for TAG, *264*, 272–73

Gagliostro, Vincent, 327
Gallagher, Kathleen (aunt), 321–22
Gallo, Robert, 145–46, 178
Gay and Lesbian Community Services Center, 196, 199, 219, 245, 375
Gay and Lesbian Pride Marches, 74, 136, *168*
gay men, gay sex, 49–50, 84, 195–97, 222, 259, 366–67, 398–99
  activism and, 26, 31, 39, 41, 58, 62–63, 72, 74–76, 79–80, 100, 115–16, 124, 133, 136, 141–43, 162, 169–74, 185, 187, 373–76
  AIDS and, 20, 68, *108*, 109, 113–16, 118–20, 124–29, 131–39, 141–53, 162, 169–75, 181, 197, 200, 237, 320, 373–76, 391, 396
  books on, 39–40, 56, 75–76, 109–10, 113

gay men, gay sex (*cont.*)
Bucks County scene of, 131, 169–70
Clinton and, 277–79, *324,* 325–26,
331–32
closeted, 9–11, 15–16, 20, 25–26, 31,
33–34, 41–42, 54–63, 85, 98, 101–3,
110, 114–15, 122, 130–31, 133, 143,
158, 164, 204, 207, 225, 267–71,
276–77, 280
coming out of, 41, 61–62, 73, 80, 100,
110–12, 114–15, 134, 174–75, 185,
240–41, 270, 277, 280, 399
condom use by, 35, 137–38, 147–49, 166,
175, 221, 227–28, 311, 313, 335–37, 393
in Congress, 55–58, 240
cruising of, 17, 28–29, 33, 38, 67, 71–72,
75, 105, 160, 320, 336, 393
deaths of, 109, 113–14, 116, 118–20,
124–25, 131–35, 138, 149–51, 162,
173–74, 191–92
Democratic National Conventions and,
267–68
demonstrations and, 114, 188, 196–97, 231
discrimination and prejudice against, 10,
17, 40–41, 57, 60, 74, 88, 100–101,
105, 128–29, 195, 227
films based on, 74, 279, 300
fund–raising and, 57, 101–3, 105, 107,
122, 188–90, 201
Gendin and, 336–39, 374–76
Helms and, 20, 148–49, 254–56, 258
HIV and, 159, 166, 221, 247, 320,
335–38, 393–95
homophobia and, 20, 30, 57, 142, 164,
191–92, 197, 225, 247, 254–55, 271,
273, 286, 309, 364
Hudson and, 158–59, 165
hypocrisy about, 17, 57–58
injuries and pain in, 30, 35, 37
jokes and slurs on, 11, 15–17, 30, 70, 357
KS and, 118, 315, 320–21, 350
Los Angeles scene of, 204, 320
marriages of, 14, 54–55, 57
as mentally ill, 100, 115, 128, 215
in military, 41, 215, 277, 279–80, 326, 331
New York scene of, 10, 25, 36, 38–39, 55,
57, 66–67, 69–75, 85–88, 97, 106, 109,
121–22, 129, 131, 134, 160, 163, *168,*
275–76, 329, 377
O'Connor on, 227–28
older, 54–58, 61
online meetings and, 336, 393

openly, 39–42, 45, 55, 63, 75, 92, 103–4,
122, 125, 128, 130–31, 157, 240–41,
247–48, 278, 328–30, 332
outing of, 56, 81, 101
plays based on, 186, 201, *264,* 266–67,
269–73, 276, 279–80, 284
politics and, 20, 26, 55–60, 63, 65, 70–71,
74–76, 79–81, 83, 93, 100–107, 109–11,
115–16, 119, 122, 124, 126, 128–29,
133, 136, 148–49, 155–56, 162, 166,
169–74, 195, 237, 240, 267, 270
POZ and, 286, 289–90, 293–94, 297, 300,
305–6, 308–12, 378, 388
prohibition of, 187–88, 196
promiscuity of, 125–26, 129–30, 132, 134,
136, 139, 142, 147, 149, 174, 339
sexually transmitted diseases of, 72–73,
116–19, 134
shame of, 10, 31–32, 357
stereotypes of, 15–16
Strub's businesses and, 155–57
Strub's congressional campaign and, 240,
243–48
Strub's education and, 27–30, 34–35
and Strub's relationship with Misove,
161–62
Strub's sexuality and, 9–11, 15–17, 20,
25–39, 41–42, 45, 49, 59–63, 69,
71–73, 75, 80–81, 85–87, 98, 104,
110–12, 114, 118, 120, 132, 147–48,
155, 166, 174–75, 185, 199, 232–33,
240–41, 243, 245–48, 267–68, 275–77,
320, 357, 367, 399
Vidal on, 103, 385–86
violence and, 30, 36–37, 63, 70, 74, 88,
97, 125, 128–29, 356
Washington scene of, 10–11, 15–16,
28–40, 45, 54–58, 63, 69, 71, 73
White House meeting of, *22,* 40
Gay Men's Health Crisis (GMHC), 127–28,
132, 143, 173–75, 204, 231
fund–raising of, 119–20, 156–58, 175,
185, 283
HIV prevention and, 136–38, 247
Rest in Peace list of, 173–74
Gay Rights National Lobby, 100
Gebbie, Kristine, 325–26
Geffen, David, 256, 280, 300, 302
Gendin, Stephen, 290–93
activism of, 199, 371–76
ACT UP and, 203–4, 241, 252, 308,
374–75

CPS and, 252–54
death of, *370,* 371–80, 386
demonstrations and, 199, 203, 308, 374
McDowell's relationship with, 338–39
medications taken by, 253, 295–96, 361, 372–73
POZ and, 295–96, 298–302, *304,* 307–8, 313, 336–39, 361, *370,* 372, 374–77, 379, 388
sexuality and, 336–39, 374–76
Strub's congressional campaign and, 241, 245
Strub's relationship with, 199, 251, 290–91, 348, 371–73
Gentleman from Maryland, The (Bauman), 56
Georgetown, 27–29, 34, 87
Georgetown Grill, 27, 33
Georgetown University, 5, 62, 68
Strub's enrollment at, 26–29, 31, 46, 56, 58, 75, 81, 121
Georgia, 8, 103, 187
Gilman, Ben, 239, 242, 248
Gingrich, Newt, 248, 327
Glenn, John, 25
Goldstein, Leonard, 285
Goldwater, Barry, 19, *288,* 289
Gonsalves, Gregg, 235–36
"Good Luck, Bad Luck," 126–27
Gore, Al, 332–33
Gore Vidal's American Presidency, 385
Gorman, Greg, *288,* 290, 301, 319
Gran Fury, 221
Gravel, Gisele, 12
Gross, David, 204
Gruen, Julia, 221, 223, 225

Hail Marys, 2, 229
Hanks, Tom, 279, 300
Hardgraves, Walter, 224–25
Hardwick, Michael, 187–88, 196
Haring, Keith, 2, 190
ACT UP and, 220–25, *226,* 227
AIDS and, 170, 220–21
HIV of, 220–23
prices of artworks of, 220, 222–25
Swenson's relationship with, *218,* 220–21
Harrington, Mark, 235–36
Hattoy, Bob, 329
Clinton and, 268–69, *274,* 278, 326–27, 330, 332–33
Democratic National Convention and, 267–69, *274*
POZ and, 290, 326

Hawkins, Ashton, 244
Hayes, Robert:
AIDS and, 149–52
death of, 149, 151, 156, 162
Strub's first meeting with, 85–86
Heckler, Margaret, 145–46, 149
Helms, Jesse, 19–20, 373
demonstrations and, 20, *250,* 256–58
homophobia of, 20, 254–55
TAG and, 255–56
Helms Amendment, 148–49
hepatitis, 72, 87, 92, 113, 134
Hernandez, Tito, 87, 132
Hershman, Rob, 88
Heston, Charlton, 158
HHV–8, 362
Higgins, Tom, 277
Hinson, Jon, 56–57
Hirsch, Michael:
PWAC and, *168,* 171, 175, 185–86
Strub's meeting with, 171–72, 174
Hitt, Scott, 245, 330–31
HIV (human immunodeficiency virus), 134, 184, 271
Clinton and, 277, 325, 327, 330–32
CPS and, 252–53, 261
criminalization of, 392–98
demonstrations and, 198, 231, 256
diagnoses of, 145, 220, 235, 262, 287, 290, 335–36, 347
discovery of, 145–46, 149, 158, 175
empowering people with, 291–92, 396
females with, 328, 394–95, 397
funding for, 188–89, 277
of Gendin, 253, 300, 338, 373
of Haring, 220–23
Helms and, 148, 254–56
KS and, 159, 315–17, 320
of Misove, 210, 214
PCP prophylaxis and, 181–82
photos of naked people with, 387–88
POZ and, 285–87, *288,* 289–97, 302, 305–6, 308, 310, 312, 335–38, 344, 387–88
prevention of, 136–37, 148, 227–28, 231, 247, 255–56, 291–92, 296, 327, 330–32, 335, 339, 396
prisons and, 312–13, 394–97
proposed quarantine of people with, 188–90
sex with, 115, 328, 335–39, 393
stigmatizing of, 292, 307, 320, 392–98

HIV (*cont.*)
  of Strub, 87, 165–67, 169–72, 240, 243, 276, 284, 321, 325, 347, 357, 380, 387, 392–93
  testing for, 159, 164–66, 172, 190, 253–54, 275, 394
  transmission of, 145, 225, 277, 313, 327–28, 337–39, 393–94, 396
  treatments for, 177–78, 252–53, 261–62, 286, 291–92, 294–96, 305–6, 313, 332, 336, 359, 361–63, 373–74, 380, 391, 396
  see also under safe sex, safer sex
Hochberg, David, 239–40
Hockney, David, 188, 223
Hotel Fauchère, 367
House of Representatives, U.S., 7, 110, 119, 313, 395
  gay lobbying of, 100–102, 105
  gays in, 55–58, 240
  Hochberg's political ambitions and, 239–40
  legislation on gays in, 60, 100, 105, 128
  lesbians in, 25
  Strub's campaign for, *238*, 240–48, 251, 253, 257, 265–66, 270, 343, 386
  Strub's elevator operator job and, 17–18
  see also Congress, U.S.
How to Have Sex in an Epidemic (Berkowitz, Callen, and Sonnabend), 137–38, 147, 175, 336
Huddle, 105
Hudson, Rock, 158–59, 165
Hughes, Fred, 151
human immunodeficiency virus, *see* HIV
human papillomavirus (HPV), 393
Human Rights Campaign, Human Rights Campaign Fund (HRCF), 102, 107, 122, 189, 248, 333
Humphrey, Hubert, 18

"IF YOU'RE STRAIGHT, READ THIS," 279–80
InfoPak, 252, 261, 292–93
International AIDS Conference, third *194*, 196–97
Invirase, 362
Iowa, University of, 8, 14, 47, 110, 124, 208
Iowa City, Iowa, 6, 10, 24, 49–50, *64*, 80, 91, 111, 123–24, 170, 301, 358
  Strub's childhood and adolescence in, 1, 13, 16, 232

  Strub's father and, 8–9
  Strub's speech in, 232–33
  Williams's familiarity with, 46–47, 105
Iowa City Press Citizen, 8, 232–33
Italy, 117, 342–43, *382*, 384–86

Jackson, Henry "Scoop," 19
Jagger, Bianca, 86
Javits, Jacob, 19
Jews, 188, 247, 282, 350
  anti–Semitism and, 34, 116, 270, 273
Joe Allen's, 65, 139
Johnson, Jay, 241
Johnston, Dan, 312, 397
Jones, Bill, 157
Jones, Cleve, 198, 330–31
Jordan, Barbara, 25

Kameny, Frank, 41
Kantor, MacKinlay, 312
Kaposi's sarcoma (KS), 141–42, 146, 349–52, 379
  of Callen, 222, 321, 349
  of Foulon, 173, 175
  gays and, 118, 315, 320–21, 350
  of Haring, 222, 321, 349
  HIV and, 159, 315–17, 320
  physical appearance of, 139, 144, 149–50, 152, 173, 222, *314*, 315–19, 321–22, 328, 343, 351, 361–62, 384, *390*
  psychological impact of, 316, 318–19
  of Strub, *314*, 315–22, 328, 341–43, 349–50, 361–63, 365, 384, *390*
  treatments for, *314*, 317–18, 321, 350, 361–63
Keane, Tom, 229–30, 290
Keller, Mark, 191–92
Kennedy, Robert F., Jr., 242–43, 247, 272
Kennedy, Ted, 18, 78, 85
Kentucky, 269
  Democrats in, 97–100, 104, 110
  Strub's employment in, 97–100, 103–4, 110–13, 277
Key West, Fla., 49, 320
  Strub's trips to, *44*, 48, 83–84, 107
  Williams's home in, *44*, 46, 48, 83–84, 104, 106–7
Klose, Randy, 137
KNOW YOUR SCUMBAGS poster, 220–21, *226*
Koch, Ed, 100, 128, 169
Kopay, Dave, 40–41

Kostmayer, Peter, 58, 248
Kramer, Larry, 57, 134, 169, 385
  ACT UP and, 197, 203
  AIDS call to action of, 132–33
  Gendin and, 374–75, 380
  The Night Larry Kramer Kissed Me and,
    264, 266–67, 269–73, 276, 279–80,
    284
  POZ and, 295, 328
Krim, Mathilde, 137, 211–12, 301

Lambda Legal, 76, 100, 189, 397
Landry, Ryan, 265
Latimer, Nic, 215
Lavender Scare, 54
Lazarus Syndrome, 363
Ledoux, André, 144, 156, 174
  AIDS and, 131–32
  Strub's break with, 160, 162
Leibovitz, Annie, 91, 223
Lennon, John, *82*, 88–92, 97, *264*, 272–73,
    383
Lennon, Sean, 89
Leo, Jamie, 2
Lesbian, Gay, and Bisexual Pride Rally, 232
lesbians, 34, 54, 109, 155, 170, 222, 247,
    254, 259, 268, 284, 386, 398
  activism and, 39, 187
  AIDS and, 128, 139–41, 197, 200
  Clinton and, 277–78, *324*, 325–26, 332
  closeted, 40–42, 329
  in Congress, 25
  demonstrations and, 197, 231
  fund–raising and, 188, 190, 201
  legislation on, 105, 115
  in military, 277, 279
  The Night Larry Kramer Kissed Me and,
    266, 269
  open, 39–40, 332
  politics and, 20, 63, 65, 71, 74, 76, 79–81,
    83, 101–2, 104–5, 107, 115, 128–29,
    162, 267, 329
  POZ and, 286, 293, 300, 311–12
  Strub's congressional campaign and, 240,
    243–45, 248
  Strub's opinions on, 16–17
  White House meeting of, *22*, 40
Levine, Matt, 285
Limbaugh, Rush, 280
Lincoln, Abraham, 25, 385
Lindsay, John, 77–78
Little Me, 204

Los Angeles, Calif., 188, 267, 330
  ACT UP and, 204, *218*
  AIDS and, *108*, 113, 120, 135, 141, 179,
    197, 252
  gay scene in, 204, 320
  POZ and, 289, 301
  Strub's congressional campaign and, 240, 245
  Strub's KS and, 316, 320
Lost and Found, 33–35, 49
Love, Gael, 86
Loves of Anatol, The, 319–20
lymphadenopathy, 113–14, 119
Lyphomed, 182

Mabie, E. C., 47
McAllister, Patrick, 149–50
McCaffrey, Barry, 332
McCarthy, Joseph, 19, 54, 57, 163, 341
McDonald, Joe, 132, 149, 152
McDonald Amendment, 60, 105
McDowell, Kyle "Hush":
  Gendin's death and, 371–72, 375
  Gendin's relationship with, 338–39
McFarlane, Rodger, 138
McGovern, George, 18, 26, 50
McKean, Aldyn, 223–24
McKinney, Stewart, 58
MacLeod, Bob, 244
Maddow, Rachel, 312
Marc, 65–66
Marinol, 308
Matlovich, Leonard, 41, 198
Matthews, Chris, 17
Meat Rack, 320
Medicare, *340*, 341
Memorial Sloan–Kettering Cancer Center,
    87, 113
Mendolia, Victor, 220, *226*
Merck, 362–63
Meredith, Linda, 300
Merrick, Gordon, 39
methadone, 73, 211
Meyer, Howard, 351–52
Mezvinsky, Ed, 110–12, 277
Miano, Lou, 270–71
Midnight in the Garden of Good and Evil
    (Berendt), 383–84
Milford, Pa., 364–68
  Strub's activities in, 366–68, 379–80
  Strub's home in, 366, 372, 377, 384, 397
  Suttle's move to, 397–98
Milk, Harvey, 63, 69–70, 88, 128

Mineshaft, 67, 134
Misove, Michael, 160–66, 179, 207–16, 317
  antiques shop of, 208–9, 215, 241, 281
  cooking of, 161–62, 183, 207, 209, 239
  cryptococcal meningitis of, 3, 210–12,
    214–15
  death of, 3, 212–16, 219, 223, 230, 239,
    241, 270, 275, 281, 351, 372, 384,
    398–99
  headaches of, 209–10
  hospitalization of, 210–12
  memorial service for, 216
  niece of, 398–99
  scent of, 214, 219
  Strub's HIV test and, 165–66
  Strub's relationship with, 161–63, 165–66,
    183–84, 187, 208–15, 275, 281
Misove, Paul, 213–14, 216
Misove, Rose, 160–61, 212–14, 216
Mr. P's, 36
Mr. Smith Goes to Washington, 367–68
Mixner, David, 188–89
Mondale, Walter, 18
Monster, 48
Montagnier, Luc, 145–46, 158
Morales, Xavier, *274,* 326, 329, *390*
  business of, 280–81
  letter to Strub's parents by, 349
  POZ and, 287, 295, 298–99, 310–11, 318
  property hunting of, 364–66
  sexuality of, 275–76, 280
  Strub's break with, 376–77, 399
  Strub's first meeting with, 275–76
  Strub's KS and, *314,* 318, 320–21
  and Strub's marriage to O'Donnell, *340,*
    341–42
  Strub's relationship with, 276, 280–81,
    287, 298–99, 301, 347–49, 364–67,
    372, 376–77, 384, 399
Moral Majority, 10, 101–3, 105, 128
Moree, Monique, 394–95, 397
Morgan, David, *390*
Morgan, Scott, 204
Morrissey, Francis X., Jr., 270–71
Moscone, George, 63
Munson, Thurman, 77
mycobacterium avium–intracellulare (MAI),
  146, 308

Nall, Jim, 87
  AIDS and, 152–53
  death of, 149, 153, 162

Strub's meeting with, 38–39
Strub's relationship with, 39, 49
Strub's visits with, 49, 65, 67–68
Napolitano, Andrew, 270–71
National Association of People with AIDS,
  173, 196–97
National Cancer Institute, 118, 145–46,
  182
National Conservative Political Action
  Committee (NCPAC), 57
National Gay and Lesbian Task Force
  (NGLTF), 40, 100, 122, 156
  and fund–raising, 189, 201, 280
  and gays in military, 279–80
National Gay Rights Advocates (NGRA),
  180, 198, 201, 240
  fund–raising and, 188–89
National Institutes of Health (NIH), 145,
  151, 179–81, 236, 295, 326
National March on Washington for Lesbian
  and Gay Rights, 79–80, 83
Navarro, Ray, 2
Nazis, 195, 380
Near, Holly, 79
needle–exchange programs, 277, 327–32
Neupogen, 350
New St. Marks Baths, 71–72, 85–86, 109
New York City, 13–14, *64,* 65–79, 109–10,
  162, 189, 204, 207–8, 222, 227, 244,
  259, 292–93, 342, 351, 364, 395, 399
  ACT UP and, 195–97, 199, 203, 265
  AIDS and, 119–20, 126–27, 130, 132,
    134–36, 138–39, 141–42, 144, 147,
    150–52, 155–56, 159, 165, 169–72,
    174–75, 184, 186, 203, 207
  comparisons between Washington and, 10,
    65, 68–69, 71, 73, 86
  crime in, 24, 73
  Democratic National Conventions in,
    23–25, 55, 84–85, 267–68
  demonstrations and, 1–2, 70–71, 74,
    169–71, 195–96, 225, 228–31
  fiscal crisis of, 24–25
  gay politics and, 65, 70–71, 74–76, 103
  gay scene in, 10, 25, 36, 38–39, 55, 57,
    66–67, 69–75, 85–88, 97, 106, 109,
    121–22, 129, 131, 134, 160, 163, *168,*
    275–76, 329, 277
  Gendin and, 371–72, 376
  GMHC fund–raising and, 157–58
  Lennon's assassination and, *82,* 88–92, 97
  Misove and, 211, 214–16

Morales and, 281, 349
The Night Larry Kramer Kissed Me and, 266–67, 269–73
POZ and, 287, 293, 301, *346*
Sonnabend's practice in, 73, 116–18, 318
Strub's illnesses and, 87, 164, 316, 318, 362
Strub's living accommodations in, 68–69, 73–74, 78, 88, 97, 118, 146, 207, 267–68, 276, 376–77
Strub's meeting with Williams in, 104–7
Strub's move to, 68, 70–72, 113, 163
and Strub's move to Pennsylvania, 367–68
Strub's part–time jobs in, 69, 85
and Strub's visits with Nall, 49, 65, 67–68
violence against gays in, 88, 97, 129
New Yorker, The, 294, 298
New York Native, The, 109, 113–14, 118, 120, 124, 126–27, 129–30, 132, 135, 171, 177, 254, 285
New York Political Action Committee (NYPAC), 75–76
New York Post, 170–71
New York Times, The, 26, 40, 58, 75–76, 145, 207, 263, 271, 278
demonstrations and, 195–96, 230–31
and gays in military, 279–80
POZ and, 290–91
New York University, *64*, 69, 121
New York University Medical Center, 190, 350
Night Larry Kramer Kissed Me, The (Drake), *264*, 266–67, 269–73, 276, 279–80, 284
Ninth Circle, 69, 121, 163, 377
Nixon, Richard, 8, 27, 57, 68
No on 64 campaign, 188–90
Normal Heart, The (Kramer), 169, 266
Northrop, Ann, 202, 375
Norvir, 362
Nureyev, Rudolph, 386
Nye, Frank, 6

O'Connor, John Cardinal, 1–2, 227–29
on AIDS, 228, 231
demonstration and, 2, 220, *226*, 229, 231, 242
on homosexuality, 227–28
O'Donnell, Doris, 164, 347, 377
POZ and, 343–44
Strub's marriage to, *340*, 341–43
Vidal's relationship with, 342–44, 384

O'Hara, Scott, 287, 293
O'Leary, Jean, 40–41, 209, 268, 329
demonstrations and, 197–98
fund–raising and, 188–89
Strub's congressional campaign and, 240–41, 245, 247
and White House meeting of gay and lesbian leaders, *22*, 40
Onassis, Jacqueline Kennedy, 92, 244
"1,112 and Counting" (Kramer), 132–33
Ono, Yoko, 271–73, 280
husband's assassination and, 89–91, *264*
The Night Larry Kramer Kissed Me and, *264*, 272–73
Ortho Pharmaceutical, 308
Osborn, Torie, 188, 245
Outweek, 225, 292

Pacino, Al, 74
Palisades, N.Y., 301, 364
Palumbo Hotel, 343
Pasteur Institute, 145–46, 158
Patrick, Stephen, 348–49
Peebles, Brad, *304*, 377–78
Penn+Schoen, 155
Penn School, 232
Pennsylvania, 24, 92, 121, 239
Democrats in, 110, 119, 277
Strub's employment in, 110–12, 114, 119
Strub's move to, 367–68
pentamidine, 182
People With AIDS Caucus, 141–44
People With AIDS Coalition (PWAC), 136, *168*, 171–75, 177–79, 222, 235
fund–raising of, 171, 185–87
Living Room of, 171, 175
Strub's work with, 174–75
Pérez–Feria, Richard, 290, 294, 298
Perot, Ross, 278, 331
Perret, Edmund, 45–48, 83, 105
Perrin, Marlene, 232–33
Petoniak, Steve, 157, 204
Petrelis, Michael, 2
pharmaceutical companies, 180–81, 254–55, 261–62, 376
generic medications and, 332
POZ and, 295, 297–300, 305–8, 380
Philadelphia, 279, 300
Phillips, Kevin, 246
physician–assisted death, 348
Pier, Nathaniel, 164–65, 169
AZT and, 176–77

Pier, Nathaniel (*cont.*)
  death of, 178, 236
  Strub's prognosis and, 165, 177, 235–36
Pier House, *44,* 83–84
Piermont, N.Y., 208–9, 212, 219, 239,
    301–2, 364
Pike County, Pa., 364–66
Plague, The (Camus), 117
pneumocystis carinii pneumonia (PCP), 146,
    159
  prevention of, 181–82, 296, 308
  of Strub, 289–91
Politics of the Rich and Poor, The (Phillips),
    246
Polka–Dot Dilly, The (Strub and Gallagher),
    321–22
Positively Naked, 387
POZ, 142, 252, 289–302, *304,* 305–13, *346,*
    347–48, 368, 383–88
  advertising in, 286, 295, 297–302, 305–8,
    310, 362, 380
  business models and plans of, 285–86,
    301, 306
  celebration of sex in, 335–39
  Clinton and, 290, 325–27, 330, 332
  contributors to, 286–87, *288,* 289–90,
    293, 295, 297, 301, 312
  diverse communities addressed by,
    309–10
  finances of, 285, 291, 297–302, 305–6,
    310, 318, 377–78, 386
  first anniversary of, 298, 328
  Gendin's death and, *370,* 372, 374–77,
    379
  launch of, 280, 282, 284–87, *288,* 289,
    291, 312, 347, 387
  naming of, 285
  photo of people with HIV on cover of,
    387–88
  prisons and, 312–13, 397
  sale of, 386–87
  Strub's columns in, 293, 313, 319, 325,
    344, 378–79, 392, 398
  Strub's C–SPAN interview and, 328–29
  Strub's depression and, 378–79
  Strub's KS and, 318–19
  subscriptions to, 131, 287, 302, 310
  tenth anniversary of, 387–88
  treatments and, 294, 297, 305, 361–63
  Vidal and, 343–44
POZ en Español, 310–11
Prelude, 170

Presidential Advisory Council on HIV/AIDS
    (PACHA), 245, 330–31
prisons, 98, 270
  HIV and, 312–13, 394–97
Privacy Project '82, 102
Project Inform, 197, 253–54
Proposition 64, 188–90
protease inhibitors, 306, 359, 361–64,
    373–74, 388
Prunty, Jim, 49–50
Pustil, Ronnilyn, 374
PWA Health Group, 178–79

Quick, Ernest, 224

Radical Rites Press, 14
Rafsky, Bob, 319, 325
Ramrod shooting, 88, 97, 129
Rapoport, Paul, 76
Rascals, 45
Reagan, Nancy, 151, 158, 335
Reagan, Ronald, 10, 19, 68, 246
  AIDS and, 116, 144–45, 151, 158,
    197–98
  gay politics and, 101–2
  presidential campaign of, 85, 88
  presidential election of, 88, 97, 102, 128
Real Health, 311
Redden's Funeral Home, 213–14, 372
Reese, Matt, 97–98
Reilly, Adam, *108,* 109–10, 112
reproductive rights, 2–3, 14, 16, 19, 102,
    139, 231
Republicans, Republican Party, 10, 12–13,
    85, 185, 239, 252, *288,* 289, 295, 310,
    327
  closeted gays and, 55–59
  gay politics and, 102–3
  HIV criminalization and, 395, 397
  Strub's congressional campaign and, 244, 247
  Strub's political beliefs and, 23–24
Resistance Conspiracy Case, 312
Restaurant Florent, 387–88
Reuben, David, 10
Rhoades, Nick, 393–97
Ribavirin, 180
Rich, Frank, 291
Riggio, Len, 311
right–to–die movement, 260
Robinson, David, 202
Robinson, Paul, 76
Roche, 180, 307, 362

Rockland County *Journal News,* 243, 245–46, 248
Rodale, Inc., 300–302
Rogers, Roy, 383–84
Rolling Stone, 223, 272
Rolo–dead files, 191
Rolonda, 375–76
Rondinaia, La, 343, *382,* 384
Roosevelt Hospital, 73, *82,* 90, 190, 207
Rosett, Jane, *168*
Ross, Ty, *288,* 289–90, 310
Russo, Vito, 72, *108,* 121, 167, 284, 319, 391
  AIDS and, 169–71
  biography of, 112–13
  book written by, 109–10, 113
  on coming out, 110–12
  Strub's relationship with, 110–14, 371

safe sex, safer sex, 339
  AIDS and, 137–38, 142, 148, 220, 338
  barebacking and, 335–38
  condoms and, 1–2, 35, 137–38, 147–49, 160, 166, 175, 220–21, *226,* 227–28, *250,* 251, 256–57, 291, 313, 335–38, 393–94
  demonstrations and, 1–3, 220–21, 230, *250,* 251, 256–57, 311
  HIV and, 115, 148, 227–28, 247, 291–92, 296, 313, 335–38, 393–94
St. Mary's Church, 3, 232
  Strub as altar boy at, 1, 13, 233
  Strub's nephew's baptism at, 231
St. Patrick's Cathedral:
  demonstration at, 1–2, *226,* 228–32, 242, 247, 290, 357
  Masses at, 1–2, 228–29, 242
St. Patrick's Day parade, 227
St. Vincent's Hospital, 190–91
  Misove's death and, 212–13
  Misove's meningitis and, 210–11
same–sex marriage, 14, 57, 398
Sanford, Terry, 24
San Francisco, Calif., 52, 63, 267, 293
  AIDS and, 120, 135, 141–42, 147, 197, 208
  demonstrations and, 69–70, 197
  gay scene in, 10, 70
  HIV testing and, 253–54
  Russo in, 113–14
Sarandon, Susan, 220, 271
Save Our Children campaign, 128
Scarce, Michael, 337–39

Schaire, Jeffrey, 262
Schiavi, Michael, 112–13
Schmalz, Jeffrey, 278
Schoofs, Mark, 290
Scott, 68–70, 73
Scott, Marcia, 330
Sean O. Strub, Inc., 131
Senak, Mark, 173
Senate, Iowa State, 23–24, 395
  Strub as page at, *4,* 6, 26
Senate, U.S., 19, 57, 77, 103, 121–22, 255, 258
  legislation on gays in, 148–49
  Strub's elevator operator job and, 5–7, 11–15, 17–18, 20, 31–33, 42
  see also Congress, U.S.
Senior Action in a Gay Environment (SAGE), 156, 259
seroconversion, 87, 337–39, 372
sero–positioning, 336
Sero Project, 395–98
sero–sorting, 336
Sessums, Kevin, 256, *288,* 289–90, 301
Sevcik, Jeffrey, 114
Sex Panic!, 338, 375
Sex Positive, 138
Shalala, Donna, 326–29, 333
  needle–exchange programs and, 327–29, 331–32
  outing of, 329
  POZ and, 328–29
shark–cartilage slurry, 321
Sheen, Martin, 220
Shields, Mark, 282
Shulman, Marvin, 223–25, 256, 280
Signorile, Michelangelo, 225, 337
Silence=Death logo, 3, 195–96, 201, 220, 230, 241, 327
Simon, John, 320
Six–Day War, 188
Sloan, Amy, 186–87
Slowik, George, 298
Smith, David, 333
Smith, Jerry, 40
Smith, Rupert, 149–50
Snyder, Dick, 367, 380
Socarides, Richard, 330
Social Security, 341
Soldiers', Sailors', Marines', Coast Guard, and Airmen's Club, 215–16
Sonnabend, Joseph, 175–79, 335–36, 398
  AIDS and, 118, 125, 127, 129–31, 136–38, 147, 159, 175, 235–36

Sonnabend, Joseph (*cont.*)
 AZT and, 73, 177, 253
 background of, 73, 116–17
 conflict between GMHC and, 137–38
 KS and, 118, 317–18, 350
 letters and cards received by, 399–400
 Misove and, 210–12
 PCP prophylaxis and, 181–82
 PWAC and, 175, 178
 PWA Health Group and, 178–79
 on safe sex, 137–38, 147, 175, 339
 sexually transmitted infections treated by,
  116–18
 Strub's relationship with, 379–80
Spitz, Mark, 9
Staley, Peter:
 ACT UP and, 199–201, 203, 252, 255
 demonstrations and, 256–58
 TAG and, 255–56
State Department, U.S., 54, 332
Steers, Hugh, 344
Steinbrenner, George, 77
Steinem, Gloria, 103, 156
Stennis, John, 19–20
Sterling Forest, 242–43, 247–48
Sternglass, Ernest, 135–36
Stoddard, Tom, 75–76, 88, 90
Stone, Roger, 57
Stonewall Inn, Stonewall riots, 45, 70–71,
  114–15, 126, 170, 231
Stop the Church! action, 223, *226,* 228–32
Strub, Carl Francis, Jr. (father), 5–6, 8–10,
  20, 27, 97, 170, 230–33, 359
 Misove's meeting with, 208–9
 son's arrest and, 198–200
 son's education and, 5, 77, 79, 81, 356
 son's homosexuality and, 10, 42, 61–62,
  73, 80–81, 112, 399
 son's illnesses and, 348–49
 son's mouse trapping and, 123, 283
Strub, Carl Francis, Sr. (grandfather), 9, 47
Strub, Carl Francis, III (brother), 9, 231
Strub, Elizabeth Jane O'Brien (mother), 5–6,
  9–10, 20, 27, 97, 123, 170, 208, 230,
  232, 359
 children's book written by, 321–22
 son's arrest and, 198–99
 son's education and, 5, 79, 356
 son's homosexuality and, 10, 42, 61–62,
  73, 80–81, 112
 son's illnesses and, 87, 348–49
Strub, Gilbey (sister), 167, 170

Strub, Joseph (nephew), 231
Strub, Megan (sister), 42
 brother's KS and, *314,* 317–18
 and brother's marriage to O'Donnell, *340,*
  341–42
 brother's relationship with, 167, 170,
  348–49, 384, 387
 Misove and, 210–13
 POZ and, 294, 297–302, *304,* 307, 318,
  377–78, 387
Strub, Missi (sister), 366
Strub, Sean O'Brien:
 activism of, 26, 31, 62–63, 74–76, 79–81,
  83, 91, 93, 100, 104–5, 110–11, 115,
  119, 122, 124, 129, 133, 155–56, 166,
  169–71, 185–90, 192, *194,* 196–99,
  201–5, 219, 222–24, 237, 239–40,
  242–44, *250,* 253, 255–58, 262, 267,
  270–71, 278, 283–84, 291, 367,
  391–96
 alcohol consumed by, 16, 30–31, 55, 59,
  75, 105–6, 384–86
 ambitions of, 5–8, 10–11, 13–14, 17–18,
  20, 24, 41, 68, 104, 163, 199, *238,*
  239–48, 251, 253, 257, 265–66, 270,
  282, 343, 386, 392
 anger of, 210, 213, 271, 372, 399
 arrest of, 41, *194,* 198–200, 203
 businesses of, 131, 155–58, 162–64, 167,
  170, 185, 187–88, 199–201, 204–5,
  214, 241–42, 247, 251–54, 259, 261–
  62, 266–67, 273, 278, 280–81, 283–87,
  290–301, *304,* 305–13, 318–19, 321,
  324, 325–30, 335–38, 347–48, 355,
  367–68, 376–79, 384, 386–87
 childhood and adolescence of, 1, 6–8, 10–
  16, 23–26, 30, 35, 41, 47, 53, 123–24,
  202, 232–33, 283, 293, *354,* 355–58
 coming out of, 61–62, 73, 80, 110–12,
  114, 174–75, 185, 241, 277, 399
 congressional campaign of, *238,* 240–48,
  251, 253, 257, 265–66, 270, 343, 386
 death threats of, 273
 diet of, 118, 183–84
 education of, 1, 5, 8, 14, 18, 24, 26–31,
  34–35, 46, 56, 58, 62, 68, 75, 77, 79,
  81, 85–87, 92, 97, 121, 155, 187,
  232–33, 312, *354,* 355–58, 392, 399
 elevator operator job of, 5–7, 11–15,
  17–20, 26, 31–33, 42, 58
 entrepreneurship of, 123–24, 201, 237,
  291, 392

fears and anxieties of, 149, 155, 159, 163, 175, 181, 357, 391–92
finances of, 6, 25, 30, 36, 38, 48, 68–69, 85, 91, 97, 123–24, 131, 156, 170, 201, 208, 214, 251, 283–85, 297–98, 301, 364–66, 377, 392
grieving of, 192, 212–13, 219, 223, 372, 376
health consciousness of, 183–84, 190–91
illnesses of, 3, 72–73, 87–89, 92, 97, 113–14, 119–20, 125, 131–32, 146–47, 149, 153, 155, 160, 164–67, 169–72, 176–77, 183–85, 208, 235–36, 240, 243, 247, 271, 276, 284, 289–91, 294, 297, 300–302, 308, *314,* 315–22, 325, 328, 341–43, 347–50, 355–59, 361–63, 365, 367–68, 371–72, 376–80, 384, 387, *390,* 392–93
improving health of, 362–65, 371, 377, 379
life insurance policies of, 285, 297
loneliness and alienation of, 41, 63, 275
marriage of, *340,* 341–43
medications taken by, 176–79, 183, 223, 237, 253, 262, 308, *314,* 350, 355, 361–64, 380
mentoring of, 16, 39, 53–54, 99, 111, *168,* 251, 281–82, 293, 341, 371
mice trapped by, 123, 283
mind–body connections of, 183–84
mortality of, 3, 284–5, 290, 297–98, 300, 318, *340,* 341–42, 348, 350, 352, 355, 363–64, 366, 368, 371, 377, 392
nakedness of, 387–88
naming of, 9
physical appearance of, 11, 24, 27, 29, 40, 45–46, 48, 66, 77, 91, 171, 198, 298, 300, *314,* 315–19, 321–22, 328, 343, 347, 350, 356–57, 384, *390*
political beliefs of, 9, 14, 16, 23–24, 49, 76, 84–85, 87–88, 94, 97, 109–10, 119, 121–22, 185, 240, 277–78, 282
politics as obsession of, 6, 46, 49, 53, 75, 185, 283
poppers and marijuana used by, 7, 84, 112, 134
pride of, 79, 199, 230, 283, 289, 299, 357, 366, 377–78
prognosis of, 165, 177, 235–36
property hunting of, 364–66
rape of, 36–37
reading of, 5, 11, 18, 36, 39–40, 45,

117–19, 132–33, 150, 171–72, 176, 203, 236, 253, 312, 357–58
religious beliefs of, 1–2, 10, 13–14, 16, 26, 76–77, 80, 165, 177, 183, 202, 221, 229–33, 242, 356–58, 372, 399
restaurant purchased by, 124, 283
secrecy of, 9, 20, 26, 34, 42
self–hatred of, 35, 356
sexual abuse of, 30, 35, 66, 88, *354,* 355–59
sexuality of, 9–11, 15–17, 20, 25–39, 41–42, 45, 49, 59–63, 69, 71–73, 75, 80–81, 85–87, 98, 104, 110–12, 114, 118, 120, 132, 147–48, 155, 166, 174–75, 185, 199, 232–33, 240–41, 243, 245–48, 267–68, 275–77, 320, 357, 367, 399
shame of, 10, 31–32, 35, 37, 39, 62, 66, 169, 183, 233, 356–57, 387–88
social life of, 13, 16–17, 36, 40, 45–46, 49, 59–61, 63, 65–67, 75, 85–88, 122, 134, 160–61, 163, 174, 275
speeches of, 232–33, 244–46, 391
stigmatizing of, 275, 319, 358, 391–92
stress of, 289, 363, 377–78
suicidal thoughts of, 348, 379–80
survival sought by, 237, 239
wardrobe of, *4,* 11, 13–14, 32, 40, *194,* 198, 200, 242, 298, 308
weight loss of, 113, 308, *390*
will of, 167
Strub, Trip (brother), 123
Strub/Collins, 162–64, 167, 214
 ACT UP and, 199–201, 204–5
 clients of, 156–58
 Strub's activism and, 185, 187–88
 and Strub's relationship with Misove, 162–63
Strub's Store for Everybody, 9, 47
Studds, Gerry, 55–56, 58, 240
Studio 54, 13, 65–67, 85–87, 134, 164
Suares, J. C., 290, 294, 298, 383
Sullivan, Andrew, 328
Summers, David, 186
Supreme Court, U.S., 8, 19, 277
 gay sex prohibition and, 187–88
Surviving AIDS (Callen), 236–37
Sustiva, 380
Suttle, Robert, 394–95, 397–98
Sutton, Burleigh, 208
Swenson, Swen, 204, *218,* 219–21, 272, 280

Taylor, Elizabeth, 19, 198, 271, 328
T–cells, 296–97, 308, 347
Teles, Rubens, 241
testosterone replacement therapy, 308
Thurmond, Strom, 19–20
Time, 41, 198, 384
Totem 89 (Haring), 223–25
Tower, John, 13
Treatment Action Group (TAG), 255–58, 264, 272–73, 295, 362, 376
Treatment and Data Digest, 252
Trinity (Uris), 18
Tucker, Gary, 83–84
Tunick, Spencer, 387–88

Udall, Morris, 6, 14, 24
Uncle Charlie's, 38, 160, 329
Uris, Leon, 18

Valenzuela, Tony, 337–39
Vidal, Gore:
    on gays, 103, 385–86
    O'Donnell's relationship with, 342–44, 384
    political ambitions of, 121–22, 343, 386
    Strub's KS and, 343, 384
    Strub's visits with, 342–44, 382, 384–86
Vietnam War, 8, 26, 41, 89, 110, 246
Village Voice, The, 130, 290
Viola, Tom, 267, 269
viral loads, 315, 347, 362, 393
Visit to a Small Planet (Vidal), 386
voter registration, 51, 99–100, 119, 276

Walters, Barbara, 264, 272
Wang, An, 78
Warhol, Andy, 86, 149–52, 222, 267, 383
Washington, D.C., 5–8, 48–51, 76, 78, 92, 104, 109, 122, 164, 241, 282, 301, 332, 368, 385
    AIDS and, 145, 196–98, 274
    comparisons between New York and, 10, 65, 68–69, 71, 73, 86
    Crangle's job offer and, 58–59, 62
    crime in, 27, 33

demonstrations and, 188, 194, 197–200, 250, 256–58
    gay politics and, 79–80, 83, 100, 103
    gay scene in, 10–11, 15–16, 28–40, 45, 54–58, 63, 69, 71, 73
    O'Donnell–Vidal relationship and, 342–43
    power in, 14, 61, 86
    Strub's departure from, 68, 85, 113
    Strub's elevator operator job and, 5–7, 11–15, 17–20, 26
    Strub's living accommodations in, 14–15, 26, 36–37
Washington Blade, 39–41, 63
Washington Post, The, 51–52, 59, 332
wasting, 141–42, 144, 152, 259, 379
Watergate scandal, 8, 25, 110
Watters, Sam, 286
"We Know Who We Are" (Callen and Berkowitz), 124–26
Wessel, John, 230
Westchester County, N.Y., 214, 239, 242
Westerman, Max, 64, 69, 350, 377
    on Cohn, 163–64
"Whatever Happened to AIDS?" (Schmalz), 278
White, Dan, 63, 69–71
White, Ryan, 256
white blood cells, 178, 350
Whitehorn, Laura, 294, 312
Wildwood, 75
Williams, Tennessee:
    gay politics and, 83, 103–7, 122
    Strub's visits with, 44, 46–48, 83–84, 104–7
Wilson, Robert W., 270–71
Women's Health Action and Mobilization (WHAM), 228
Woolley, Robert, 244–45
World War II, 9–10, 105, 117
Wyatt, Schuyler, 83–84

York, Dick, 386

Zamora, Pedro, 310, 326
Zingale, Daniel, 333
Zonana, Victor, 32

An Interview with Sean Strub

In February 2014, Sean Strub spoke with Charity Nebbe for Iowa Public Radio's Talk of Iowa *program. This interview has been edited for clarity and length.*

CN: You grew up in Iowa City, where you became interested in politics. You became a page in the Iowa State Senate, and then your interest in politics ended up taking you to Washington, D.C. What were your hopes and dreams as a teenager when you thought about your political career?

SS: I didn't think about it far into the future. I thought I was supposed to be successful. I was supposed to go to college. But I think that as a gay person—not even understanding yet that I was a gay person—it precluded me from having much of a vision of my future, because I didn't see anyone like me represented in any of the institutions or the cultural context I grew up in. But politics was very immediate and very exciting. I was a news junkie at an early age, and my internal life was tied to what was going on in the media. That attracted my interest, and I had a sense of commitment to social change that I absorbed growing up so near the University of Iowa campus.

CN: When you went to Washington, D.C., as a teenager, you chose to focus on politics, and a career in politics, almost in a way to avoid the subject of sexuality. You weren't familiar with other gay people, and didn't have a community to turn to; it strikes me that spending time in the Capitol, in Washington, D.C., is a very strange place to start to learn about your sexuality.

SS: It is. I arrived in Washington in the spring of 1976, just after Watergate and the Vietnam War. Everywhere in Washington was plastered with the bicentennial celebration logo, and there was a lot of excitement. Jimmy Carter was running for president, promising, "I will never lie to you," a novel concept in national politics at the time. So it kind of fed into this idealism I had. As a political junkie, by then working in the U.S. Senate, running a "Senators Only" elevator, it was like getting a contact high everyday.

I think I had initially substituted political ambition for political purpose. I'd been exposed to all sorts of social change movements growing up, antiwar protests, civil rights protests, and, to a very great extent, feminism. That was a part of me. But I almost disconnected that from the ambition I took with me to Washington. Then starting to understand that I was attracted to men, and coping with that, and my Catholic background, while every day being in the presence of some of the most powerful men in the country, it was a very unusual coming out experience.

The first gay men I met were also working very close to the concentrations of political power in the country, elected and senior officials in both parties. At that time there wasn't an ideological divide socially among the closeted gay circles in Washington. Initially I met no lesbians. It was only gay men, almost entirely white gay men, and their political ideology didn't matter. You'd go to a party and there'd be extreme right-wingers who by day were spewing antigay homophobic nonsense, but in the evening they were socializing privately in great secrecy with people on the left. As I started to get to know this circle, and became part of it, I also started reading the *Washington Blade*, a gay paper in Washington, and became more conscious of the gay rights movement. It was then kind of at the edge of the body politic, not taken seriously by most of the central players in a national political process, but it was there and I was aware of it. And as I followed it more, the disconnect between the milieu I came out into, and this political movement that I felt so drawn to, started to grow.

CN: You spent a couple of years at Georgetown University, and then you transferred to Columbia in New York City. You had been visiting New York quite a bit, and the gay community in New York was *very* different from the gay community in Washington, D.C. What was it that you saw in New York and experienced in New York that made you want to be a part of it?

SS: The out gay community in Washington was very small and very much apart from the gay circles I first became familiar with. In New York I was meeting all of these out gay people who were totally integrated into their professions, their careers. They didn't care who knew they were gay and that was very exciting to me, including some of the political people like Ethan Geto, who ran the campaign against Anita Bryant's "Save Our Children" effort to overturn the Miami-Dade County, Florida, Human Rights Ordinance, in 1977. He ran this campaign as an openly gay man. That was a revelation to me—something I couldn't have imagined in the circles I was part of in Washington.

CN: Can you put in perspective for us, for people who don't know about the politics of the late '70s and early '80s, how very different it was at that time to think about coming out?

SS: I write in *Body Counts* that most of the gay men I first met in Washington were so deeply closeted that I believed they were prepared to kill themselves rather than to have their sexual orientation publicly known. It was not so long from the purges of the 1950s and early '60s, when people by the hundreds, by the thousands actually, were fired from the State Department and other government agencies for being gay, or suspected of being gay. Many of them did commit suicide. So that was still very fresh in the consciousness in Washington, which back then was essentially still a Southern city with the social conservatism that implies.

I thought coming out meant giving up my political ambitions and any hope of running for office. It meant separating myself from most of the friends I grew up with, the people I knew in grammar school in Iowa City, and then junior high school, and at the Jesuit boarding school in Wisconsin I attended, many of whom were afraid, disgusted, angry, or just distanced themselves from me. That was painful, and in some ways it still remains painful, particularly when I see groups of friends who I know remain good friends with each other today, yet I was no longer a part of that circle after I came out.

I knew coming out was going to hurt my parents, and to do something that you were conscious was going to hurt someone else was very difficult. My mom is no longer living, but my dad a few years ago said something really beautiful to me, one of the most beautiful things he's ever said to me, which was that he thought that my coming out of the closet made him a better person and made our family a better family. But that's in hindsight. Back then it was very difficult. It was very lonely.

CN: In New York you were present for the beginning of what turned into an epidemic. You write about the early ideas of what HIV, what AIDS, was and not just what was heard in the media, but also the things that you were talking about with your friends, and your own private fears about it. There was so much that wasn't known. Can you give us an idea of what it was like to be there, to be in this community and starting to see this disease emerge?

SS: It was terrifying, but when it became terrifying varied by person. When the very first reports came out, a lot of people thought, "Well, it's a handful of people, it's five people, it's forty-three people, there are a lot of gay men in the world." Or, it was people who were promiscuous, whatever that means. I've learned over the years that "promiscuous" is generally defined as anyone who has more sex than you.

People would find ways to distance themselves from those they felt were getting sick. In my circle there were people who were in total denial, who wouldn't talk about it and even resented it if it was brought up in a social context, like at a dinner party. Then there were people who were obsessing over AIDS, were so terrified with every cough and mosquito bite—they were sure that that was the beginning of the end for them. In those very earliest days I swung from one extreme to the other, but I was more than anything else curious. I wanted to know and understand what this was about.

I saw health care in political terms from when I was twelve or thirteen years old and was first exposed to activism around reproductive rights, so it was easy for me to see AIDS in political terms as well. I already had a good sense of how little concern the government and others had about the health of gay men.

CN: I was really struck by what you wrote about doctors who were trying to figure out what AIDS was, and how it was transmitted, and who it would affect. You even personally knew a number of dif-

ferent doctors with incredibly different theories about how people could get AIDS. And a lot of this was political at the time as well— this was a time when gay politics were very contentious. So how did you even try to make sense of what it was and what it meant to you?

SS: I made sense of it by just learning, immersing myself in it, and listening to all sorts of different views and opinions, whether it was about causation or treatment, or whatever. One of the central debates was whether this was a previously undiscovered pathogen (suspected to be a virus) and that once exposed to it you were going to die, or whether it was a result of repeated assaults on one's immune system, the multifactorial theory. A lot of gay men at the time had had so many sexually transmitted diseases. There was such an explosion of gay male hypersexuality in the '70s, and the commercial sex establishments, the bathhouses and so on, that many gay men were getting sexually transmitted infections at a phenomenal rate, and treating them quite casually. And there was a view that this was having a cumulative effect, resulting in the breakdown of one's immune system.

Then a new virus—HIV—was discovered in 1984, but it was those behaviors of gay men that had created an incredibly efficient ecosystem for transmitting pathogens. I include myself as part of that. To a certain extent the epidemic is a public health consequence of the repression that gay men had faced for so long. You cannot take any part of society and stigmatize it, criminalize it, give it fewer chances in life, tell it that it is sick, define it as mentally ill (as all homosexuals were, until 1973), and treat it so poorly, without ultimately having some kind of public health consequence. After the Stonewall riots in 1969 a sort of new era of sexual liberation came into being. This new community at its core was a sexual liberation movement where sexual communion became synonymous with liberation.

Yet at the same time many of us knew very little about our bodies. There was virtually no health care that was specifically for gay men. When the epidemic hit it was a real challenge because this newfound sexual freedom was incredibly important, yet any suggestion that we were doing anything that could somehow have contributed to the epidemic, or facilitated its spread, was incredibly contentious. Even using the word "promiscuity" in relation to the epidemic risked accusations of being "sex-negative."

A lot of the gay community leadership and the initial AIDS organizations were unwilling to recognize this; everything about the epidemic was politically contentious and difficult. The first "Safer Sex" materials from Gay Men's Health Crisis were focused on identifying if your partner might have AIDS. It would say, "Take a shower with your partner before having sex, and check and see if he has any spots" (the red or purple lesions that were a sign of Kaposi's sarcoma, an AIDS-related cancer). In a GMHC brochure, condoms weren't mentioned until the seventh item on a list of ten things you can do to reduce your risk of getting AIDS.

CN: You contracted HIV very early on in this epidemic. You suspected it long before you actually knew. What was going through your mind when you suspected that you were infected, but you didn't know?

SS: When I read the first article in the summer of 1981 that described symptoms shared by a group of gay men who'd gotten sick and died, I had all of those symptoms: swollen lymph glands—the year before I'd been at Sloan Kettering, because my lymph glands were grotesquely and mysteriously swollen—night sweats, and weight loss. At that age my weight fluctuated all the time, I didn't pay much attention to it and just thought I sweat a lot. But when I read those three symptoms in that article I got this feeling in the pit of my stomach that this had something to do with me. Then I found that lots of my friends had those same symptoms.

But in those first few years AIDS was people who were dying, who were very, very sick, who had no immune system left, and were generally dead within weeks of their diagnosis. I remember doctors telling me and others that because we were not dying, it meant we still had an immune system, that our bodies were fighting back. We didn't necessarily see the disease as progressing from our lesser symptoms. There was even the suggestion that because we had these mild symptoms it meant we wouldn't get AIDS because our bodies were able to control the infection. So there's tremendous confusion, and of course stigma and fear. Literally people afraid to touch you. I write in *Body Counts* about incidents like being at an all-gay dinner party in the Village. When one of the guys who was rumored to have AIDS used the bathroom, the host discreetly took the hand towels out of the bathroom and replaced them. After the guests left I stayed and helped clean up, and the host used a separate sink of super hot water for that guest's dishes and utensils. That was a part of our daily life. You'd run into someone—the deaths were coming at such a rate that if I saw someone on the street I hadn't seen in a while my first reaction was relief they're still here. Then if we started talking, and maybe we had a mutual friend I hadn't seen in a while, I'd be afraid to ask, because sometimes you'd say, "Hey, have you seen Joe?" and you'd hear, "Oh, didn't you hear? Joe died." This was happening all the time. We were going to more funerals and memorial services than birthday parties. And you didn't even have time to grieve because you were so quickly on to the next death. There were times when I would go visit someone in the hospital—there were separate AIDS wards generally—I would walk along and read the names of other patients in that wing, because inevitably there would be someone else I knew.

CN: You knew you were living with HIV, and at some point you had sort of a change of mind-set, which led to your magazine, *POZ*. People were living with HIV, you had seen a lot of people dying with AIDS, but what was it that made you think, wait a minute,

**we're still here, I'm still here, there are other people who have to live
with this disease, and I need to be doing something for them?**

SS: When the test came out in 1985, and I was officially diagnosed,
my doctor held my hand across his desk, he had tears in his eyes, and
he said, "Sean, these days you can have two good years left." That
was optimistic, hopeful news. That was the best thing he thought
he could tell me. And at that point I believed that. I sold my house
and prepared to die. But a few weeks later, I got involved with the
People with AIDS Coalition in New York, a network of people with
AIDS that was formed to help each other, be each other's support,
and create the services that we needed, whether it was health care or
social support, research, buyers' clubs—we formed the first buyers'
club.

My doctor, the health care establishment, and the media was
telling me I should expect to die. But then I started meeting other
people with AIDS who were leading vibrant lives. Yes, they were
dealing with a very serious life-threatening illness, and many of
them ultimately did die, but they were also falling in love and
breaking up, pursuing their careers, paying their rent, raising their
families, going to school, starting businesses, and many of them
were engaged in advocacy and activism to help other people with
AIDS. I was drawn to that and found them to be people who were
leading the most vital and, I would even say, important lives of
anyone I knew. So I migrated toward them, and eventually became
kind of an evangelist with other people who were diagnosed, saying, "Don't believe that this necessarily means you're going to die,
you have a lot of life to live, you're alive right now, realize that, act
on that," and that's what ultimately led me to start *POZ* magazine.

**CN: The world today is very different than it was in 1980, and 1985,
and you have expressed in other interviews frustration with how
little young people even know about AIDS, and about this time. In**

writing this book, in talking with people, in meeting with young people, what do you want people to know that you don't think is being talked about?

SS: Well, first and foremost the epidemic rages on. A senior epidemiologist at the Centers for Disease Control a few months ago released data that shows that among college-age gay men today half of them will have HIV by the time they're fifty at the current rates of seroconversion. Of college-age gay men of color today, half of them will have HIV by the time they're thirty-five. This is masked by the fact that the epidemic overall in the United States is largely static, but the heterosexual transmission has declined and the gay male transmission has increased, particularly with young gay men, and especially with young gay men of color.

We're in this "look back" moment where there's all this cultural production around the epidemic, exhibits, and films and books, and a concern I have is that they sometimes convey the feeling that the epidemic is over. It isn't.

Second, I think that a lot of the things we did in the very beginning of the epidemic, pre–ACT UP, were incredibly effective and we need to go back to those strategies. It was the self-empowerment movement of people with AIDS themselves, largely modeled after the women's health movement in the '60s and the '70s. A lot of those ideals—a "peer-to-peer" model, supporting networks of people with HIV to empower people with HIV, the principle of engaging people with HIV meaningfully in all aspects of policy making and service delivery, serving on the boards of provider organizations—those principles that were so important early in the epidemic have largely faded away. The "peer-to-peer" service delivery network we created has incrementally moved back toward the more traditional paradigm of "benefactor-victim." Taking our focus off empowering people with HIV is one major reason why stigma has increased. Stigma is one of the biggest obstacles to reducing the rate of HIV transmission.

At the same time we have to recognize that the consequences of HIV are profoundly different today than they were twenty-five years ago. We have to respond to the epidemic that is right now, not the epidemic that was. Too often the message to young gay men is either, "Oh, it's horrible, the most awful thing, life's over," or, "It's no big deal, you just pop a pill and you forget about it." The reality is somewhere in between. Getting diagnosed with HIV is a life-changing event. You don't want to get this virus. It's a lifelong health challenge, it's expensive, it's time-consuming, it's stigmatizing beyond belief, and it complicates intimate relationships in ways one can't possibly understand unless they've gone through it. But we need to convey that message in a way that also affirms queer sexuality and isn't shame- or fear-based.